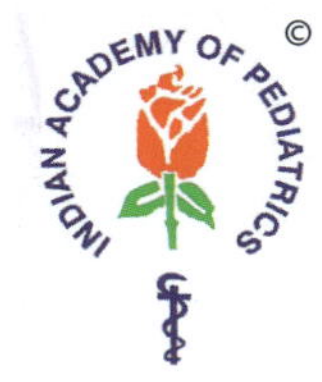

IAP National Treatment Guidelines

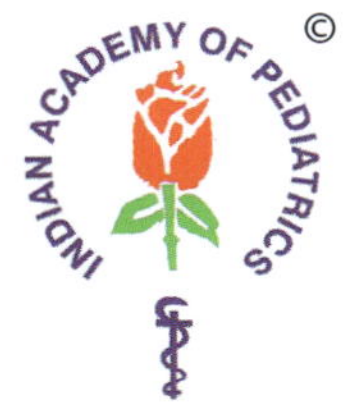

IAP National Treatment Guidelines

Editors-in-Chief

GV Basavaraja
MD DNB FIAP
Professor
Department of Pediatrics
Indira Gandhi Institute of Child Health
Bengaluru, Karnataka, India
IAP National President, 2024

Vasant M Khalatkar
MD PGDID FICMCH
Consultant
Pediatrician and Neonatologist
Khalatkar Hospital
Nagpur, Maharashtra, India
IAP National President, 2025

Executive Editors

Yogesh N Parikh
MD
Associate Professor
Department of Pediatrics
Government Medical College
Surat, Gujarat, India
Secretary General, IAP (2024–2025)

Atanu Bhadra
DCH
Medical Superintendent
ESI Hospital
Asansol, West Bengal, India
National Treasurer, IAP (2024–2025)

Academic Editors

Arun Bansal
MD FRCPCH FCCM FAMS
Professor
Department of Pediatrics
Advanced Pediatric Centre
Postgraduate Institute of Medical
Education and Research
Chandigarh, India

Vinod H Ratageri
MD DCEH
Professor and Head
Department of Pediatrics
Karnataka Medical College and Research Institute
Hubballi, Karnataka, India

Vishnu Mohan PT
MD PGDMLS PGDHM
Fellowship in Neonatology
Senior Consultant
Department of Neonatology
Aster Malabar Institute of Medical Sciences
Kozhikode, Kerala, India

Sheikh Minhaj Ahmed
MD DNB MNAMS FIAP
Fellowship Pediatric Critical Care
Consultant Pediatric Intensivist
Lilavati Hospital and Research Center
Mumbai, Maharashtra, India

Suresh Kumar Angurana
MD DM
Additional Professor
Department of Pediatrics
Postgraduate Institute of Medical
Education and Research
Chandigarh, India

Mihir Sarkar
MD
Professor
Department of Pediatrics
Government Medical College
Kolkata, West Bengal, India

Foreword
Sunit C Singhi

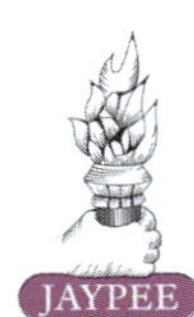

JAYPEE BROTHERS MEDICAL PUBLISHERS
The Health Sciences Publisher
New Delhi | London

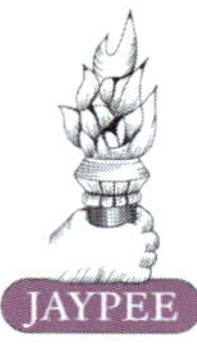

Jaypee Brothers Medical Publishers (P) Ltd

Headquarters
EMCA House, 23/23-B
Ansari Road, Daryaganj
New Delhi 110 002, India
Landline: +91-11-23272143, +91-11-23272703
+91-11-23282021, +91-11-23245672
e-mail: jaypee@jaypeebrothers.com

Corporate Office
4838/24, Ansari Road, Daryaganj
New Delhi 110 002, India
Phone: +91-11-43574357
Fax: +91-11-43574314
e-mail: jaypee@jaypeebrothers.com

Overseas Office
JP Medical Ltd.
83, Victoria Street, London
SW1H 0HW (UK)
Phone: +44-20 3170 8910
e-mail: info@jpmedpub.com

EU GPSR Authorised Representative
Logos Europe, 9 rue Nicolas Poussin
17000, La Rochelle, France
Phone: +33 (0) 6 67 93 73 78
e-mail: contact@logoseurope.eu

Website: www.jaypeebrothers.com
Website: www.jaypeedigital.com

Inquiries for bulk sales may be solicited at: jaypee@jaypeebrothers.com

IAP National Treatment Guidelines

First Edition: **2026**

ISBN: 978-93-6616-365-9

Printed in India

Dedicated to

The children, whose innocence and resilience inspire our every endeavor
And to the tireless Pediatricians across the nation, whose unwavering commitment, clinical acumen, and compassion save young lives each day

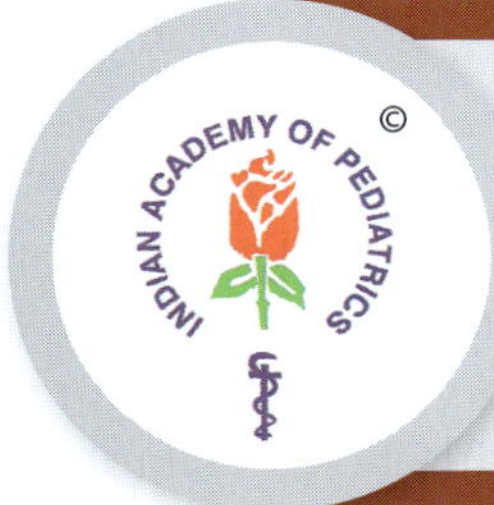

About the Editors

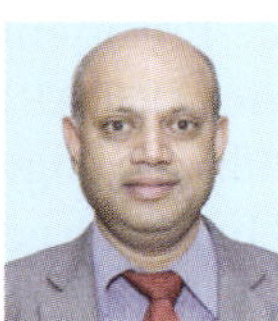

GV Basavaraja MD DNB FIAP is currently Professor, Department of Pediatrics, and Head, Pediatric Intensive Care Unit, Indira Gandhi Institute of Child Health, Bengaluru, Karnataka, India. He is a recognized Teacher of Pediatric Critical Care and an astute Clinician. He is the National President of Indian Academy of Pediatrics (IAP) 2024, National General Secretary, IAP (2021–2022), National Chairperson, IAP—Intensive Care Chapter, 2021. He is the recipient of many orations, and resource person for more than 20 IAP modules. He has been on the Editorial Board of Indian Pediatrics, *Journal of Pediatric Critical Care*, and *Journal of Pediatric Infectious Disease* and has more than 100 publications and book chapters.

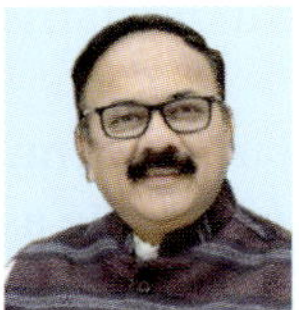

Vasant M Khalatkar MD PGDID FICMCH PG Diploma in Pediatric Infectious Disease is a distinguished figure in Indian Pediatrics, currently serving as the National President of the Indian Academy of Pediatrics (IAP) for 2025. With a career spanning decade, he is the Director, Consultant, and Owner of Khalatkar Hospital, Nagpur, Maharashtra, India, for Mother and Child, and serves as Director and Consultant at "Colours Children Hospital" in Nagpur, a 100-bedded tertiary care pediatric and maternal care facility.

A dedicated clinician and academician, his extensive experience includes numerous leadership roles such as National Chairperson for Pediatric Neurology (2022) and Pediatric Infectious Diseases Chapter (2023), and Vice President of the International Society of Tropical Pediatrics. He has also been actively involved in research, participating in phase III and IV clinical trials for vaccines and medications.

He is an author and editor, with publications including the *Textbook of Ped. Infectious Diseases, Child Neurology & Beyond*, and *Colour Book of Pediatrics*. He has received multiple national and state awards from the IAP for his contributions to child health initiatives. Driven by the principle of "Friendship First", his dream is to serve children, colleagues, and the country through CIAP and do charity to the unreached children.

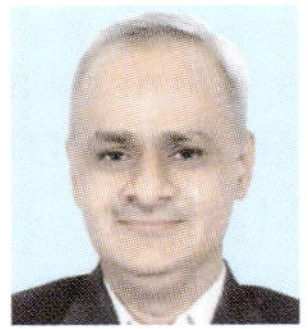

Yogesh N Parikh MD currently serves as the Hon. Secretary General of the Indian Academy of Pediatrics for 2024–2025. He is a former Professor and Head, Department of Pediatrics, PDU Government Medical College and KT Children Hospital, Rajkot, Gujarat, India, and is presently Associate Professor, Department of Pediatrics, Government Medical College, Surat, Gujarat.

He has held numerous prestigious positions, including National Vice President of the IAP (West Zone) in 2023 and President of the Academy of Pediatrics, Gujarat State, in 2021. He has been an Executive Board Member of Central IAP for multiple years and has coordinated significant national projects like the NC ECD IAP-JJ project (2021–23) and the IAP NRP FGM Program (2018–19, 2021). His contributions extend to the National Neonatology Forum (NNF) as an Executive Board Member (2019).

An accomplished academician, he has over 30 scientific publications and presentations in national and international conferences and indexed journals. He was honored with a prestigious travel award for his research at the Congress of the Asian Society for Pediatric Research in Tokyo (2005) and received an award for establishing a "1000 days facility" by the Government of Gujarat. He is a recognized MCI/NMC Assessor, a UG-PG-DNB Examiner for various universities, and has served on the advisory boards of the *Indian Journal of Practical Pediatrics* and *Indian Pediatrics*.

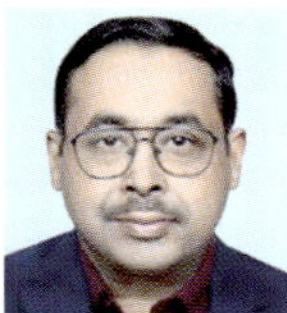

Atanu Bhadra DCH is a distinguished Pediatric Intensivist and Senior Consultant based in Asansol, West Bengal, India. He currently holds the significant position of Medical Superintendent, ESI Hospital, Asansol. A prominent figure in the Indian Academy of Pediatrics (IAP), he serves as the National Treasurer for CIAP (Central IAP) for the term 2024–2025. He is also entrusted with the crucial role of Organizing Secretary for the National Pedicon in 2026.

His commitment to the field of pediatrics is further evidenced by his numerous accolades and leadership positions. He is a Fellow of the Indian Academy of Pediatrics (FIAP) and was the National Scientific Convener for the Presidential Action Plan in 2023. In 2021, he served as the Vice President of CIAP (East Zone). His extensive involvement with the West Bengal Academy of Pediatrics (WBAP) includes his current role as Secretary and past roles as Joint Secretary and Secretary of the Pulmonology Chapter. He has also been an Executive Board Member of CIAP in 2014, 2019, and 2020, and has chaired the IAP Coalfield Branch. He is a recipient of the Purbanchal Award, recognizing his contributions to Pediatrics in the region.

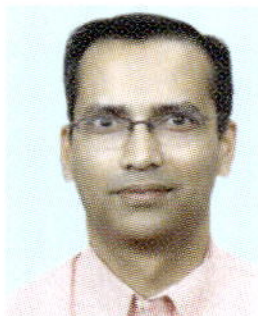

Arun Bansal MD FRCPCH FCCM FAMS is currently Professor of Pediatric Emergency and Intensive Care at the Advanced Pediatric Center, Postgraduate Institute of Medical Education and Research (PGIMER), Chandigarh, India. He is an eminent academician and clinician with extensive experience in pediatric emergency medicine and pediatric intensive care.

He currently serves as the Chairperson of the Pediatric Intensive Care Chapter of the Indian Academy of Pediatrics (IAP), and Dean of the Indian College of Pediatrics. Internationally, he represents India as the Treasurer of the World Federation of Pediatric Intensive and Critical Care Societies (WFPICCS), a testament to his leadership in advancing global pediatric critical care.

With over 200 peer-reviewed publications and 50 book chapters to his credit, he is widely recognized for his contributions to the field. He has been instrumental in the development of numerous IAP modules and national clinical guidelines. He is a regular invited faculty at national and international scientific meetings and has played a key role in organizing major pediatric intensive care conferences across India.

A Fellow of the Royal College of Physicians and Surgeons of Canada (FRCPC), the American College of Critical Care Medicine (FCCM), the National Academy of Medical Sciences (FAMS), and the Indian Academy of Pediatrics (FIAP), he is highly regarded for his commitment to medical education, clinical excellence, and health systems development. He continues to mentor future leaders in pediatric critical care through his academic, clinical, and policy leadership roles.

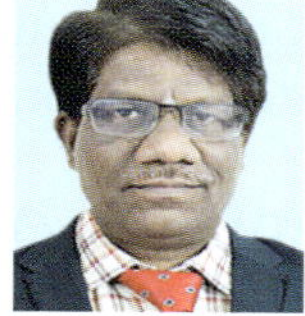

Vinod H Ratageri MD DCEH is currently Professor and Head, Department of Pediatrics, Karnataka Medical College and Research Institute, Hubballi, Karnataka, India. He obtained his postgraduate (MD) in Pediatrics from prestigious All India Institute of Medical Sciences, New Delhi. His field of interest is pediatric critical care and pulmonology, vector-borne diseases and environment and child health. He was awarded Diplomat in Environment and Child Health in 2007 by International Pediatric Association (IPA) at Athens, Greece. He is actively involved in research activities, currently working/having three ongoing projects including WHO ACTION III trial. He received Satya Gupta Award (1999) for best Paper and Best Teacher Award (2023) from IMA Karnataka. He has published 80 plus scientific papers and presented papers at many national and international conferences. He has contributed many chapters in various pediatric textbooks. Under his guidance many postgraduates successfully completed thesis. He has been the faculty in many national and international conferences and resource person for several IAP modules. Served as Member of IAP COVID Task Force and Member of Task Force for prevention of 3rd wave by Government of Karnataka.

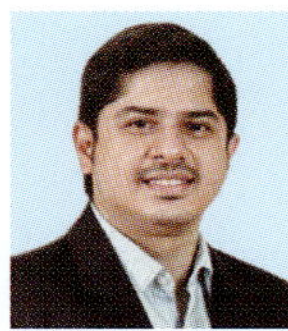

Vishnu Mohan PT MD PGDMLS PGDHM Fellowship in Neonatology is currently working as Senior Consultant, Department of Pediatrics and Neonatology, Aster Malabar Institute of Medical Sciences, Kozhikode, Kerala, India. He is an alumnus of Pushpagiri Institute of Medical Sciences, Tiruvalla, Kerala and Dr Mehta's Children's Hospital, Chennai. His area of interest is neonatal resuscitation and neonatal sepsis. He is actively involved in research and postgraduate training. He has published several scientific papers and presented papers at many national and international conferences. He has contributed many chapters in various pediatrics and neonatology textbooks. He has been a guide for postgraduate thesis since the last 10 years. He has been a faculty in many national and international conferences and resource person for several IAP modules. He is actively involved in activities of Indian Academy of Pediatrics serving as the Editor of Pediatric Companion, the Secretary of IAP Medical Education Chapter and National Convenor for the NRP FGM Project.

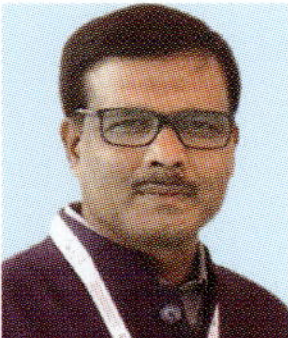

Sheikh Minhaj Ahmed MD DNB MNAMS FIAP Fellowship Pediatric Critical Care is a Full-time Pediatric Intensivist, Lilavati Hospital and Research Center, Mumbai, Maharashtra, India. He is a Postgraduate Medical Teacher, Guide to DNB Pediatrics students and a recognized Teacher at the College of Pediatric Critical Care India.

He is a prolific contributor to pediatric literature, he has publications in journals and textbooks, including roles as Editor for *IAP Updates and Guidelines Pediatric Critical Care 2024* and Associate Editor for the *Textbook of PICU Protocol 2024* and the *Journal of Pediatric Critical Care*. He is national faculty for Pediatrics and Pediatric Critical Care, and National Trainer for various CAIP modules including NRP, EPIC, and TaSK. His organizational responsibilities include being an Executive Board Member for the Pediatric Intensive Care Chapter (2022–23) and Scientific Convener for MAHA IAP 2025.

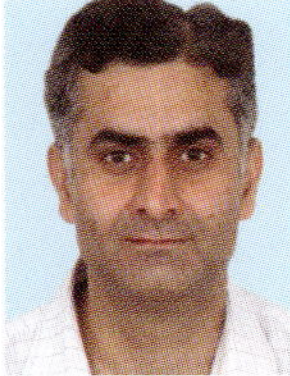

Suresh Kumar Angurana MD DM is working as Additional Professor, Division of Pediatric Critical Care, Department of Pediatrics, Advanced Pediatric Centre (APC), Postgraduate Institute of Medical Education and Research (PGIMER), Chandigarh, India. He graduated from Government Medical College, Jammu, and completed MD (Pediatrics) and DM (Pediatric Critical Care) from PGIMER, Chandigarh. He is having several fellowships including FIMSA, FCCP, FRCPCH, and FICCM. He is very astute clinician and teacher. His clinical and research interests include pediatric mechanical ventilation, restrictive maintenance fluid strategies, neurocritical care, point-of-care ultrasonography, bronchoscopy, hemophagocytic lymphohistiocytosis (HLH) in pediatric intensive care unit (PICU), and gut microbiome and probiotics in PICU. He is a well-known researcher with 225 publications in national and international journals. His research covered areas including probiotics in critically ill children, COVID-19 and MIS-C, point-of-care ultrasound, restrictive maintenance fluid therapy, and status epilepticus. He had won several awards including Dr Ritu Gupta Oration 2024, NAMS Dr Tulsi Das Chugh Award 2022, ICMR Dr HB Dingley Award 2019, Prof D Subrahmanyam Gold Medal 2018, and Major General Amir Chand Gold Medal 2012. He is actively involved in several IAP activities including IAP Chandigarh branch, pediatric intensive care chapter, IAP ALS and BLS group, pediatric emergency medicine, and IAP UG and PG quizzes.

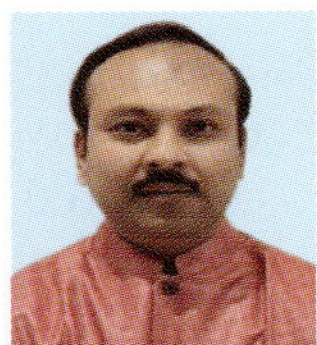

Mihir Sarkar MD is currently Professor, Department of Pediatrics and Head of PICU Unit of Government Medical College, Kolkata, West Bengal, India. He is a recognized Teacher at the College of Pediatric Critical Care. He has vast experience in pediatric critical care and emergency over the last 15 years. He is associated with PG teaching for 10 years. He has special interest in simulation-based education for nurses and residents. He has been in editorial board of *Journal of Pediatric Critical Care*. He has authored more than 45 publications in international and national journals.

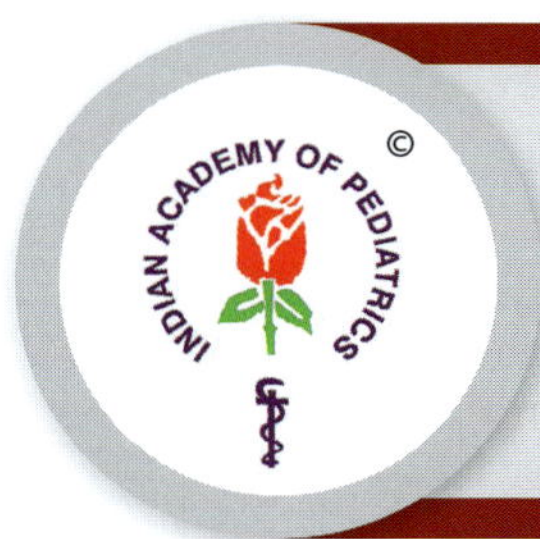

Contributors

Aakash Chandran
Agni Sekhar Saha
Anita Sharma
Arun Bansal
Ashish Simalti
Ashwini Chityala
Atanu Bhadra
Bal Mukund
Bela Verma
Bharat Choudhary
Chandrika R Doddihal
Chetan Ginigeri
Chirag Sethi
Daisy Khera
Debdatta Mukhopadhyay
Deepankar Bansal
Devajit K Sharma
Gomathy Srividya V
GV Basavaraja
Harini Chowdary Jaladi
Indumathy Santhanam
Jaidev MD
Jason Dsouza
Javed Ismail
Jayashree Muralidharan
Karthik Narayanan
Karthi Nallasamy
Kaustabh Chaudhuri
Kavitha TK
Kiran Anand
Krishna Mohan R
K Sathishkumar
Lokesh Kumar
Lokesh Lingappa
Lokesh Tiwari
Madhu PK
Madhusudan S
Mallanagouda M Patil
Manjula Anand
Meghana Tiwary
Mihir Sarkar
Moumita Samanta
Mounika Reddy
Mullai Baalaaji AR
Namrata Das
Narayanan Parameswaran
Nitesh Upadhyay
Poovazhagi V
Rajeev Redkar
Rajeshwari Nataraj
Ramesh Rajesh Pol
Rashmi Kattimani
Rashna Dass Hazarika
Remya R Pai
Renu Suthar
Reshmi Mishra
Rohit Bhowmick
RV Dhakshayani
Sai Charan
Sasidaran Kandasamy
Sasmita Devi Agrawal
Shalu Gupta
Sharada Sathishkumar
Sheikh Minhaj Ahmed
Sibabratta Patnaik
Sivamurukan Palanisamy

Sneh Yadav

Suchitra Ranjit

S Shanthi

Sumita Mishra

Suresh Kumar Angurana

Swathi Rao

Syed Ahmed Zaki

Thangavelu S

U Vijaya Kumar

Vasant M Khalatkar

Vidya Lakshmi BK

Vinitha KA

Vinod H Ratageri

Vishnu Mohan PT

Vivin Abraham

Vykunta Raju KN

Yankappa N

Yogesh N Parikh

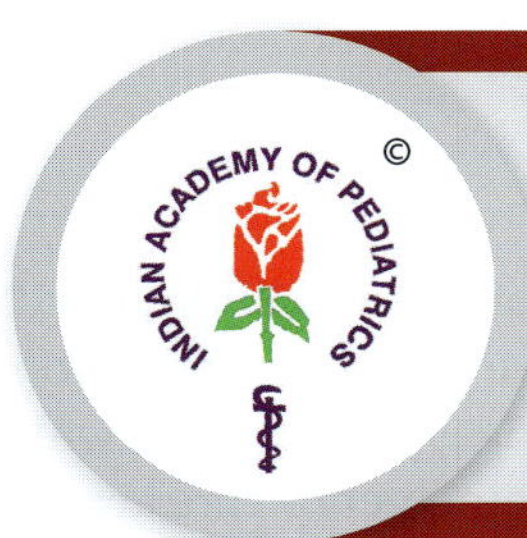

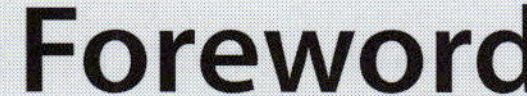

Foreword

Strengthening of Pediatric Emergency Care in India

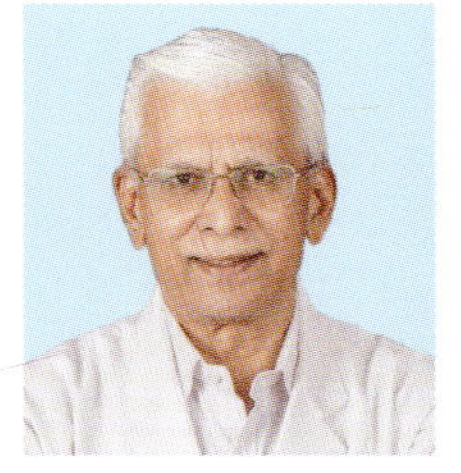

It gives me immense pleasure to write this foreword for the *IAP National Treatment Guidelines*. The guidelines are a result of a commendable initiative by Dr GV Basavaraja, IAP National President, 2024, under Presidential Action Plan, supported by current President, Dr Vasant M Khalatkar and an accomplished team of editors and academic editors. Publication of these national guidelines marks a key moment in the evolution of care of sick children and practice of Pediatric Emergency Medicine (PEM) in India. In a country where over 40% of the population is under the age of 18, the development and standardization of pediatric emergency protocols is not just timely—it is imperative.

Undoubtedly, some excellent text and protocols devoted to PEM in India are available. However, there are significant disparities, because of varying levels of resources, training, and adherence to varying protocols. While urban areas may have access to specialized care, rural regions often lack basic emergency services. The introduction of National Treatment Guidelines marks a significant step toward rectifying this imbalance and offers a crucial framework to bridge these gaps. This in turn can help to standardize care protocols and ensure that every child, regardless of location or socioeconomic status, is offered uniform, timely and appropriate care when faced with a life-threatening situation. This approach aligns with the National Health Mission's operational guidelines, which emphasize strengthening pediatric care at district hospitals.

I understand that the guidelines will provide evidence-based protocols that address specific needs, covering a spectrum of emergencies from trauma and febrile illnesses to respiratory distress and poisoning. By providing a structured approach to management, including that for critical toxicological exposures, these guidelines have the potential to significantly reduce preventable morbidity and mortality among children. One of the strongest aspects of the guidelines is their emphasis on clarity of terminology and definition and use of flowcharts for issues related to management. The inclusion of poison-specific management protocols is particularly commendable, considering that unintentional poisoning remains a significant cause of hospitalization in children, especially in rural areas with limited access to prompt care.

The standardization of care facilitated by these guidelines will have a profound impact on the quality and consistency of pediatric emergency services nationwide. It will promote a more systematic approach to diagnosis, treatment, and referral, thus reducing the risk of errors and ensuring that best practices are followed across all health-care settings. This will also enable more effective monitoring and evaluation of outcomes, however, the implementation of these guidelines presents a number of challenges. This includes ensuring the availability of essential medicines and making pediatric medicines affordable and accessible. Infrastructure deficiencies, especially in rural and tribal regions, must be addressed to support the sophisticated care algorithms proposed. Moreover, periodic revision of these guidelines based on emerging data and surveillance from poison control centers will be essential to maintain their relevance and effectiveness. Leveraging technology, such as artificial intelligence and telemedicine, can enhance the reach and efficiency of pediatric emergency services, especially in underserved areas.

To end, I believe that the book represents a significant investment in the health and future of India's children and a landmark advancement in care of sick children. This initiative, poised to standardize PEM care protocols across the nation, addresses a critical gap in pediatric emergency medicine. By addressing existing challenges and aligning with national health objectives, these guidelines have the potential to significantly improve pediatric emergency care across the country and promises to enhance the outcomes of sick children.

Sunit C Singhi
MBBS MD FIAP FAMS FISCCM FICCM FCCM
Professor Emeritus, Former Head, and Senior Professor
Department of Pediatrics and Advanced Pediatrics Centre
Postgraduate Institute of Medical Education and Research
Chandigarh, India
Professor, Senior Consultant and Head
Department of Pediatrics
Amrita Institute of Medical Sciences
Faridabad, Haryana, India

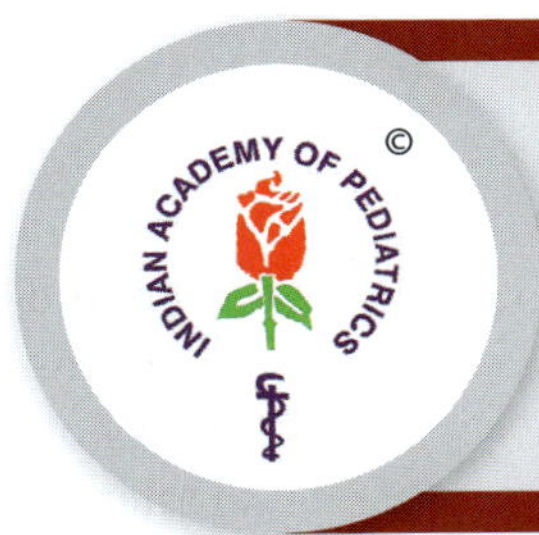

From President's Desk

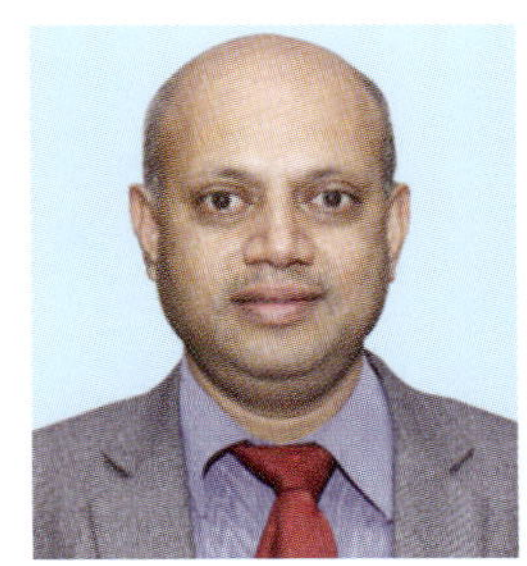

It is with great pleasure that I introduce *IAP National Treatment Guidelines*, a comprehensive, structured, and user-friendly resource designed to serve postgraduate students, teaching faculty, and practicing pediatricians. This pioneering publication aims to bridge the gap between theory and practice by offering clear, evidence-based guidelines on managing pediatric emergencies and toxicology cases.

The first issue covers 50 of the most common topics encountered in clinical practice, meticulously curated and authored by renowned experts in the field. The peer-reviewed content ensures accuracy, relevance, and practicality, making it an invaluable reference for healthcare professionals dedicated to improving pediatric emergency care.

I would like to extend my sincere appreciation my Co-editor-in-chief, Dr Vasant M Khalatkar, whose visionary leadership has been instrumental in bringing this project to fruition. Thanks, are also due to the Executive Editors, Drs Yogesh N Parikh and Atanu Bhadra for their support and guidance during this project.

Thanks to the Academic Editors, Drs Arun Bansal, Vinod H Ratageri, Vishnu Mohan PT, Sheikh Minhaj Ahmed, Suresh Kumar Angurana, and Mihir Sarkar, whose collective efforts have ensured the publication's quality and relevance.

I am confident that this book will serve as a reliable and practical tool, enhancing the quality of pediatric emergency and toxicology care across the region. May it inspire continued learning, collaboration, and excellence in this vital area of pediatrics.

With Regards

GV Basavaraja
MD DNB FIAP
Professor
Department of Pediatrics
Indira Gandhi Institute of Child Health
Bengaluru, Karnataka, India
IAP National President, 2024

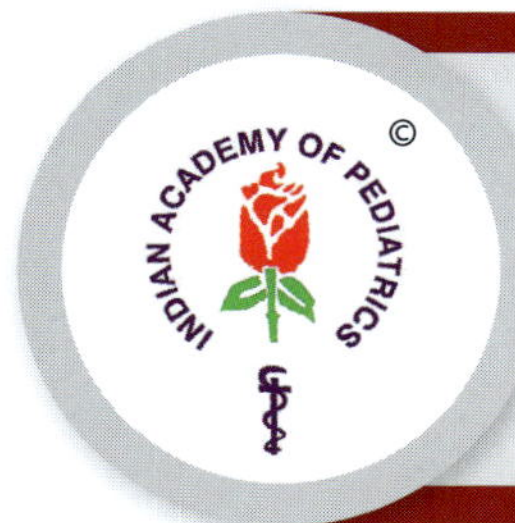

From President's Desk

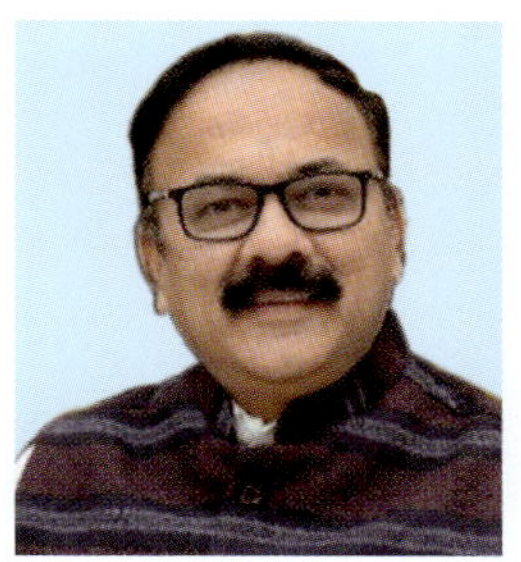

It is with immense pride and satisfaction that I extend my heartfelt congratulations to the editorial team and contributors of the *IAP National Treatment Guidelines*. This comprehensive reference represents a major milestone in standardizing the management of pediatric emergencies across the country.

Pediatric emergency care is a critical component of child health services, where timely recognition and evidence-based interventions can be lifesaving. The inclusion of toxicology—a field often underrepresented yet of growing significance—adds valuable depth to this volume. These guidelines bring together national expertise, practical algorithms, and context-specific recommendations that are not only scientifically robust but also feasible for use across diverse healthcare settings, from urban hospitals to rural health centers.

This initiative reflects the IAP's continued commitment to strengthening pediatric healthcare delivery through knowledge dissemination, skill enhancement, and clinical standardization. I am confident that this book will serve as an indispensable tool for pediatricians, emergency physicians, medical students, and frontline health workers.

I extend my heartfelt appreciation to the Co-Editor-in-Chief, Dr GV Basavaraja whose visionary leadership has been pivotal in bringing this significant project to the completion. I would also like to acknowledge the invaluable contributions of the Executive Editors, Drs Yogesh N Parikh and Atanu Bhadra for their crucial role in maintaining the quality, relevance, and depth of this publication.

My sincere thanks to the Academic Editors, Drs Arun Bansal, Vinod H Ratageri, Vishnu Mohan PT, Sheikh Minhaj Ahmed, Suresh Kumar Angurana, and Mihir Sarkar for their unwavering dedication to advancing the field of pediatric emergency medicine. Their scholarly contributions are truly commendable.

I commend the dedicated efforts of all involved in this endeavor and urge all healthcare professionals to adopt these guidelines in their clinical practice. Together, let us continue striving toward excellence in pediatric care, ensuring a safer and healthier future for our children.

Through this endure let's complete our moto to "Serve children, Colleagues and Country".

Warm regards

Vasant M Khalatkar
MD PGDID FICMCH
Consultant
Pediatrician and Neonatologist
Khalatkar Hospital
Nagpur, Maharashtra, India
IAP National President, 2025

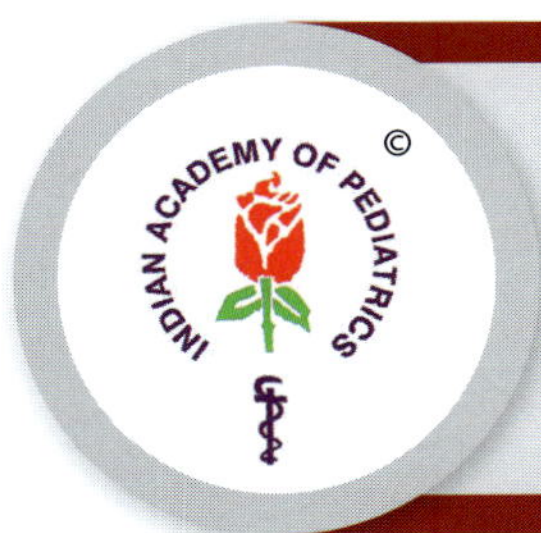

From Honorary Secretary General' Desk

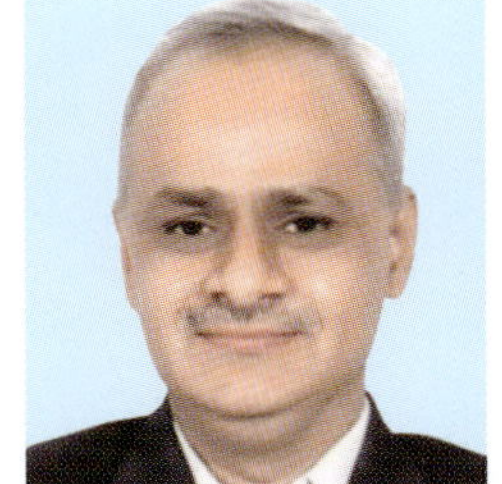

The *IAP National Treatment Guidelines* represents a groundbreaking initiative in pediatric care, offering a comprehensive, structured, and simplified approach to managing pediatric emergencies and toxicology. In a rapidly evolving medical landscape, where timely intervention can be the defining factor between life and loss, having a standardized, expertly curated reference is not just beneficial—it is essential.

This pioneering effort, meticulously crafted for postgraduates, teaching faculty, and practicing pediatricians, serves as a beacon of knowledge, ensuring that those at the frontline of pediatric emergencies have access to the most reliable, evidence-based, and practical treatment protocols. Every page of this book reflects years of collective expertise, bringing together renowned specialists to author 50 critical topics, addressing both the breadth and depth of pediatric emergency and toxicology management.

Pediatric Medicine is not just a science; it is an art of timely decision-making, an ever-evolving discipline guided by wisdom, experience, and structured knowledge. This book bridges the gap between theoretical expertise and real-world application, empowering practitioners to make critical, life-saving choices with confidence. It represents a collective vision—one that prioritizes precision, clarity, and the highest standards of pediatric care.

This monumental work would not have been possible without the dedication and visionary leadership of the Editors-in-Chief, Drs GV Basavaraja and Vasant M Khalatkar; the Executive Editors, Drs Yogesh N Parikh and Atanu Bhadra; the Academic Editors, Drs Arun Bansal, Vinod H Ratageri, Vishnu Mohan PT, Sheikh Minhaj Ahmed, Suresh Kumar Angurana, and Mihir Sarkar, whose collective expertise has shaped this invaluable resource.

May this book serve as a cornerstone in the practice of pediatric medicine, guiding professionals toward more precise, informed, and life-saving interventions. It is more than a book—it is a commitment to excellence, a tribute to collective knowledge, and a tool that will define the future of pediatric emergency care.

With kind regards

Yogesh N Parikh
MD
Associate Professor
Department of Pediatrics
Government Medical College
Surat, Gujarat, India
Secretary General, IAP (2024–2025)

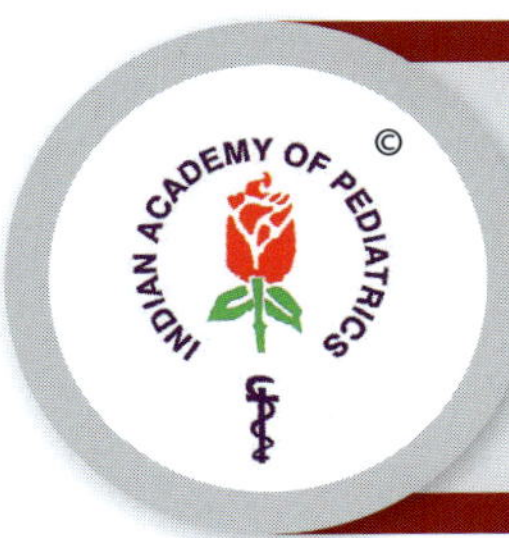

Message from the IAP National Treasurer (2024–2025)

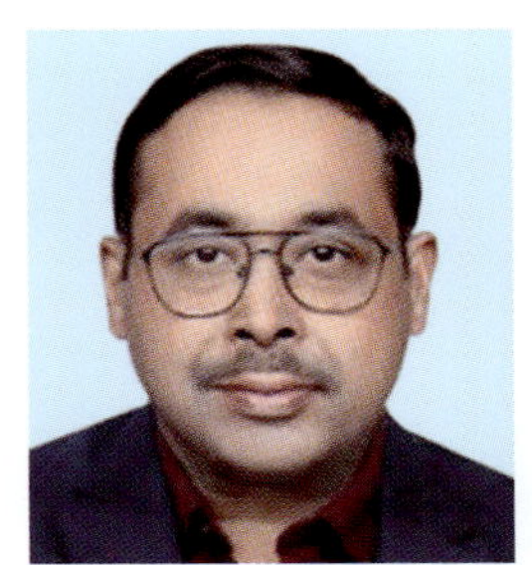

Heartfelt congratulations to the editors, authors, and contributors of the *IAP National Treatment Guidelines*. This comprehensive resource will undoubtedly benefit postgraduate students, teaching faculty, and practicing pediatricians. Kudos to the entire team for their meticulous work in creating a valuable guideline for the medical community.

"Special appreciation to the editorial team led by Drs GV Basavaraja and Vasant M Khalatkar, along with the Executive Editors, Academic Editors, for their exceptional leadership and dedication to this project."

Atanu Bhadra
DCH
Medical Superintendent
ESI Hospital
Asansol, West Bengal, India
National Treasurer, IAP (2024–2025)

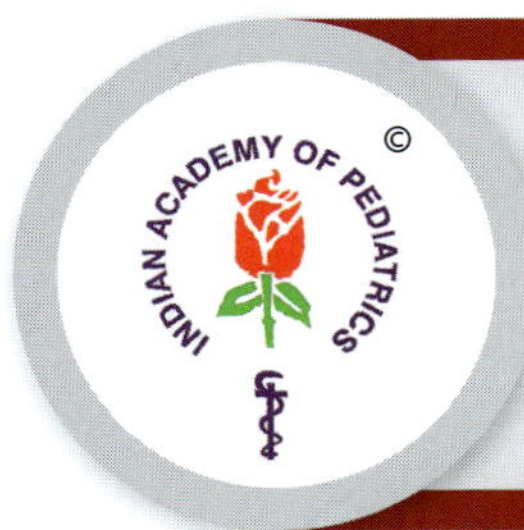

Preface

Pediatric emergencies demand precision, speed, and sound clinical judgment—traits that must be backed by standardized, evidence-based protocols. The *IAP National Treatment Guidelines* have been meticulously conceived as a national resource to empower pediatricians, emergency physicians, and frontline healthcare providers across India in delivering uniform, timely, and effective care to every child in need.

In a country as diverse as ours, where healthcare delivery spans from tertiary urban centers to remote rural clinics, the need for structured and contextually relevant emergency guidelines is pressing. This volume responds to that need. By combining the latest evidence with pragmatic recommendations tailored to India's unique epidemiological and healthcare landscape, these guidelines aim to bridge the gap between medical knowledge and real-world practice.

This compendium includes over 50 high-yield topics authored by a distinguished panel of national experts, ensuring both depth and breadth. The inclusion of pediatric toxicology as a dedicated section acknowledges the growing burden of toxic exposures and poisoning, especially in under-resourced regions, and aims to provide life-saving clarity in such scenarios.

Special care has been taken to ensure clarity of definitions, logical structuring of clinical algorithms, and consistency in therapeutic approaches. These features, combined with flowcharts and concise guidance, make the book not just a reference, but a reliable companion in the emergency room.

The creation of this publication has been a collaborative and inclusive effort. From the vision of the IAP leadership to the scholarly dedication of the editorial and author teams, every page reflects a shared commitment to improving pediatric outcomes. The guidelines are also aligned with broader national goals of strengthening emergency pediatric services at district and sub-district levels.

This book is more than a publication—it is a testament to the pediatric fraternity's resolve to serve children with compassion, competence, and consistency. It is dedicated to the countless children whose resilience inspires us daily and to the pediatricians whose tireless commitment makes a difference, one emergency at a time.

We hope that this volume not only guides critical clinical decisions but also catalyzes continued learning, system-wide improvement, and a culture of excellence in pediatric emergency care.

Editorial Team
IAP National Treatment Guidelines

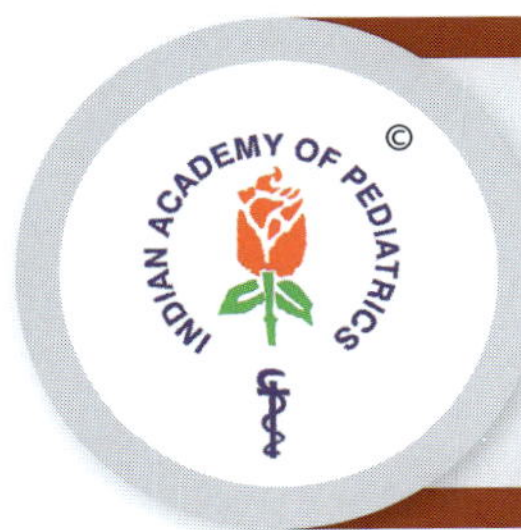

Acknowledgments

This endeavor, the *IAP National Treatment Guidelines* for pediatricians, has been a journey of collective passion and expertise, driven by a shared commitment to the well-being of children.

We are profoundly grateful to the Indian Academy of Pediatrics (IAP) leadership, including Dr Vasant M Khalatkar, IAP National President, 2025; Dr GV Basavaraja, IAP National President, 2024; Dr Neelam Mohan, President-Elect, IAP, 2025; Dr Yogesh N Parikh, Secretary General, IAP (2024–2025); and Dr Atanu Bhadra, National Treasurer, IAP (2024–2025), for entrusting with this vital project and for their unconditional support throughout its development.

We are immensely indebted to all the expert contributors who have generously shared their invaluable knowledge, clinical experience, and precious time to meticulously craft each chapter. Their rigorous efforts in synthesizing complex information into practical, evidence-based guidelines form the very bedrock of this publication.

Accolades to the editorial team, whose tireless work in coordinating, editing, and harmonizing diverse contributions was pivotal in shaping this book into a cohesive and accessible. The editorial team's commitment to excellence is deeply appreciated.

We are thankful to Shri Jitendar P Vij (Group Chairman), Mr Ankit Vij (Managing Director), Mr MS Mani (Group President), Mr Sabyasachi Hazra (Director—Professional Publishing, Marketing, and Business Development), Mr Naman Singh (Development Editor), and the publishing team at M/s Jaypee Brothers Medical Publishers (P) Ltd, New Delhi, India, for their professionalism and dedication in bringing this project to reality.

This book is a resource forged by many, for the benefit of many. It is dedicated to empowering pediatricians and all frontline healthcare providers with the most current and effective strategies to manage pediatric emergencies and toxicological challenges. We hope these guidelines will foster greater confidence, improve patient outcomes, and ultimately contribute to the well-being of every child under their care.

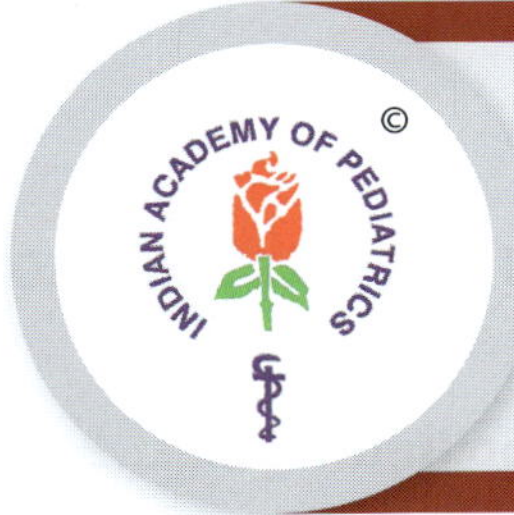

Contents

1 Section

General

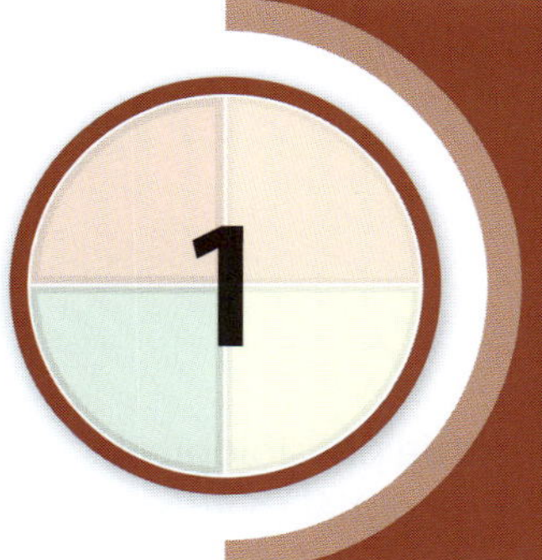

Approach to Triage in Pediatric Emergency Room

Suresh Kumar Angurana, Shalu Gupta

LEARNING OBJECTIVES

- Systematic approach to recognition of a sick child using the "ABCDE" approach (Airway, Breathing, Circulation, Disability, and Exposure)
- Understanding the importance of functional or physiological impairment rather than definitive diagnosis in an emergency set-up
- Application of interventions for stabilization depending on physiological status

A CRITICALLY ILL CHILD

A critical illness exists when impending or existing organ malfunction threatens or interferes with viability of cellular function. This may be a result of any severe illness, disease, or injury as:

- Fever with altered consciousness, toxicity, body temperature >40°C, and hypothermia
- Accident/trauma with loss of consciousness, or bleeding, blunt abdominal/chest trauma, burns, fire-smoke inhalation, drowning, and foreign body
- Respiratory distress, slow/irregular breathing, stridor, and obstructed airway
- Unconsciousness, convulsion, and sudden paralysis
- Severe diarrhea and/or vomiting
- Suspected poisoning, snake bite, scorpion, and other stings
- Acute bleeding
- Postoperative
- Sudden worsening of a previously known illness

WHY SYSTEMATIC ASSESSMENT OF A SICK CHILD IS NEEDED?

Early recognition of sick children is important, because children usually have very little physiological reserve and they progress very rapidly into irreversible organ system damage. It is essential to adopt a systematic approach and focus on identification of functional impairment of organ systems (e.g., respiratory distress, respiratory failure, or shock) to direct the lifesaving intervention(s) to make up for child's inability to compensate physiologically.

RAPID ASSESSMENT: PHYSICAL EXAMINATION

Critical care is generally equated with high technology and equipment. However, the recognition of critical illness and provision of early care depend entirely on the use of eyes, ears, and hands by "ABCDE" assessment approach **(Table 1)**. This includes *evaluation/assessment* of the patient, *identification* of the physiological derangement, and institution of appropriate *interventions* based on the physiological derangement *(E-I-I cycle)*. At any step, if there is any life-threating situation, the appropriate interventions should be directed before proceeding to the next step.

TABLE 1: Components of ABCDE assessment.

A	Airway	To assess if airway is open
B	Breathing	To assess oxygenation and ventilation
C	Circulation	To assess adequacy of tissue perfusion
D	Disability	To assess intactness of central nervous control of all vital functions
E	Exposure	To look for surface findings

Assessment of Airway

Is it clear and breathing comfortable? Or any sign of airway obstruction (stridor), secretions? Look for movements of the chest and abdomen, and listen for air movements and breath sounds.

Assessment of Breathing

Assessment of breathing includes evaluation of respiratory rate, respiratory efforts, chest expansion and air movements, lung and airway sound, and oxygen saturation (SpO_2).

- *Respiratory rate:* Whether slow, fast (>60 breaths/min), irregular **(Table 2)**?
- *Respiratory effort:* Is work of breathing increased (tachypnea, retractions, grunting, head-bobbing, and see-saw breathing), decreased, or absent?

- *Chest expansion and air movements:* Is the chest expansion adequate with each breath?
- *Lung and airway sounds:* Air entry on auscultation good and equal or any added sounds?
- *Oxygen saturation:* SpO_2 of <90% suggests inadequate oxygenation.

TABLE 2: Normal respiratory rates for different age groups.

Age group	*Normal respiratory rate range*
Infant (<1 year)	30–60 breaths/min
Toddler (1–3 years)	24–40 breaths/min
Preschooler (4–5 years)	22–34 breaths/min
School age (6–12 years)	18–30 breaths/min
Adolescents (13–18 years)	12–16 breaths/min

Assessment of Circulation

The circulatory system is designed to meet body's oxygen and nutrient demand. Adequacy of circulation depends on cardiac output (COP) and blood pressure (BP). COP is determined by stroke volume (SV) and heart rate (HR); SV depends on myocardial contractility, preload (volume of blood coming to right side of heart) and after load, or systemic vascular resistance (SVR) (resistance to forward flow of blood). Assessment of adequacy of circulation includes:

- HR and rhythm
- Pulses (both central and peripheral pulses)
- Capillary refill time (CRT)
- Skin color and temperature
- BP
- Urine output

Heart rate: It is an important determinant of COP as COP = HR × SV. Tachycardia suggests a compensatory effort to meet circulatory needs. It is an early and sensitive indicator of impending circulatory decompensation. HR >180 beats/min in children <5 years and HR >220 beats/min in infants may indicate a tachyarrhythmia (e.g., SVT). It should also include obtaining an electrocardiography (ECG) to identify abnormal rhythm, especially in cases with very fast pulse rate (>200–220 beats/min), and irregular or absent pulse. Age-wise limits of HR are provided in **Table 3**.

TABLE 3: Age-wise normal heart rate range on children.

Age group	*Normal heart rate range*
Newborn to 3 months	85–205 beats/min
3 months to 2 years	100–190 beats/min
2–10 years	60–140 beats/min
>10 years	60–100 beats/min

Palpation of pulse: This should be done over carotid (central) [older children] and brachial pulse [for infants]. A good pulse examination gives information about SV, BP, and SVR. Weak or absent carotid pulse indicates poor SV/COP, requiring immediate intervention. A poor peripheral pulse volume is an early sign of hypovolemia than hypotension and suggests critical loss of vital organ perfusion.

Capillary refill time: This is assessed by rapidity of filling of cutaneous capillary bed after blanching the skin of distal extremity (foot/hand) with pressure of examiner's thumb. It should be performed at a neutral thermal environment (i.e., room temperature) and extremity must be lifted slightly above the level of heart. Normal CRT is ≤2 seconds. Increased CRT indicates poor skin perfusion and low COP.

Skin color and temperature: In a well-perfused child, the skin color and temperature should be similar over trunk and extremities; and mucus membranes, nail beds, palms, and soles should be pink. In cases with low COP, cooling of skin begins from peripheries (fingers and toes) and extends proximally. Cool or clammy extremities indicate low COP; pale, blue, or mottled skin indicates ischemia; and cyanosis suggests slow flow through skin or hypoxemia.

Blood pressure: BP is dependent on COP and SVR. A fall in BP reflects decreased COP. Hypotension is a late sign of circulatory decompensation as BP may be maintained till late in shock state inspite of a fall in COP because of compensatory vasoconstriction and tachycardia. Therefore, even mild hypotension must be treated quickly, because it signals decompensation and imminent cardiopulmonary arrest. Accurate BP measurement requires a proper size cuff. The length of the bladder cuff should be 80–100% of arm circumference, width at least 40% with lower end of the cuff around 2–3 cm above the antecubital fossa. Hypotension is defined by threshold of systolic BP for age as shown in **Table 4**.

TABLE 4: Systolic blood pressure cut-off in children to define hypotension.

Age group	*Systolic blood pressure threshold*
Term neonates (0–28 days)	<60 mm Hg
Infants (1–12 months)	<70 mm Hg
Children (1–10 years)	<70 + [age (in years × 2)] mm Hg
Children >10 years	<90 mm Hg

Assessment of Disability/Central Nervous System Function

It is the quick evaluation of neurological function and brain perfusion in ill or injured child. These signs include level of consciousness, muscle tone, and pupillary response. Common causes of decreased consciousness in children include encephalitis, meningitis, poor cerebral perfusion, traumatic brain injury, hypoglycemia, drugs, hypoxemia, and hypercarbia.

The assessment of level of consciousness can be done by using Glasgow Coma Scale (GCS) **(Table 5)** or AVPU Pediatric Response Scale **(Table 6)**. The integrity of brainstem should be assessed by examination of pupils (size, reaction to light), respiratory pattern, and motor response and posture **(Table 7)**. Always include bedside measurement of blood glucose at this stage of evaluation.

TABLE 5: Glasgow Coma Scale.	
Eye opening	***Best motor response***
4 Spontaneous 3 To verbal command 2 To pain 1 No opening	6 Obeys verbal command (>2 years) 5 Localizes pain 4 Flexion withdrawal (>6 months) 3 Flexion—decorticate (<6 months) 2 Extension—decerebrate 1 No response
Best verbal response	
≤3 years	***≥4 years***
5 Smile, interacts 4 Crying, consolable 3 Inconsistently consolable 2 Inconsolable, restless 1 No response	5 Oriented, converses 4 Disoriented, converses—words 3 Inappropriate words—vocal sounds 2 Incomprehensible speech 1 No response

TABLE 6: AVPU Pediatric Response Scale.

Score	*Description*
A	Alert and active
V	Responsive to verbal commands
P	Responsive to painful stimuli
U	Unresponsive

TABLE 7: Neurological signs seen with brainstem involvement at different levels.

Central nervous system level	*Pupils*	*Doll's eye movement*	*Respiratory pattern*	*Motor response*
Thalamus	Small reactive	Variable	Cheyne-Stokes	Normal response
Midbrain	Midposition fixed	Absent	Hyperventilation	Decorticate
Pons	Pinpoint fixed	Absent	Apneustic	Decerebrate, flaccid
Medulla	Small reactive	Present	Ataxic	No posturing flaccid

Assessment of Exposure

It includes head-to-toe examination to note fever, any temperature difference between trunk and extremities, evidence of trauma, bleeding, burns, bruises, petechiae, purpura, and rash. Take precautions to avoid cold stress or hypothermia and maintain cervical spine precautions (while turning the child with suspected head and neck injury).

CATEGORIZATION OF PHYSIOLOGICAL STATUS AND SIGNS OF LIFE-THREATENING CONDITIONS

At the end of ABCDE assessment, it is possible to arrive at a reasonable physiological categorization **(Table 8)**. Depending on abnormal findings, the life-threatening conditions can be identified and life-saving intervention should be executed **(Table 9)**.

TABLE 8: Physiological categorization.

1.	Stable	Normal airway, breathing, and circulation
2.	Respiratory distress	Abnormal work of breathing
3.	Respiratory failure	Marked increased work of breathing, cyanosis, and gasping
4.	Compensated shock	Poor perfusion and normal blood pressure
5.	Hypotensive shock	Poor perfusion and hypotension
6.	Primary brain or systemic dysfunction	Includes CNS problems (increased ICP, impaired consciousness or coma, and status epilepticus) or systemic manifestations

(CNS: central nervous system; ICP: intracranial pressure)

TABLE 9: Signs of life-threatening conditions.

System	*Life-threatening conditions*	*Life-saving interventions*
Airway	Complete or severe airway obstruction	Oxygen by NRM, airway suctioning, opening the, cervical spine stabilization, bag and mask ventilation, endotracheal intubation, and positive pressure ventilation
Breathing	Apnea, significant increased work of breathing, and bradypnea	Oxygen by NRM, bag and mask ventilation, endotracheal intubation, and positive pressure ventilation
Circulation	Absence of palpable pulses, poor perfusion, hypotension, bradycardia, and arrhythmia	Vascular access (IV or intraosseous), volume expansion, vasoactive drugs infusion, and blood transfusion
Disability	Unresponsiveness, decreased level of consciousness, seizures, and raised ICP	Seizure control, control of ICP, and correction of metabolic derangements (hypoglycemia and hypocalcemia)
Exposure	Significant hypothermia, bleeding, petechiae, or purpura consistent with septic shock, and significant injury	Control of temperature, bleeding, and drainage of abscess

(ICP: intracranial pressure; IV: intravenous; NRM: nonrebreathing mask)

SECONDARY ASSESSMENT

The secondary assessment includes focused history (SAMPLE) and focused examination. The components of focused history are given in **Table 10**.

TABLE 10: Components of focused history (SAMPLE).

S	Signs and symptoms	• Cough, tachypnea, and increased respiratory efforts • Altered sensorium/decreased consciousness • Fever, diarrhea, vomiting, poor feeding, and lethargy • Bleeding
A	Allergies	Any history of drug allergy (like penicillin)
M	Medications	Last dose and type of medications (e.g., last antiepileptic-type/dose/whether missed or not)
P	Past medical history	• Past surgery • *Past medical events:* Asthma, diabetes, hypertension, arrhythmia, and heart disease
L	Last meal	The time when the last solid/liquid was taken
E	Events	Events leading to current illness or injury (gradual or sudden)

Airway and Breathing Stabilization

If airway is unstable (patency cannot be maintained, or excessive secretions), the interventions include head tilt and chin lift (jaw thrust in suspected cervical spine injury), suctioning, and placement of an oropharyngeal airway. If patient is in respiratory distress or hypoxic, 100% oxygen with a nonrebreathing mask (NRM) should be started. If breathing efforts are not good and or chest expansion is inadequate, use bag and mask ventilation with 100% oxygen, followed by endotracheal (ET) intubation and bag-tube ventilation. The indications for ET intubation and tracheostomy or a cricothyrotomy are given in **Box 1**.

BOX 1: Indications for endotracheal intubation and tracheostomy or cricothyrotomy.

Indications for endotracheal intubation

- Functional/anatomic airway obstruction
- *Loss of protective airway reflex:* Aspiration is a risk (GCS <8)
- Inadequate CNS control of ventilation
- Excessive work of breathing
- Prolonged respiratory support is anticipated

Indications for tracheostomy or cricothyrotomy

- Endotracheal intubation is difficult or the tube patency is difficult to maintain because of secretions, infection, or bleeding
- *Upper airway obstruction:* Diphtheria
- Vocal cord paralysis
- Facial/upper airway burns, trauma

(CNS: central nervous system; GCS: Glasgow Coma Scale)

Circulatory Support

If tachycardia and poor perfusion (compensated shock) or hypotension (hypotensive shock) are present, following measures are needed:

- **Establishment of a vascular access:** Establish a large peripheral vein. Often intravenous (IV) line may take time to establish because of collapsed veins. Intraosseous route should be used in case establishing an IV line is difficult.
- **Volume expansion:** Administer 10–20 mL/kg normal saline or Ringer's lactate boluses as fast as possible till pulse volume improves followed by close monitoring and reassessment for response to fluid boluses or evidence of fluid overload. Further boluses are indicated depending on clinical status. Children with hemorrhagic shock require blood after initial crystalloid administration.
- **Vasoactive therapy:** Administration of vasoactive drugs such as adrenaline or noradrenaline as IV infusion is required for fluid-refractory shock. The goal of immediate therapy is to achieve a normal HR, normal CRT, warm peripheries, well palpable pulses, normal sensorium, normal urine output, and normal BP.
- **Management of arrhythmia:** Rhythm disturbances can lead to hemodynamic compromise. Obtain ECG in all patients with arrhythmia who are in shock (unstable rhythms). A defibrillator is often required. The treatment depends on type of rhythm and hemodynamic status.
    - Ventricular tachycardia (VT) with palpable pulse requires immediate synchronized cardioversion (0.5–1 joule/kg), while pulseless VT requires defibrillation/unsynchronized shock (2 joules/kg). Drugs indicated for VT are amiodarone (5 mg/Kg) IV or lidocaine 1 mg/kg IV or ET route.
    - Ventricular fibrillation should be treated with defibrillation (2 joules/kg).
    - Supraventricular tachycardia which is unstable requires immediate synchronized cardioversion (0.5–1 joule/kg), while stable SVT can be treated with adenosine (0.1 mg/kg/dose, IV two-syringe technique) that can be repeated to a maximum dose of 12 mg.
    - *Bradycardia, asystole:* Epinephrine is the drug of choice. Atropine is reserved for vagally mediated bradycardia. External pacemaker may be required in refractory cases.

Central Nervous System Protection

In any child with coma, seizures, altered sensorium, or increased intracranial pressure (ICP), the following interventions should be instituted:

- Ensure adequate airway and breathing, and manage circulatory impairment and hypotension.
- *Seizure control:* Midazolam or diazepam may be repeated every 5 minutes for 2–3 doses followed by phenytoin 20 mg/kg IV.
- Treat hypoglycemia with glucose (25%) 2 mL/kg or (10%) 5 mL/kg IV stat.
- Treat hypocalcemia with IV calcium gluconate (10%) 1–2 mL/kg under cardiac monitoring.

- Control ICP to maintain adequate cerebral perfusion pressure by:
  - Head-end elevation, head in midline
  - Fever control
  - Sedation, minimal stimulation
  - Preprocedure sedation, analgesia is a must; ET suction requires additional ET lidocaine.
  - Avoid urinary catheter block and bladder fullness as it can increase ICP.
  - Hyperventilation for acute surge in ICP
  - Mannitol 0.25–0.5 g/kg IV or 3% saline (10 mL/kg) for acute surge in ICP

KEY MESSAGES

- Children quickly lapse into irreversible organ system damage, because they have very little physiological reserve. Therefore, early recognition of a sick child is extremely important.
- A systematic stepwise "ABCDE" approach enables quick recognition of a sick child.
- "ABCDE" algorithm can be easily performed by clinical examination and does not require high technology or advanced monitors.
- The aim is to identify the physiological derangement rather than specific diagnosis.
- Based on physiological status, interventions such as oxygen, fluids/vasoactive drugs, intubation, positive pressure ventilation, and defibrillation need to be prioritized.
- Team approach with clear individual roles and responsibilities is important during stabilization process.

SUGGESTED READING

1. Angurana SK, Jindal A, Singhi S, Jayashree M. Pediatric cardiopulmonary resuscitation and stabilization. In: Singhi SC, Jayashree M (Eds). PGIMER Management Protocols in Emergency Medicine, 3rd edition. The Indian Journal of Pediatrics; 2020. pp. 13-30.
2. Gouin S, Gravel J, Amre DK, Bergeron S. Evaluation of the Paediatric Canadian Triage and Acuity Scale in a pediatric ED. Am J Emerg Med. 2005;23(3):243-7.
3. Jayashree M, Singhi SC. Initial assessment and triage in ER. Indian J Pediatr. 2011;78:1100-8.
4. King C, Dube A, Zadutsa B, Banda L, Langton J, Desmond N, et al. Paediatric Emergency Triage, Assessment and Treatment (ETAT)—preparedness for implementation at primary care facilities in Malawi. Glob Health Action. 2021;14(1):1989807.
5. Kumar S, Singhi S. Recognition and stabilization of the critically ill child. In: Singhi S, Jayashree M, Lodha R (Eds). PGI-AIIMS Pediatric Critical Care Nursing Manual. 2016.
6. WHO. (2005). Emergency Triage Assessment and Treatment (ETAT) course. [online] Available from https://www.who.int/publications/i/item/9241546875 [Last accessed January, 2024].

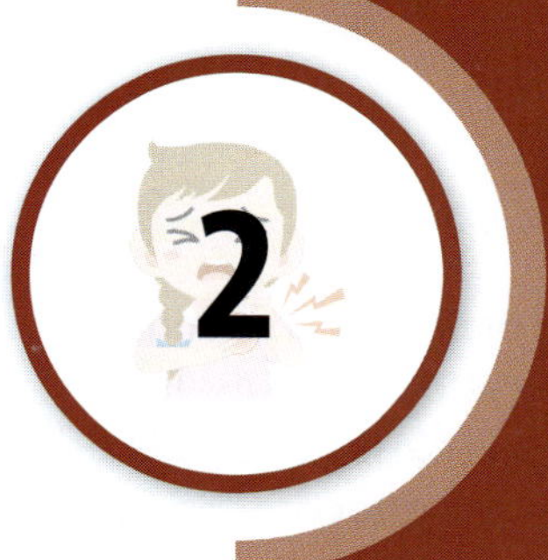

2 Cardiopulmonary Arrest

Lokesh Tiwari

DEFINITION

In a monitored setting such as pediatric intensive care unit (PICU), one may quickly identify cardiopulmonary arrest based on cardiac rhythm and respiratory effort; however, in an unmonitored setting, a practical, operational definition of cardiac arrest is when a person is unresponsive with absent or abnormal breathing. Palpation for the presence or absence of a pulse is not reliable as the sole determinant of cardiac arrest and the need for chest compressions; hence, in out-of-hospital cardiac arrest (OHCA), a lay rescuer should not delay starting CPR in a child with no "signs of life" such as movement and coughing. Healthcare providers should consider assessing the presence of a pulse as long as the initiation of CPR is not delayed more than 10 seconds.[5-7]

INCIDENCE

Cardiac arrest is a major international public health problem. The estimated annual incidence of emergency medical services-treated cardiac arrest is 30.0–97.1 individuals per 100,000 population. The brain starts to die after 3–5 minutes following the circulatory arrest, and overall survival rates often are 2–10%. Chances of survival after cardiac arrest are reduced by 10% every minute, but this may improve to 2–3% per minute with immediate and effective cardiopulmonary resuscitation.[1] The incidence of in-hospital cardiac arrest (IHCA) is reported as 2.8–12.6 events per 1,000 children in developed countries with survival at discharge of 45–50%.[2]

As there are no cardiopulmonary resuscitation (CPR) registries or central reporting process in India, the actual incidence and outcome of pediatric IHCA remain unknown. Single-center studies show an event rate of IHCA ranging from 67 to 83.7 per 1,000 infants and children admitted to the hospital with survival at discharge of 1.8–14%.[3,4]

TYPES OF RHYTHMS IN CARDIAC ARREST

Pediatric IHCA most often occurs in the setting of progressive respiratory failure or shock, and initial cardiac arrest rhythms are nonshockable, i.e., bradycardia with poor perfusion, asystole, or pulseless electrical activity (PEA). Shockable rhythm, i.e., ventricular fibrillation (VF), and pulseless ventricular tachycardia (PVT) account for approximately 10% of CPR events in children and have better outcomes than primary PEA and asystole.[2]

MANAGEMENT

The science behind CPR is continually and extensively reviewed by International Liaison Committee on Resuscitation (ILCOR).[8] Management of cardiopulmonary arrest in infants and children is depicted in three important steps **(Flowchart 1)**:

- Basic comprehensive life support or initiation of CPR
- Transition from basic comprehensive to advanced life support
- Postcardiac arrest management bundle

Basic Comprehensive Life Support or Initiation of Cardiopulmonary Resuscitation

There are three tiers of CPR depending upon the site of incidence, i.e., IHCA versus OHCA, number and proficiency of rescuers, local protocols and availability of equipment.[9]

1. *Tier 1: Hands-only CPR:* Applicable in out-of-hospital settings with a lay rescuer having limited basic life support (BLS) skills with emphasis on chest compressions only till further help arrives
2. *Tier 2: Compressions and breathing CPR:* Consists of a skilled BLS rescuer initiating CPR with a compression–ventilation ratio of 30:2 in adults/adolescents or 15:2 in infants and children till medical help is available.
3. *Tier 3: Multirescuer-coordinated CPR:* Denotes a systematic approach where multiple lifesaving actions such as compressions, ventilation, and defibrillation are performed simultaneously by multiple skilled rescuers using effective team dynamics. There should be a smooth transition from basic comprehensive to advanced life support.

Steps

A lay person or those who are not trained in pediatric CPR should assess for scene safety and initiate chest compressions following C-A-B sequence with compression to ventilation ratio of 30:2 (same as adults) in a child who is unresponsive and has no breathing or who is only gasping. A healthcare provider who is trained in pediatric CPR should follow the steps as given in **Table 1**.[9,10]

Flowchart 1: Algorithmic approach to management of cardiopulmonary arrest.

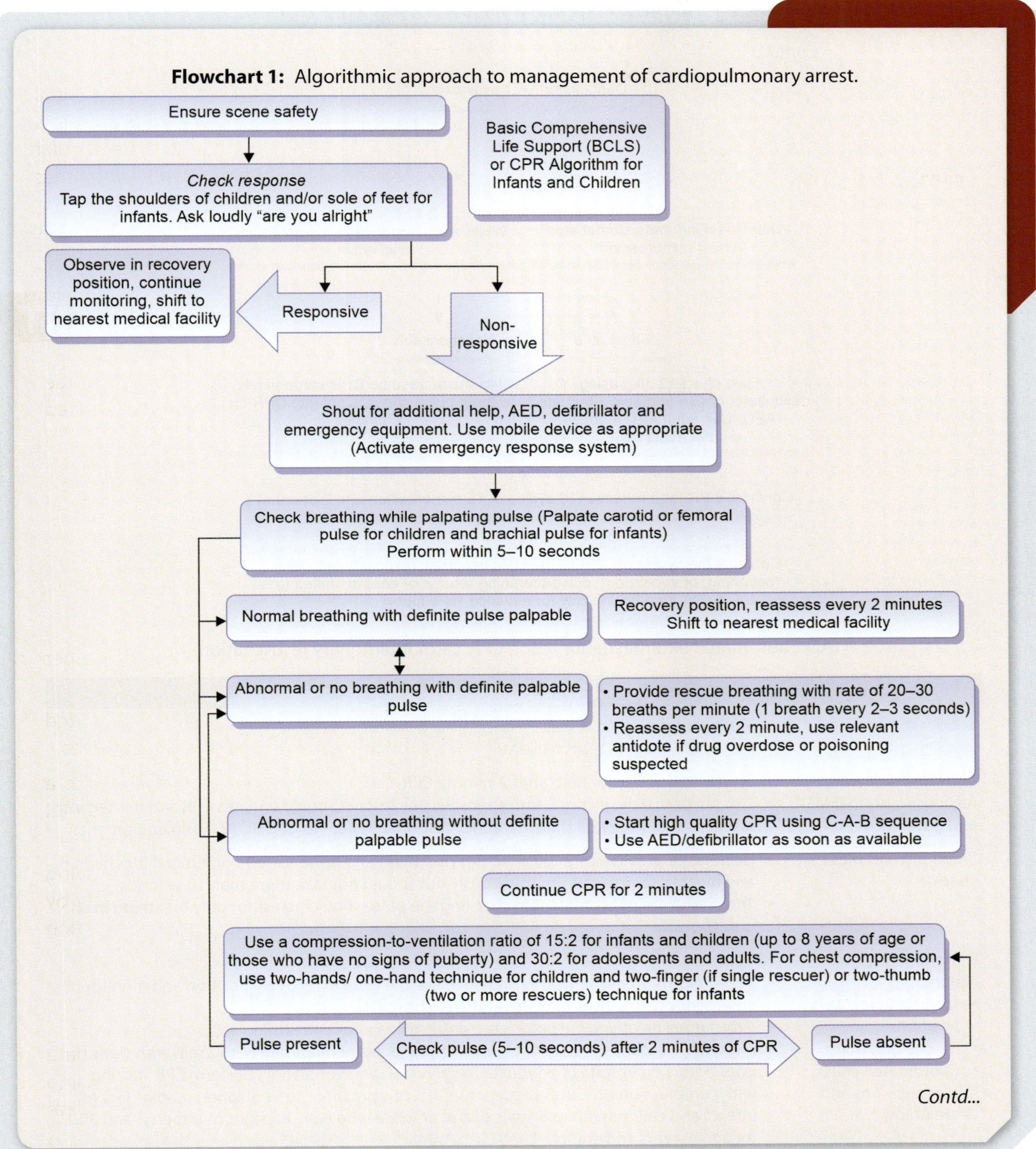

Contd...

Contd...

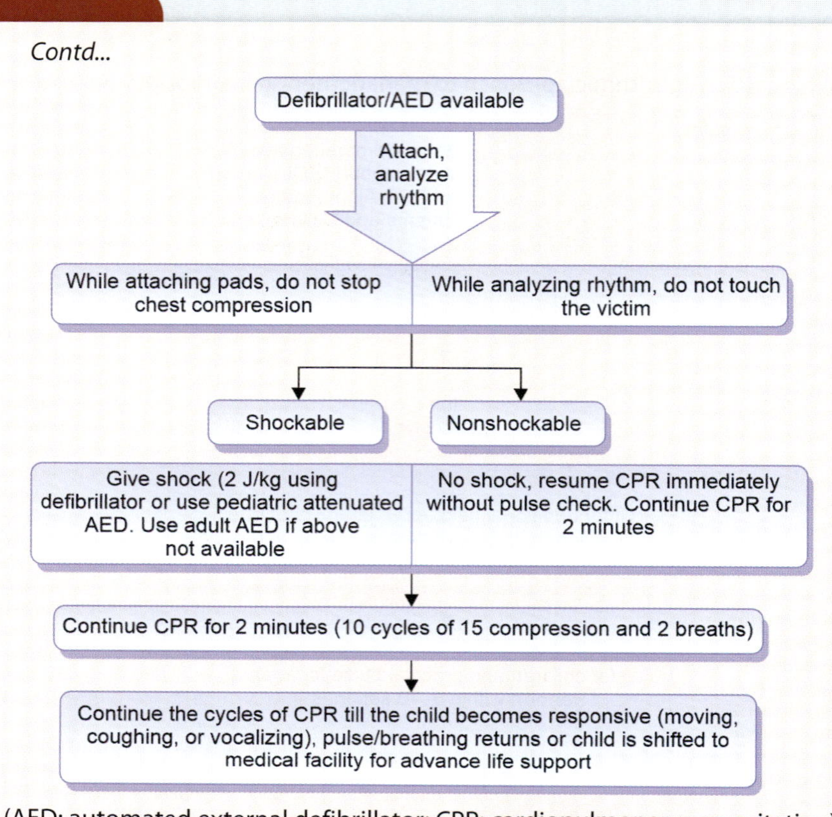

(AED: automated external defibrillator; CPR: cardiopulmonary resuscitation)

TABLE 1: Steps in Pediatric CPR.	
Scene safety and assessment	• Verify that the scene is safe • Assess the child for responsiveness
Activate emergency response system (EMS) and get AED	• *Single rescuer:* Call for help after 2-minute CPR • *Two rescuers:* If the victim is unresponsive, one rescuer should initiates CPR and the second rescuer should activate the emergency response system to gets an AED and equipment
Breathing and pulse check	• Health care providers should check for breathing and pulse (carotid or femoral for children and brachial for infants) simultaneously but should not take more than 10 seconds • Those who are not confident in checking the pulse should assess for only breathing in an unresponsive victim
Determine the next action: • Monitor in recovery position • Rescue breathing • Coordinated chest compressions and breathing	Next action: • *If breathing is normal and pulse present:* Place the child in recovery position and monitor till emergency help arrives or child is taken to hospital • *If no normal breathing but pulse is present:* Provide rescue breathing • If within 10 seconds you do not feel a definite pulse or heart rate is ≤60/min with signs of poor perfusion in spite of adequate oxygenation and ventilation, perform CPR starting with compressions in C-A-B sequence with a compression- to-ventilation ratio of 15:2 for infants and children (up to 8 years of age or those who have no signs of puberty) and 30:2 for adolescents and adults

Contd...

Contd...

Attempt defibrillation with AED	• Use an AED/manual defibrillator as soon as it is available • The rescuers should switch roles (to avoid a rescuer's fatigue) after every 2 minutes (compressors goes to ventilation; ventilation to compressor) or after every 10 cycles typically when an AED is analyzing the rhythm so that CPR quality is not affected
Resume high-quality CPR	• After shock delivery or if no shock is advised by AED, resume high-quality CPR immediately for about 2 minutes till prompted by AED for next rhythm check • Continue until ALS providers take over or victim is responsive

Transition from Basic Comprehensive to Advanced Life Support

Refer to **Flowchart 2**.

Flowchart 2: Transition from basic to advance comprehensive life support for a child with cardiopulmonary arrest.

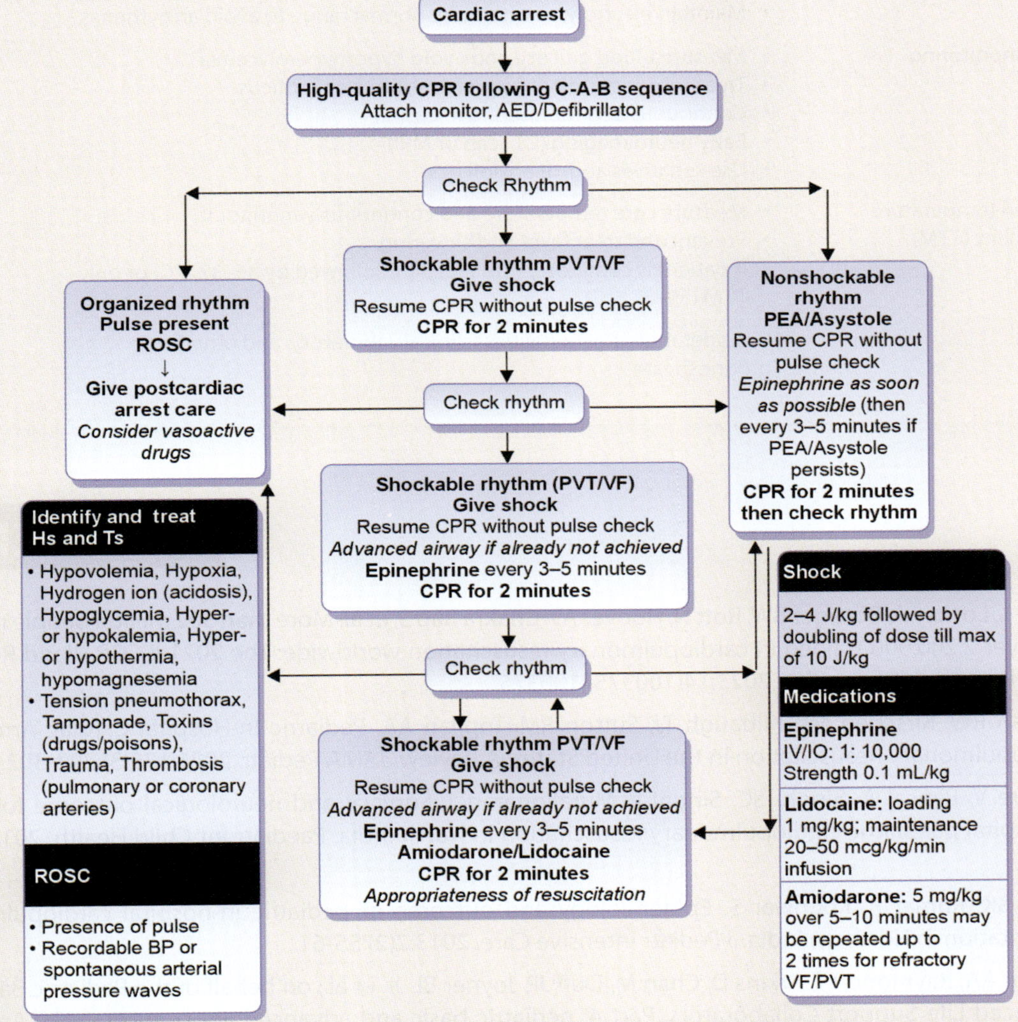

(AED: automated external defibrillator; CPR: cardiopulmonary resuscitation PEA: pulseless electrical activity; ROSC: return of spontaneous circulation)

Postcardiac Arrest Management Bundle

Refer to **Table 2**.

TABLE 2: Postcardiac arrest management bundle for infants and children.

Evaluate	*Identify and Intervene*	*Tick box*
A and B: Oxygenation and ventilation	• *Measure oxygenation:* Target SpO_2 94–99% • *Measure target $PaCO_2$:* Avoid hyper- or hypocarbia	
C: Circulation	• Set specific hemodynamic goals and review daily • Use fluid bolus with or without inotropes to maintain systolic BP > 5th percentile for age • Monitor urine output, serum lactate, $ScVO_2$, and arterial blood pressure to guide therapy • Maintain electrolytes within the normal range to avoid arrhythmias	
D: Neuromonitoring	• Measure blood glucose and avoid hypo/hyperglycemia • Treat seizures and nonconvulsive status epilepticus • Continuous EEG monitoring if feasible • Early neuroimaging (CT scan or MRI) • Use sedatives and/or anxiolytics	
E: Targeted temperature management (TTM)	• Measure core temperature and continuously monitor it • Prevent and treat fever and shivering • If patient is comatose, TTM (32–34°C followed by 36–37.5°C) or only TTM (36–37.5°C)	
Prognosis	Consider multiple modalities (clinical, laboratory, and other) to prognosticate	

REFERENCES

1. Tiwari L, Lockey A, Böttiger BW, Rott N, Hoover AV, Chakra Rao S, et al. More than 302 million people reached and over 2,200,000 trained in cardiopulmonary resuscitation worldwide: The 2021 ILCOR World Restart a Heart initiative. Resusc Plus. 2023;14(100375):100375.
2. Morgan RW, Kirschen MP, Kilbaugh TJ, Sutton RM, Topjian AA. Pediatric In-Hospital Cardiac Arrest and Cardiopulmonary Resuscitation in the United States: A Review. JAMA Pediatr. 2021;175(3):293-302.
3. Rathore V, Bansal A, Singhi SC, Singhi P, Muralidharan J. Survival and neurological outcome following in-hospital paediatric cardiopulmonary resuscitation in North India. Paediatr Int Child Health. 2016;36(2): 141-7.
4. Singh SK, Kumar R, Koonwar S. Epidemiology and outcome of pediatric in-hospital cardiopulmonary resuscitation in Northern India. J Pediatr Intensive Care. 2013;2(2):55-61.
5. Topjian AA, Raymond TT, Atkins D, Chan M, Duff JP, Joyner BL Jr, et al.; on behalf of the Pediatric Basic and Advanced Life Support Collaborators. Part 4: pediatric basic and advanced life support: 2020 American

Heart Association Guidelines for Cardiopulmonary Resuscitation and Emergency Cardiovascular Care. Circulation. 2020;142(suppl 2):S469-S523.

6. Tiwari L, Jindal A, Gupta V, Taneja LN, Garg R, Edara LR, et al. Concept proposal for IRCF national CPR Registry and update on resuscitation guidelines for infants and children. J Pediatr Crit Care. 2022;9:48-54.
7. Olasveengen TM, Semeraro F, Ristagno G, Castren M, Handley A, Kuzovlev A, et al. European Resuscitation Council Guidelines 2021: Basic Life Support. Resuscitation. 2021;161:98-114.
8. International Liaison Committee on Resuscitation (ILCOR). ILCOR scientific evidence evaluation and review system. American Heart Association, American Stroke Association. [Last accessed February, 2024].
9. Taneja LN, Tiwari L. BLS for Professionals, 3rd edition. New Delhi: Indian Academy of Pediatrics ALS BLS Group; 2018.
10. Tiwari L, Jindal A, Gupta V, Taneja LN, Garg R, Edara LR, et al. Concept proposal for IRCF national CPR Registry and update on resuscitation guidelines for infants and children. J Pediatr Crit Care. 20229:48-54.

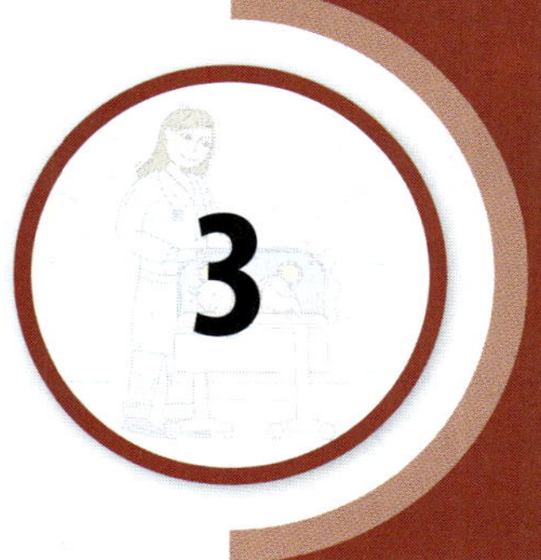

3 Rapid Sequence Intubation: Guideline

Agni Sekhar Saha

INTRODUCTION

- Rapid sequence intubation (RSI) refers to a coordinated, sequential process of planning, sedating, and paralyzing to quickly achieve a safe and favorable condition to perform intubation in emergency situations, often outside the operation theatre.
- There is evidence showing both higher success rates[1] and lesser complications[2] with RSI than not using it. The whole process of RSI starts once decision to intubate is taken. It can be divided into eight steps: Preparation, preoxygenation, physiologic optimization and premedication, sedation, paralysis, positioning including airway protection, intubation with proof, and postintubation management.
- In most cases, the entire process should take <10 minutes. This chapter will not cover the actual process of intubation or management of difficult airways.

PREPARATION

Preparation includes a focused history and examination of the patient, forming a team, and checking the equipment. Relevant points in history are given in **Table 1**.

TABLE 1: Important points in history taking and their significance.

Point	*Significance*
Previous history of difficult intubation or anesthesia.	High risk of complications, get senior help.
History of snoring or noisy breathing	Potential upper airway issues
History of asthma	May develop bronchospasm, prefer ketamine

History should also focus on possible contraindications for succinylcholine (See later), allergies, and time to last enteral intake.

EQUIPMENT CHECKLIST

- Bag and mask (or T-piece breathing circuit)
- Suction catheter (flexible and Yankauer of appropriate size)
- Two laryngoscopes (primary and back up)—should be checked
- Oral airways
- Endotracheal tubes (ETT) of appropriate size and one size smaller (preferably cuffed) and fixation for ETT—cuff should be checked
- Stylets, bougies, and laryngeal mask airways of appropriate size
- Ventilator with circuit

Standard monitoring should include heart rate, Oxygen saturation, ECG, respiratory rate, blood pressure (BP), and end-tidal CO_2. The child should have at least one and preferably two working intravenous access.

TEAM

There should be at least 3 members as detailed in **Table 2**.

TABLE 2: Team members and their roles.

Team member	*Role*
Intubator	Maintain airway, bag mask ventilation (BMV), intubate, and maintain ETT
Assistant	Monitor, cricoid pressure, give medication, assist, and back-up intubator
Nurse	Administer medication, supply instruments, fix ETT, and call for help

ETT: endotracheal tubes

If difficulty is anticipated, then additional personnel with more experience/skill may be needed.

Ideally, all personnel involved should wear standard personal protective equipment including N95 masks, gloves, gowns, and eye protection. They are paramount if there is a possibility of serious communicable droplet infection. In that case, a high-efficiency particulate air (HEPA) filter should also be attached to the bag and mask.

PREOXYGENATION

Preoxygenation should start the moment a decision to intubate is taken **(Flowchart 1)**. The idea is to replace nitrogen in patient's lungs with oxygen to create a reservoir of oxygen so that more time is available for intubation.

Flowchart 1: Algorithmic approach to preoxygenation.

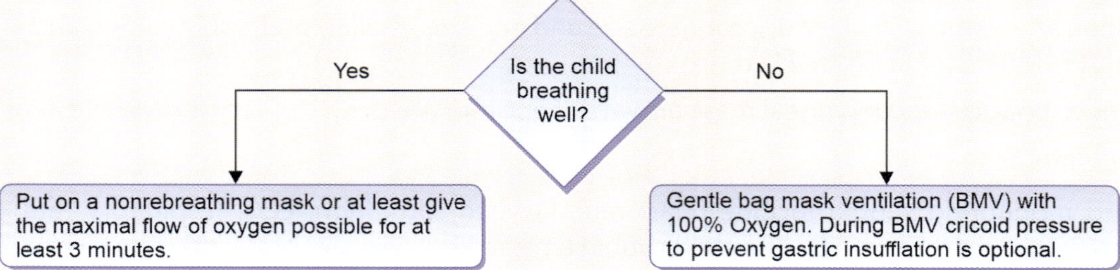

In a spontaneously breathing child, oxygen through nasal cannula may be continued @ 1 L/kg/min (maximum 15 L/min) while the child is given sedation and paralysis. This is called apneic oxygenation, evidence for which is equivocal.[3,4]

FOCUSED PHYSICAL EXAMINATION AND PHYSIOLOGIC OPTIMIZATION

Features associated with difficult airway:

- Small mouth
- Short neck
- Short mandible
- Cleft palate
- Prominent occiput
- Facial trauma or burn
- Child with hoarseness/stridor
- Child sitting in a typical tripod posture with/without drooling

Such features warrant senior personnel. Sometimes, it may in such cases. Other important physical findings are given in **Table 3**.

TABLE 3: Physical findings and steps for optimization.

Physical findings	Steps for optimization (If the condition permits)
Cardiovascular instability	Give fluid bolus, keep fluids ready; may even start inotrope infusion
Features of raised intracranial pressure	Give mannitol or 3% saline bolus depending on the blood pressure
Bronchospasm	Avoid atracurium and thiopentone, prefer ketamine.

PREMEDICATION

Atropine premedication is not routine. It can be considered in the following situations:

- Infants less than a year[5]
- Succinylcholine in children <5 years
- Repeat dose of succinylcholine
- Patients in shock, as they tolerate bradycardia poorly

If given, the mydriasis may hamper neurologic assessment. Atropine may also subsequently mask the bradycardic response to hypoxia. So, close monitoring becomes even more important.

SEDATION AND RELAXANTS

Rapid sequence intubation warrants rapid induction of sedation and amnesia. Use of a relaxing agent is an integral part of RSI. It increases success rate and reduces complications. There are many agents for sedation and paralysis **(Table 4)**. However, only a handful are recommended for RSI. Following are the agents with their prominent features:

TABLE 4: Agents for sedation and paralysis.

Name	*Dose mg/kg*	*Onset (seconds)*	*Duration (minutes)*	*Hypotension*	*Raised intracranial pressure (ICP)*	*Special property*
Etomidate@	0.3	15–40	10–12	OK	OK	See@
Midazolam	0.2–0.3	120–180*	30–40	No	OK	Antiseizure
Ketamine$	2	45–60	10–20	OK#	OK+	Analgesia
Propofol&	1–1.5	15–45	5–10	No	OK	Antiseizure
Thiopentone	3–5	20–30	5–10	No	OK	Antiseizure
Fentanyl	1–5 µg	30-60	30–45	No	OK	Chest-wall rigidity
Succinylcholine^	1–2	30–60	4–6	OK	±	Bradycardia
Rocuronium%	1	30–60	30–40	OK	OK	

@ Etomidate is contraindicated in septic shock—either proven or suspected, as it can cause short-term adrenocortical suppression.

* Midazolam takes longest time to act even with a dose of 0.2–0.3 mg/kg. It is often underdosed, making the time of onset even longer.

$ Ketamine may cause bronchodilation by endogenous catecholamine release making it ideal for patients with bronchospasm/severe asthma.

Ketamine increases BP by endogenous catecholamine release making it ideal for cardiovascularly unstable patients. However, ketamine itself has negative inotropic action. So, if a child is catecholamine depleted, i.e., needing inotrope infusion, then ketamine should be avoided.

+ Ketamine was thought to cause raised ICP. However, subsequent studies have found it to be untrue. It is still contraindicated in open globe injury.

& Propofol infusion can cause propofol syndrome in small children and is contraindicated. But it can be used as an induction agent.

^ Succinylcholine is the most suited relaxant because of its short duration of action unless there are contraindications, which are as follows:

- >48 hours after polytrauma, significant burn, or acute denervating injury (e.g., spinal cord trauma, stroke, etc.)
- Hyperkalemia with ECG changes
- Chronic neuromuscular or myopathic conditions (e.g., cerebral palsy, Duchenne muscular dystrophy, etc.)
- Family history of malignant hyperthermia
- Extensive muscle injury with rhabdomyolysis
- Increased ICP is a relative contraindication.

% Rocuronium (or all other paralytic agents) except Succinylcholine has a much-prolonged duration of action, which is not ideal, in case intubation becomes difficult. However, sugammadex (Dose: 16 mg/kg) reverses rocuronium within 3 minutes and should be readily available if rocuronium is used. Sugammadex can cause arrhythmia, so electrocardiographic (ECG) monitoring is mandatory.

Algorithm for choosing sedative agents is given in **Flowchart 2**.

Flowchart 2: Algorithm approach to choosing sedative agents.

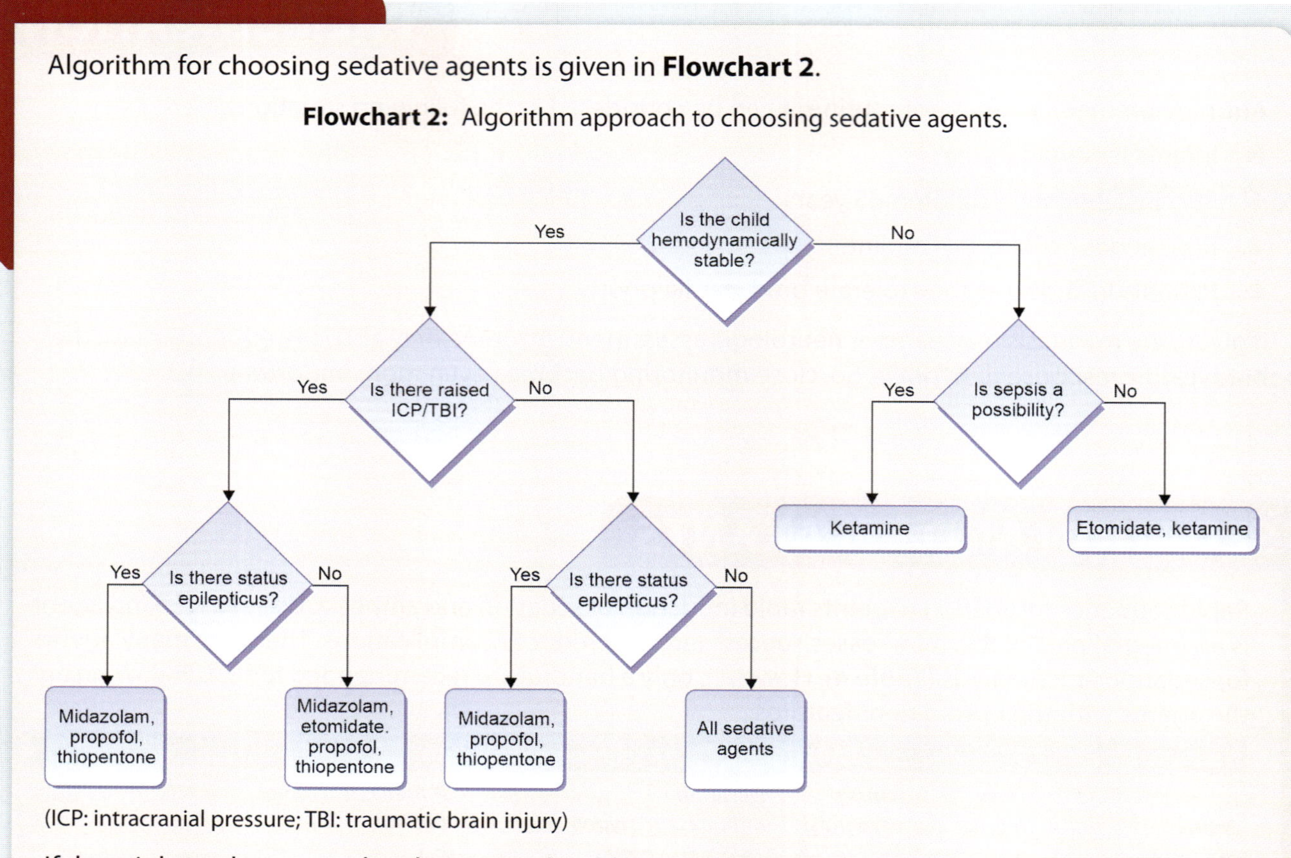

(ICP: intracranial pressure; TBI: traumatic brain injury)

If there is bronchospasm, then ketamine should be preferred. Thiopentone and atracurium should be avoided for potential histamine release.

PROOF OF INTUBATION AND POSTINTUBATION MANAGEMENT

Following intubation, placement should be confirmed clinically, through end-tidal CO_2 and a chest X-ray. Immediately after intubation, an infusion of sedation and analgesia ± relaxants should be started. In hemodynamically stable patients, a benzodiazepine (usually midazolam) and an opiate (morphine or fentanyl) is a popular combination. In unstable patients, ketamine infusion may work both as a sedative and analgesic.

CONTRAINDICATION

Cardiac arrest is the only absolute contraindication for RSI. Once administered, sedation and paralysis abolish both airway protective reflexes and spontaneous respiration making rapid establishment of a secure airway absolutely vital. Therefore, patients in whom bag mask ventilation is difficult or patients having features suggestive of difficult airway may warrant a different approach. Reduced doses of sedation may be used. Relaxants are often omitted so that patient keeps breathing. This is called "awake intubation" and is also often practiced in patients with very unstable hemodynamics.

Note: Historically, the expression RSI was used to describe the approach to intubating a subject who may not have an empty stomach. Applying cricoid pressure and avoiding bag-mask ventilation (BMV) were supposed to be the main focal points. However, subsequent studies showed no significant difference in risk of aspiration with or without cricoid pressure.[6] Moreover, it may make visualization of glottis difficult. Hence, cricoid pressure is now considered optional.

REFERENCES

1. Pallin DJ, Dwyer RC, Walls RM, Brown CA 3rd; NEAR III Investigators. Techniques and trends, success rates, and adverse events in emergency department pediatric intubations: A report from the National Emergency Airway Registry. Ann Emerg Med. 2016;67(5):610-15.
2. Li J, Murphy-Lavoie H, Bugas C, Martinez J, Preston C. Complications of emergency intubation with and without paralysis. Am J Emerg Med. 1999;17(2):141-3.
3. Vukovic AA, Hanson HR, Murphy SL, Mercurio D, Sheedy CA, Arnold DH, et. al. Apneic oxygenation reduces hypoxemia during endotracheal intubation in the pediatric emergency department. Am J Emerg Med. 2019;37(1):27-32.
4. Overmann KM, Boyd SD, Zhang Y, Kerrey BT. Apneic oxygenation to prevent oxyhemoglobin desaturation during rapid sequence intubation in a pediatric emergency department. Am J Emerg Med. 2019;37(8):1416-21.
5. Jones P, Dauger S, Denjoy I, Pinto da Costa N, Alberti C, Boulkedid R, et al. The effect of atropine on rhythm and conduction disturbances during 322 critical care intubations. Pediatr Crit Care Med. 2013;14(6):e289.
6. Birenbaum A, Hajage D, Roche S, Ntouba A, Eurin M, Cuvillon P, et. al; IRIS Investigators Group. Effect of cricoid pressure compared with a sham procedure in the rapid sequence induction of anesthesia: The IRIS randomized clinical trial. JAMA Surg. 2019;154(1):9-17.

4

Approach to Multisystem Trauma

Bal Mukund

INTRODUCTION

- Pediatric trauma is an emerging epidemic worldwide. According to data from West, pediatric trauma comprises up to 25% of all trauma.[1] Detailed data from developing countries is lacking; however, National Crime Record Bureau Data in 2022 revealed a total death of 40,637 in age <18 years, and majority resulted from road traffic accidents.[2]
- Blunt injury accounts for 90% of all pediatric trauma. Polytrauma is defined as injury to more than one anatomical region.[3] Children are more predisposed to multisystem injury when blunt force is applied to relatively small body, however fortunately, the majority of polytrauma cases are mild to moderate in severity.
- A protocolized approach as suggested by Advance Trauma Life Support (ATLS) is based on trimodal death distribution. The first peak occurs immediately within minutes and is only amenable to prevention of injury, the second peak occurs within minutes to hours and during this "golden hour", a rapid assessment and timely treatment will decrease mortality and morbidity.
- Third peak, which takes days to week, requires dedicated and definitive care to mitigate delayed mortality. The unstable pediatric patients refer to children who have abnormal vital signs due to disruption in vital functions or due to injuries of critical nature. It is important to have knowledge of vital signs by age and gender.

INJURY CLASSIFICATION

There are multiple ways to classify trauma, and hence multisystem trauma also may be classified similarly. These are used to predict morbidity and mortality, require diagnostic evaluation, and treatment, and prognostication. The classification is based on body region involved—local versus multisystem, mechanism—penetrating versus blunt, and severity which may be mild, moderate, or severe.

Injury type: The types of injury vary from penetrating trauma like sharp objects, gunshots, and stab wounds to blunt trauma due to falls and motor vehicle accidents. Penetrating trauma on organ sites are more likely to result in significant organ injuries. Further, they can be classified for injury severity on the basis of vital signs, Glasgow coma scale for brain injury, and severity of organ injury for other organs **(Box 1)**.

BOX 1: Physical findings or high-energy impact associated with critical injury.

Vital signs and level of consciousness:
- Glasgow coma scale <13
- Shock-compensated or decompensated
- *Respiratory rate:* Lower or higher than normal for age

Evidence of high-energy impact:
- Falls >10 feet or >2–3 times height of child
- High-risk auto crash-intrusion >12 inches from occupant site or >18 inches from any site
- Ejection of any grade or death in same passenger compartment
- Vehicle data consistent with high-risk injury or vehicle rollover
- Significant auto/car speed >64 kmph or pedestrian run over or thrown
- Extrication time >20 minutes
- Automobile-induced pedestrian injury with >8 kmph

Anatomy of injury:
- Airway trauma with respiratory distress, anterior neck tenderness, or deformity
- Chest trauma with persistent tachycardia, tenderness or respiratory distress, and deformity
- Abdominal distention or tenderness with persistent tachycardia
- Two or more proximal long-bone fracture
- Pelvic fracture
- Crushed, deformed, degloved, or mangled extremity
- Open or depressed skull fracture
- Penetrating trauma to head, neck, chest, abdomen, or proximal extremity
- Amputation proximal to wrist or ankle
- Paralysis

INITIAL APPROACH

The primary goal in polytrauma management in children lies in rapid assessment, deducing management priorities, and institutional critical lifesaving intervention. For this, the clinician needs a systemic approach as defined in ATLS and Advance Life Support (ALS) manual. They include primary survey and rapid stabilization of vital functions like airway, breathing, circulation, and disability (mentation). During the same time, any resuscitation required should be instituted. A secondary survey will include postresuscitation vitals monitoring, use of other adjuvants, and initial laboratory tests. This will be followed by transition to definitive care.

Primary survey (including resuscitation) ⟹ Secondary survey ⟹ Definitive care

It is emphasized that critical management should be guided according to ALS manual where assessment and management would occur simultaneously during primary survey. Any threat to life should be stabilized first during primary survey before going to next priority area. In case of further deterioration during these steps, appropriate intervention should be instituted before going to definitive care. To improve outcomes in pediatric multisystem trauma, it is essential to identify such injuries and offer rapid treatment by a multidisciplinary team.

Primary Survey

Assessment and Management

The sequence of primary survey is guided by ATLS/ALS manual and shall include:

A. Airway assessment and maintenance with cervical spine stabilization

B. Breathing and ventilation

C. Circulation and hemorrhage control

D. Disability evaluation for neurological status

E. Exposure—complete visual examination and prevention of hypothermia

Upon arrival of the patient, clinicians should place the appropriate monitors; obtain vital signs like pulse, respiratory rate, oxygen saturation, blood pressure, and temperature (based on age-appropriate cutoffs of vital signs as per ALS manual); and provide supplemental oxygen. It is imperative for the clinician to assess pediatric vital signs and a readily available reference of normal values for age should be available in triage area. When multiple clinicians are present, evaluation and management go side by side like intravenous (IV) placement may precede chest tube placement even though breathing precedes circulation in primary survey.

A—Airway Assessment and Management: It includes assessment of patency and any presence of foreign body or any evidence of facial injury, such as mandibular or tracheal/laryngeal injury, which can cause airway obstruction. Any child who can cry or speak verbally is unlikely to have potential airway obstruction. It requires a constant evaluation as a child may experience potential airway loss subsequently after arrival due to complications resulting from above-mentioned injury. It is important to restrict motion at cervical spine during airway management. Any child with multisystem trauma, motor vehicle collision, head and neck trauma, anatomically remote distracting injury, or anatomical predisposition for such trauma as Down syndrome should always be assumed to have cervical spinal injury. A padding under shoulder and back and stiff collar are recommended along with avoidance of head tilt, chin lift maneuver during opening of airways. It is also important to suction the secretions, assess requirement of oropharyngeal or supraglottic airways or urgent cricothyroidotomy as it may be required. Indications of endotracheal intubations are severe head injury with Glasgow Coma Scale (GCS) ≤8, hemorrhagic shock unresponsive to initial fluids or potential significant airway trauma, flail chest with inadequate chest wall movement, significant laryngeal trauma, significant pulmonary contusion, and inhalation injury.

B—Breathing Assessment and Management: It requires close inspection of nose and thorax. Clinician should evaluate for tracheal deviation, subcutaneous emphysema, use of accessory muscles, and signs of trauma in neck and thorax. Full evaluation requires all steps to be followed like in ATLS manual. Bedside ultrasonography may be utilized to diagnose pneumothorax or hemothorax. These may impair ventilation, and hence should be suspected early in polytrauma children. Management requires the administration of high concentrations of oxygen through an appropriate inteface and bag and mask/tube ventilation if there is bradypnea or requires intubation. If these do not improve the vital signs, clinician must suspect and use a needle thoracocentesis or chest tube for pneumothorax. Use of gas analysis if readily available is recommended.

C—Circulation Assessment and Management: The most common cause of shock in polytrauma patient is volume loss, and hence, early recognition and management are recommended. In early phase of shock, while it is compensated, the fall in blood pressure may not be apparent, while in hypotensive shock, the blood pressure drops and cause hypotension. In nonresponders, a cardiac tamponade should be suspected and bedside ultrasonography may be helpful in the diagnosis. Due to the physiologic reserve, blood pressure may be maintained despite a loss of up to 45% of the circulating blood volume. The trauma patient who is cool and tachycardic may be in shock until proven otherwise. Other signs of shock include delayed capillary refill, narrowing of the pulse pressure to <20 mm Hg, skin mottling, cool extremities, decreased level of consciousness, and decrease response to pain. Any child with abdominal tenderness, pelvic pain or instability, open fracture of long bones, and spinal shock or with significant external injury will require appropriate management. Hemorrhage control, two large bore IV access or intraosseous (IO) route, and administration of crystalloid or blood along with appropriate management of trauma may be required. For uncontrolled external hemorrhage, a direct pressure or tourniquet, and clips or sutures may be required. For internal hemorrhage, hemostatic products, fibrin sealant, or IV antifibrinolytics like tranexamic acid may be tried if administered within 3 hours of trauma. Both pediatric and adult studies have found reduced mortality in uncontrolled hemorrhage with IV tranexamic acid without increase in thromboembolism only if administered within 3 hours of polytrauma.

Fluids and blood products: In compensated shock, a 10–20 mL/kg of crystalloid fluid should be given over 10–15 minutes. Ringer lactate or saline may be started but Ringer lactate should be avoided with blood in same venous access as it may induce clotting. Blood products may be required in case of poor improvement with crystalloid. A volume of 10–20 mL/kg up to 2 units of type-specific or unmatched O-negative-packed red blood cells may be transfused with inline warmer if available. When multiple blood products are used, a massive transfusion protocol which recommends fresh frozen plasma (FFP) to platelets to red cells (PRBC) in ratio of 1:1:1 should be followed, as observational study have found improved outcomes. The estimated volume trigger is dependent on weight and volume required (**Table 1**).

TABLE 1: Estimated volume trigger for massive transfusion protocol.

Group	*Weight in kg*	*Volume trigger in mL/kg*
Neonate	<5	55
Infant and child	5–25	50
School-going children	25–50	45
Adolescent	>50	40 or 6 units of PRBC

In polytrauma patients, presence of coagulopathy and requirement of blood products should be the triggers for this protocol. Children with head trauma and documented coagulopathy always warrant FFP even in absence of blood transfusion and always PRBC transfusion. A controlled hypotension approach for torso or gunshot injury is still controversial as evidence is still lacking, however, it is followed in adults. This approach may be detrimental to head injury as it may decrease cerebral perfusion. A child of polytrauma with refractory shock is generally indicative of ongoing blood losses, splenic or liver trauma, or cardiac tamponade. In cardiac tamponade, Beck's triad—distended neck veins, muffled heart sounds, and hypotension are seen. Cardiac tamponade may also result in pulse-less electrical activity. Bedside ultrasonography can easily diagnose this and help in emergency pericardiocentesis. For major vessel injury an open thoracotomy may be required.

D—Disability Assessment and Management: It requires rapid evaluation of level of consciousness by pediatric GCS in <2 years or GCS for older children. It is also important to assess pupillary reflex, gag reflex, and blood sugar. Unequal or fixed dilated pupils indicate cerebral herniation and need aggressive management for raised intracranial pressure (ICP). The tiered approach of raised ICP should be followed. The evidence for best osmolar therapy is lacking hence hypertonic saline (3%) or mannitol in standard doses may be used, though 3% NaCl has added advantage in hypotension due to positive inotropy, hence it does not exacerbate hypotension. Any child with GCS ≤12 warrants consultation by neurosurgeon and a GCS ≤8 requires invasive monitoring of ICP if available and feasible.

E—Exposure: Evaluation and management should be started after complete undressing of the child. A log roll should be used in suspected cervical spine trauma even during full examination. A detailed examination includes sphincter tone and avoidance of hypothermia is recommended. Various methods of warming by blanket, radiant warmers, warmed fluids/blood products or oxygen may be used during assessment and management.

Laboratory test: The patients should be reassessed for vital signs frequently and after each intervention. An initial sample for blood grouping, cross matching, hematocrit estimation, blood glucose, liver enzyme estimation (AST >200 IU/L or ALT >125 IU/L are highly suggestive of intra-abdominal injury in blunt trauma), blood gas, and in severe unstable children coagulogram, electrolytes, renal function test, serum amylase, and lipase should also be sent. In polytrauma the triad of coagulopathy, hypothermia, and acidosis may contribute to mortality and hence requires special attention. Screening radiographs like cross-table lateral cervical spine, anteroposterior (AP) chest, and AP pelvis may be required if indicated. A cross-table C-spine X-ray can identify only 80% of fracture, dislocation, or subluxation, hence their absence does not exclude possibility of spinal trauma.

A polytrauma child may require urinary catheterization if not suspected of urethral injury for urine output monitoring. Similarly, an orogastric or nasogastric tube should be placed as they may have gastroparesis and may decrease chance of aspiration. Nasogastric tube insertion should be avoided in oro-maxillary trauma as these patients may have fractures in cribriform plate and hence orogastric tube should be placed.

Extended focused assessment with sonography for trauma (eFAST) includes a rapid ultrasound examination of abdominal compartments; right upper quadrant, left upper quadrant, subxiphoid and pelvis, lung, and heart. The primary aim is to detect intraperitoneal fluid due to intra-abdominal injury, pneumo or hemothorax, hemopericardium, or cardiac tamponade. The importance is more in an unstable child with polytrauma as an accurate diagnosis and intervention may be lifesaving and have high sensitivity in trained hands. It is emphasized that hemodynamically unstable children with polytrauma and high probability of intra-abdominal injury always warrant an abdominal CT regardless of eFAST findings. eFAST when combined with diligent clinical examination may result in higher sensitivity and high negative predictive value.[4]

Secondary Survey

Secondary survey is systematic evaluation of trauma patients and is commenced after initial resuscitation. This requires AMPLE history, head-to-toe examination, and additional studies and investigation. In AMPLE history, allergy, medications, past medical history, last meal, and events leading to injury are asked. Clinician need to do thorough examination from head to toe. Important signs to look for are raccoon eye, Battle's signs, hemotympanum, and seatbelt sign. Adjuvant in this survey are screening radiographs, eFAST, and CT scan whenever indicated. It is important to remember that possibility of spinal cord injury may be there due to spinal cord injury without radiographic abnormality (SCIWORA) in the pediatric population; hence, in any brief or sustained sensory or motor deficit, even if screening imaging is normal, there may cervical spine injury and motion restriction must be maintained. Similarly, for head CT scan, specific indications and standard guidelines by Brain Trauma Foundation (BTF) or Pediatric Research in Emergency Departments International Collaborative (PREDICT) guidelines may be followed. Chest CT scan may be indicated to identify vascular or tracheobronchial injury, especially if screening chest radiograph shows abnormalities like wide mediastinum, obscured aortic knob, and large left hemithorax or clinically suspected of such injuries.

In unstable children, it is important to refer them to emergency, surgical, or endovascular repair rather than additional imaging study. Abdominal CT scans with contrast may be required in a hemodynamically stable polytrauma child, as they are sensitive and specific in diagnosing liver, retroperitoneal structure, and splenic injury. Alone, they are less sensitive in diagnosing pancreas, lumbar spinal, or intestinal tract injuries. In unstable child despite initial fluid resuscitation, direct operative intervention should be done as they are at high risk for significant intra-abdominal injury. In suspected intestinal injury or penetrating trauma and if child is stable then emergent laparoscopy as an alternative to laparoscopy should be considered. Fractures may be managed with splinting and orthopedic consultation. Pelvic fracture can be temporarily managed by wrapping pelvis in bedsheet at greater trochanter to reduce further bleeding. Any open wound should be managed with appropriate wound care, IV antibiotics, and analgesics. If there is potential soil contamination in would, it is advisable to cover additionally with metronidazole or clindamycin in patients with known beta-lactam hypersensitivity. The preferred regime is cefazolin and in B-lactam hypersensitive children, vancomycin is recommended. In case of freshwater contamination, piperacillin–tazobactam or levofloxacin plus metronidazole should be used. The later combination regime may also be used in sea-water contamination.

Definitive Care

A dedicated trauma center with pediatric facility is the preferred site for management and has better outcomes. In case of nonavailability of dedicated center, an adult trauma center or combined trauma center may be utilized. Unfortunately, only 50% of the polytrauma children reach within 1 hour of incident in these centers, resulting in higher mortality even in resource-rich countries. Clinicians' expert field triage and trauma should be utilized during prehospital transportation. A dedicated team of trauma surgeon, neurosurgeon, orthopedic, intensive care specialist, ENT specialist, plastic surgeon, and maxilla facial surgeon may yield better outcomes.

PROGNOSIS

The traditionally BIG score has been validated to predict mortality independently in polytrauma in children. The optimum cutoff of BIG score <16 has been taken in children with polytrauma and it indicates high probability of survival. It is independent of prehospital interventions, presence of head injury, or hypotension. Mortality increases significantly if BIG score is >16. It is calculated as BIG score = *B*ase deficit + (2.5 × *I*NR) + (15 – *G*CS). The other score used in pediatric polytrauma is pediatric trauma score (PTS) in <18 years age group. It emphasizes the importance of weight of children, airways, and GCS. It is a valid tool to predict mortality, lower the PTS is, higher the mortality risk. Mortality is 9% with a PTS >8 and with PTS ≤0, it is 100%. The minimum score is –6 and the maximum score is +12 **(Table 2)**.

TABLE 2: Pediatric trauma score (PTS) to be added and a score ≤8 indicates potentially significant trauma.

Pediatric trauma score (PTS)	+2	+1	–1
Weight in kgs	>20	10–20	<10
Airways	Patent	Maintainable	Unmaintainable
Systolic BP in mm Hg	>90	50–90	<50
CNS	Awake	+Loss of consciousness	Unresponsive
Fractures	None	Closed or suspected	*Multiple:* Closed or open
Wounds	None	Minor	Major, penetrating, or burns

KEY LEARNING POINTS

- Pediatric polytrauma is increasing worldwide and initial assessment requires primary survey and simultaneous resuscitation as per ATLS. This addresses life-threatening injury that affects breathing, circulation, and oxygenation.
- Head injury is the leading cause of mortality, especially in children with polytrauma; hence, a structured approach as in BTF or PREDICT should be followed.
- The chest, abdominal, and pelvic injuries are relatively rare but may contribute to mortality, especially chest trauma if not assessed and managed optimally.
- All patients with head trauma and road traffic injuries should be assumed to have cervical spinal injury and should be managed accordingly.
- A multidisciplinary team should be utilized for optimum management of polytrauma patient.
- BIG score and PTS may be utilized for prognostic purpose and estimation of mortality.

REFERENCES

1. Prakash Raju KNJ, Jagdish S, Kumar GK, Anandhi D, Antony J. Profile of pediatric trauma among the patients attending emergency department in a tertiary care hospital in South India. J Emerg Trauma Shock. 2020;13(1):62-7.
2. Hannon MM, Middleberg LK, Lee LK. The initial approach to multisystem pediatric trauma patient. Pediatr Emerg Care. 2022;38(6):290-8.
3. Babu A, Rattan A, Ranjan P, Singhal M, Gupta A, Kumar S, et al. Are falls more common than road traffic accidents in pediatric trauma? Experience from a Level 1 trauma centre in New Delhi, India. Chin J Traumatol. 2016;19(2):75-8.
4. Stengel D, Leisterer J, Ferrada P, Ekkernkamp A, Mutze S, Hoenning A. Point-of-care ultrasonography for diagnosing thoracoabdominal injuries in patients with blunt trauma. Cochrane Database Syst Rev. 2018; 12(12):CD012669

5 Anaphylaxis

Jaidev MD, Jason Dsouza

DEFINITION

Anaphylaxis is a severe systemic/generalized hypersensitivity reaction, which is rapid in onset and potentially life-threatening, manifesting as airway, breathing, or circulatory problems.

DIAGNOSTIC CRITERIA

Anaphylaxis is highly likely when any **one** of the following three criteria is fulfilled:

1. Acute onset of an illness (minutes to several hours) with involvement of the skin, mucosal tissue, or both (e.g., generalized hives, pruritus or flushing, swollen lips, tongue, and uvula) *and at least one of the following :*
   - Respiratory compromise (e.g., dyspnea, wheeze, stridor, hypoxemia)
   - Reduced blood pressure (BP) or associated symptoms of end-organ dysfunction (e.g., hypotonia, collapse, syncope, incontinence)
2. *Two* or more of the following that occur rapidly after exposure to a *likely* allergen (minutes to several hours):
   - Involvement of the skin or mucosal tissue (e.g., generalized hives, pruritus, or swollen lips, tongue, uvula)
   - Respiratory compromise (e.g., dyspnea, wheeze, stridor, hypoxemia)
   - Reduced BP or associated symptoms (e.g., hypotonia, collapse, syncope, incontinence)
   - Persistent gastrointestinal symptoms (e.g., crampy abdominal pain, vomiting)
3. Reduced BP after exposure to a *known* allergen (minutes to several hours):
   - *Infants and children:* Low systolic BP (age-specific) or greater than 30% decrease in systolic BP
   - *Adults:* Systolic BP of <90 mm Hg or greater than 30% decrease from that person's baseline

Low systolic blood pressure for children is defined as:

- <70 mm Hg from 1 month to 1 year
- <70 mm Hg + (2 × age) from 1 to 10 years
- <90 mm Hg for >10 years of age

SYMPTOMS AND SIGNS

The symptoms and signs are given in **Table 1**.

TABLE 1: Symptoms and signs of anaphylaxis.

System	*Symptoms*
Skin (80–90%)	• Flushing; pruritus; hives; erythema/rash; swelling of tongue, lips, uvula/palate, peri-orbital; pruritus of genitalia, palms, soles, external and auditory canals; conjunctival erythema; tearing • **Up to 20% of anaphylaxis episodes may not have skin changes**
Respiratory (70%)	• *Nose:* Pruritus, congestion, sneezing, rhinorrhea • *Larynx:* Dysphonia, tightness in throat, cough, stridor • *Lung:* Dyspnea, cough, chest tightness, wheezing, cyanosis
Cardiovascular (45%)	Chest pain, palpitation, tachy/bradycardia, arrhythmias, syncope, hypotension, shock, urinary or fecal incontinence, cardiac arrest
Gastrointestinal (45%)	Nausea, vomiting, diarrhea, crampy abdominal pain
Central nervous system (15%)	Altered mental status, feeling of impending doom, headache, and tunnel vision **Infants and young children may have sudden behavioral changes (cessation of playing, becoming clingy, crying, becoming irritable)**
Others	Metallic taste in mouth, dysphagia, uterine contractions in postpubertal female

DANGER SIGNS

- Rapid progression of symptoms
- Presence of respiratory distress (e.g., stridor, wheezing, dyspnea, increased work of breathing, retractions, persistent cough, and cyanosis)
- Signs of poor perfusion
- Abdominal pain and vomiting
- Dysrhythmia
- Hypotension and collapse

PATTERNS

- *Uniphasic:* Symptoms start usually within 30 minutes and resolve within 120 minutes.
- *Biphasic (up to 20% cases):* Recurrence of symptoms of anaphylaxis without further exposure to triggers after an initial resolution or treatment and generally occurs within 12 hours but is reported up to 72 hours.
- *Protracted:* Persistent symptoms lasting more than 5 hours and up to days or even weeks.
- *Delayed:* Initial onset of symptoms begins several hours after exposure to triggering agent.

CAUSES

The causes of anaphylaxis are as follows:

- Allergens [immunoglobulin E (IgE)-dependent immunologic mechanism]
  - *Foods:* Milk, egg, soy, wheat, peanut, tree nut, fish, shellfish, sesame, and food additives (colorants including carmine, vegetable gums, gelatin, and spices)
  - *Medications (biologics and vaccines):* Beta-lactam antibiotics, nonsteroidal anti-inflammatory drugs (NSAIDs), neuromuscular blocking agents, monoclonal antibodies, and chemotherapeutic agents
  - Insect stings (e.g., hymenoptera venom) and insect bites (e.g., kissing bugs)
  - Natural rubber latex
  - *Inhalants (rare):* Horse dander, cat dander, and grass pollen
- Immunologic triggers (IgE-independent mechanism)
  - *IgG-dependent (rare):* High-molecular-weight dextran and infliximab
  - *Coagulation system activation:* Heparin contaminated with oversulfated chondroitin sulfate
- Nonimmunologic triggers (direct activation of mast cells and basophils)
  - Physical factors (exercise, cold, heat, and UV radiation)
  - Medications (opioids and NSAIDs)
  - Radiocontrast agents
  - Alcohol (ethanol)
- Idiopathic anaphylaxis

RISK FACTORS AND COFACTORS

The risk factors and cofactors are given in **Figure 1**.

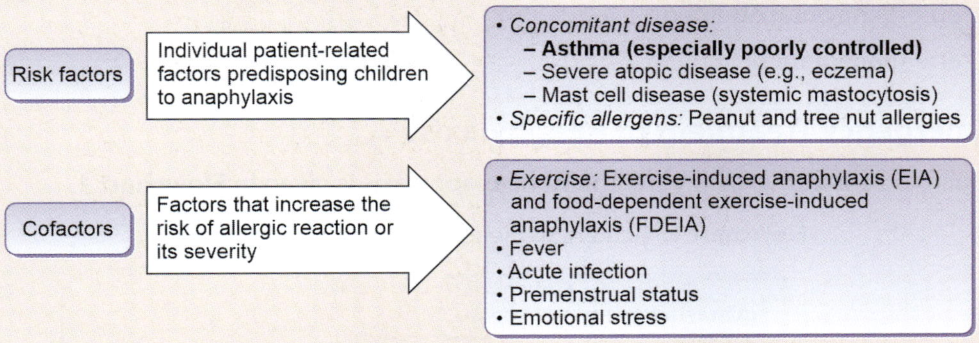

Fig. 1: Risk factors and cofactors of anaphylaxis.

DIFFERENTIAL DIAGNOSIS

Differential diagnosis of anaphylaxis includes the following:

- Common conditions:
  - Acute generalized urticaria or angioedema
  - Acute asthma
  - Syncope (vasovagal)
  - Panic attack/acute anxiety
- Postprandial syndromes:
  - Pollen food syndrome
  - Scromboidosis
  - Monosodium glutamate
  - Sulfites
- Excess endogenous histamine production: Mastocytosis/mast cell disorders
- Flush syndromes:
  - Vancomycin flushing syndrome
  - Alcohol
- Nonorganic causes:
  - Vocal cord dysfunction
  - Anxiety and panic disorder
- Other causes:
  - Shock (septic/cardiogenic/hypovolemic/distributive)
  - Hypoglycemia and pheochromocytoma
  - *Neuropsychiatric diseases:* Hyperventilation syndrome and dissociative and conversion disorder

MANAGEMENT

The management of anaphylaxis is of two types:

1. Acute/emergency management
2. Long-term management

Acute/Emergency Treatment of Anaphylaxis

The approach to acute/emergency treatment of anaphylaxis is given in **Flowchart 1**.

Flowchart 1: Acute/emergency treatment of anaphylaxis.

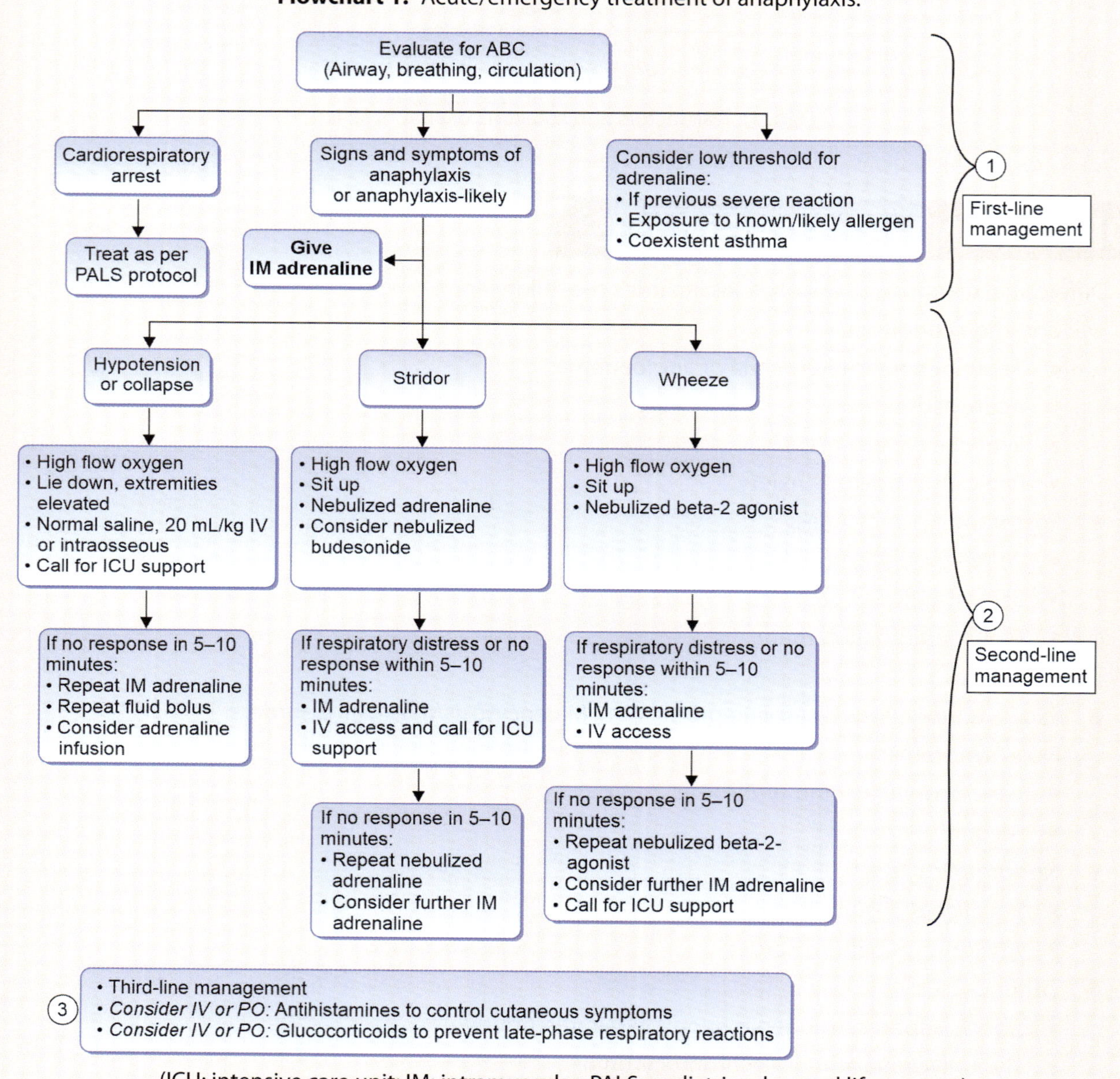

(ICU: intensive care unit; IM: intramuscular; PALS: pediatric advanced life support)

In case of urticaria or angioedema ONLY:

- Oral antihistamine
- *If coexistent asthma:* Give inhaled beta-2 agonists.
- Observe for at least 4 hours for progression of symptoms and signs as this may be an early presentation of anaphylaxis.

Drugs Used in Treatment of Anaphylaxis

Drugs used in treatment of anaphylaxis are given in **Table 2.**

TABLE 2: Drugs used in treatment of anaphylaxis.

	Dosage by age			
*Adrenaline IM (1 mg/mL of 1:1000 solution) *Site:* Mid-outer thigh	<6 months	6 months–6 years	6–12 years	>12 years
	150 mcg (0.15 mL)		300 mcg (0.3 mL)	500 mcg (0.5 mL)
Normal saline	20 mL/kg			
$Hydrocortisone (IM or slow IV) or Methylprednisolone 1 mg/kg (max 125 mg IV)	25 mg	50 mg	100 mg	200 mg
$Chlorpheniramine (IM or slow IV)	0.25 mg/kg	2.5 mg	5 mg	10 mg
$Diphenhydramine	1 mg/kg (maximum 40 mg IV)	1 mg/kg (maximum 40 mg IV)	1 mg/kg (maximum 40 mg IV)	1 mg/kg (maximum 40 mg IV)

**If* there is no response or inadequate response to IM adrenaline, injection can be repeated every 5–15 minutes. Patients usually respond to one, two, or at the most three injections.

**If* signs of poor perfusion are present and symptoms are not responding to IM adrenaline, consider IV adrenaline infusion (0.1–1 µg/kg/min)

$*Third-line* drugs that can be used for symptom control.

Long-Term/Home Management of Anaphylaxis

A three-step approach is as follows:

- *Step 1:* Discharge management
  - Adrenaline autoinjector/prefilled syringes of adrenaline
  - Educating about anaphylaxis/allergy emergency action plan
  - Medical identification (bracelets and chains)
- *Step 2:* Confirm anaphylaxis trigger(s) on follow-up (after 3–4 weeks of acute episode)
  - Allergy skin tests
  - Allergen-specific IgE levels and component testing

- *Step 3:* Avoidance and immunomodulation
    - Avoid known triggers
    - Identify medications
    - Immunotherapy (stinging insect venom immunotherapy)

KEY LEARNING POINTS

- Anaphylaxis is a potentially life-threatening condition, which may progress rapidly; hence, prompt and early recognition is essential (use clinical criteria).
- *Only* medication that treats anaphylaxis is *adrenaline.*
- Early and prompt treatment with IM adrenaline (mid-outer thigh) is *life-saving.*
- *No absolute contraindications to adrenaline* in the setting of anaphylaxis.

SUGGESTED READING

1. Muraro A, Roberts G, Worm M, Bilò MB, Brockow K, Fernández Rivas M, et al. Anaphylaxis: Guidelines from the European Academy of Allergy and Clinical Immunology (EACCI). Allergy. 2014;69(8);1026-45
2. Muraro A, Worm M, Alviani C, Cardona V, DunnGalvin A, Garvey LH, et al. EAACI guidelines: Anaphylaxis (2021 update). Allergy. 2022;77(2):357-77.
3. Simons FE. Anaphylaxis. J Allergy Clin Immunol. 2010;125(2 Suppl 2):S161-81.
4. Smith S (Ed). Advanced Paediatric Life Support: A Practical Approach to Emergencies, 7th edition. New Jersey, US: Wiley; 2023.

Section 2

Respiratory

6 Sore Throat

S Shanthi, RV Dhakshayani

INTRODUCTION

Acute pharyngitis or sore throat is one of the most common infectious diseases encountered in the outpatient department. Though most often the etiology is viral, bacterial organisms like *Streptococcus pyogenes* or group A β-hemolytic *Streptococcus* (GABHS) account for 5–30% of the episodes. They are prone to serious complications mandating early and intensive treatment.

DEFINITION

Acute pharyngitis or sore throat is the inflammation of the posterior oropharynx.

ETIOLOGY

- Viral pharyngitis is common (50–80%) and often caused by rhinovirus, influenza, parainfluenza, and adeno and coxsackie viruses. COVID-19 infection, though asymptomatic in children, causes upper respiratory infection (URI) symptoms including sore throat. Less common viral pathogens include simplex, Ebstein–Barr virus (EBV), human immunodeficiency virus (HIV), and coxsackie virus.
- Severe cases tend to be bacterial in origin and develop commonly after an initial viral infection. The most common bacterial infection is GABHS. Others include nongroup A streptococci, *Staphylococcus aureus, Haemophilus influenzae, Moraxella catarrhalis, Chlamydia pneumoniae, Mycoplasma pneumoniae, Neisseria* spp, *Corynebacterium diphtheriae*, and *Fusobacterium necrophorum.*
- Less common causes include trauma, reflux, toxins, etc. Chemicals and environmental allergens also cause acute pharyngitis. Sore throat may be a presenting symptom of serious illnesses including epiglottitis, peritonsillar abscess, retropharyngeal abscess, and Kawasaki disease (KD).

PATHOPHYSIOLOGY

Bacteria and viruses cause direct invasion of pharyngeal mucosa resulting in excess secretion and edema, causing symptoms of pain in the throat, dysphagia, odynophagia, and fever. Viruses like rhinovirus cause irritation of the throat secondary to nasal secretions.

Clinical manifestations of acute sore throat include:

- Fever
- Painful cervical adenopathy
- Pharyngeal erythema
- Tonsillar exudates
- Dysphagia
- Odynophagia
- Otalgia

Uncomplicated infectious pharyngitis, both viral and bacterial, is usually self-limited to 5–7 days, is nonprogressive, and does not have trismus or airway obstruction.

COMPLICATIONS OF BACTERIAL PHARYNGITIS

- Epiglottitis
- Otitis media
- Mastoiditis
- Sinusitis
- Acute rheumatic fever (ARF)
- Poststreptococcal glomerulonephritis (APSGN)
- Toxic shock syndrome
- Pneumonia
- Nephritis
- Meningitis

CLINICAL EXAMINATION

Clinical examination can give a clue to the underlying etiology though it may not be possible to reliably distinguish between viral, bacterial, and noninfectious pharyngitis by clinical examination alone.

TABLE 1: Clinical conditions and their corresponding symptoms.

Clinical condition	*Symptomatology*
Viral pharyngitis	Cough, rhinorrhea, conjunctivitis, headache, and rash
GABHS pharyngitis	Fever, tonsillar exudates, and cervical adenopathy
IMN	Fever, headache, myalgia, fatigue, anterior and posterior cervical lymphadenopathy, tonsillar enlargement, hepatomegaly or splenomegaly; symptoms persist up to 3 weeks; some develop morbilliform rash following amoxicillin therapy
Retropharyngeal abscess	High-grade fever, neck pain, and neck stiffness
Acute epiglottitis	High-grade fever and stridor
Lemierre's syndrome or internal jugular vein thrombophlebitis	Fever, rigors, throat pain, unilateral swelling, and tenderness at the angle of mandible
Acute retroviral syndrome	Fever and nonexudative pharyngitis
Diphtheria	Fever, chills; fatigue, sore throat; hoarseness of voice, cough; headache; dysphagia, odynophagia, difficulty in breathing, foul-smelling and blood-stained nasal discharge, diffuse lymphadenopathy—bull's neck appearance, patch in the throat on clinical examination
Quinsy/peritonsillar abscess	Fever, headache, throat pain, odynophagia, trismus, hot potato voice, otalgia, tender cervical lymphadenopathy, unilateral enlarged tonsils, and abscess on clinical examination
Scarlet fever	Fever, rash, circumoral pallor, beefy red strawberry tongue, and a fine diffuse erythematous macular-papular rash
Herpangina	High-grade fever, vomiting, headache, malaise, myalgia, poor feeding, drooling, sore throat, and dysphagia, small, tender, papular, or pinpoint vesicular lesions on an erythematous base scattered over the soft palate, uvula, and tongue

(GABHS: group A β-hemolytic *Streptococcus*; IMN: infectious mononucleosis)

Red flags indicative of a more severe disease or complication warranting hospitalization and emergent care are:

- Stridor
- Toxic appearance
- Bull neck
- Torticollis
- Neck stiffness
- Drooling of saliva
- Rapid progression
- Respiratory distress
- Trismus

EVALUATION

Clinical assessment scales help clinicians to predict bacterial etiology by appropriate selection of patients for a rapid antigen detection test (RADT). This averts an overdiagnosis of streptococcal pharyngitis and overzealous prescriptions of broad-spectrum antibiotics.

DIAGNOSTIC METHODS TO ASCERTAIN THE PRESENCE OF A GABHS INFECTION

- *Clinical scoring systems:* Centor score, McIsaac score, and FeverPAIN criteria are commonly used to assess the risk of bacterial sore throat.
- *Throat culture:* High sensitivity, specificity, and high cost; GABHS identification is based on colony morphology, Gram stain, and serogrouping; does not differentiate an acute infection from carrier state, producing false positives
- *Rapid antigen detection test (RADT):* Detects the presence or absence of Lancefield group A carbohydrate, a GABHS-specific cell-wall antigen; lateral flow immunochromatographic assay is the commonly used RDT and has high specificity.
- *Nucleic acid amplification tests:* Probe testing detects nucleic acid sequences specific to GABHS; high specificity, sensitivity, and high cost; cannot discriminate an infection from carrier state.
- Streptococcal antibody tests like ASO titer or antihyaluronidase titer are not used in the diagnosis of acute pharyngitis.

CLINICAL SCORING SYSTEMS: RISK ASSESSMENT SCORES

The Centor Score is one of the most commonly used scores in pediatric population. Modified Centor (McIsaac) score and FeverPAIN criteria are other widely used tools **(Tables 2 and 3)**.

TABLE 2: Comparison of Centor versus McIsaac scoring systems.

Centor symptom	*Point*	*Total score*	*Recommended actions*	*McIsaac Scoring System*	*Point*	*Total score*	*Recommended actions*
Tonsillar exudates	1	0–2	No testing or antibiotics	Tonsillar swelling or exudate	1	−1 to 2	No testing or antibiotics
Tender anterior cervical adenopathy	1	3	Rapid antigen test	Tender anterior cervical adenopathy	1	3	• Throat swab for culture • Delay antibiotics until culture reports • RADT in children aged 3–15 years
Absence of cough	1	4	No testing, empirical antibiotics	No cough	1	4–5	No testing, empirical antibiotics
Fever history	1			Temperature >38°C	1		
				Age			
				3–14 years	1		
				15–44 years	0		
				≥45 years	−1		

TABLE 3: FeverPAIN criteria.

Individual criteria	*Individual score*	*Composite scores*	*Likelihood of streptococcal sore throat*
Fever (during previous 24 hours)	1	0 or 1	13–18%
*P*urulent tonsils	1	2 or 3	34–40%
*A*ttend rapidly (reporting within 3 days after onset of symptoms)	1	4 or 5	62–65%
Severely *I*nflamed tonsils	1		
*N*o cough or coryza	1		

DIFFERENTIAL DIAGNOSIS OF ACUTE SORE THROAT

- Allergic rhinitis
- Gastroesophageal reflux disease
- Peritonsillar abscess
- Diphtheria
- Epiglottitis
- Herpangina—Coxsackie A virus
- Pharyngoconjunctival fever—adenovirus type 3
- Infectious mononucleosis (IMN)

INVESTIGATIONS

Total leukocyte count does not differentiate viral from bacterial pharyngitis. Lymphocytosis (>50%) or increased atypical lymphocytes (>10%) may suggest IMN.

The sensitivity of RADTs in the diagnosis of GABHS is variable between 70 and 90% and the specificity is approximately 96%. Positive RADT necessitates appropriate treatment in children.

Throat culture is the gold standard for diagnosis; it is recommended only for high-risk group.

Infectious mononucleosis caused by EBV is diagnosed by clinical picture, lymphocytosis, atypical lymphocytes, and a heterophile antibody test and is confirmed by Epstein–Barr virus serology.

Chest X-ray is not routinely needed. X-ray neck lateral view may be helpful in the diagnosis of retropharyngeal abscess. Computed tomography (CT) scan may help identify a peritonsillar or retropharyngeal abscess.

Imaging modalities used in the evaluation of septic thrombosis of internal jugular vein include ultrasound, CT neck with contrast, and magnetic resonance imaging (MRI).

TREATMENT GOALS FOR GABHS

- To provide symptom relief—analgesic and antipyretic agents like acetaminophen
- Use of appropriate antibiotics only for streptococcal pharyngitis

TREATMENT/MANAGEMENT (TABLE 4)

Antibiotics in GABHS pharyngitis shorten the duration of symptoms by 16–24 hours.

Penicillin V is the first-choice antibiotic; oral Amoxycillin is an equally effective option. A 10-day course of oral penicillin is recommended for eradication of bacterial carriage and prevention of rheumatic fever. Intramuscular penicillin is also an option.

Cephalosporins can be used in mild penicillin allergy. In patients with a history of anaphylaxis to penicillin, azithromycin or clindamycin is used. The patient is rendered noninfectious after 24 hours of antibiotics.

TABLE 4: Antimicrobial treatment of acute sore throat (GAS pharyngitis) in children.*

Choice of antibiotic	*Age of patient*	*Dose and course*†
Oral Phenoxymethyl-penicillin (I choice)	1–11 months	62.5 mg four times a day or 125 mg twice a day for 5–10 days
	1–5 years	125 mg four times a day or 250 mg twice a day for 5–10 days
	6–11 years	250 mg four times a day or 500 mg twice a day for 5–10 days
	12–17 years	500 mg four times a day or 1,000 mg twice a day for 5–10 days
Intramuscular benzathine penicillin G	Children ≤ 27 kg	600,000 U as a single dose
	Children > 27 kg	1.2 million U as a single dose
Oral amoxicillin		50 mg/kg as a single dose; max. 1–1.2 g × 10 days

*Antibiotics initiated within 9 days of onset of symptoms can prevent ARF.
†5 days treatment for symptomatic cure; 10-days course is indicated for microbiological cure.

For persons allergic to penicillin: Cephalexin—25 mg/kg/dose BD, maximum dose 500 mg/dose × 10 days (Or) Clindamycin—6–7 mg/kg/dose TDS, maximum dose 300 mg/dose ×10 days.

For persons allergic to β-lactams: Azithromycin, children: 12 mg/kg (maximum: 500 mg/dose) on day 1 followed by 6 mg/kg/dose (maximum: 250 mg/dose) OD on days 2 through 5 (Or) Clarithromycin —15 mg/kg in two divided doses for 10 days (Or) Erythromycin (preferred drug in pregnancy)—250–500 mg four times a day or 500–1,000 mg twice a day for 5 days.

Lozenges and gargles provide symptomatic relief. Acetaminophen or nonsteroidal anti-inflammatory drugs (NSAIDs) are recommended for pain and fever.

Recurrent episodes of *streptococcal pharyngotonsillitis* should be treated as individual acute episodes.

Tonsillectomy is indicated if the child has >7 episodes of tonsillitis in the previous year or > 5 episodes/year over a 2-year period, tonsillar abscess, and enlarged tonsils causing significant airway obstruction.

Peritonsillar abscess (or) Quinsy: Clindamycin 40 mg/kg/day IV TDS and Ceftriaxone 50 mg/kg/day IV OD; Piperacillin–Tazobactam or Meropenem are alternatives. Oral Amoxy clav can be used for convalescent therapy. Intraoral incision and drainage is the surgical option in children who do not respond or present with complications.

Retropharyngeal abscess: Clindamycin 40 mg/kg/day IV TDS and Ceftriaxone 50 mg/kg/day IV OD should be initiated. Vancomycin or linezolid is recommended if patients fail to respond or show features of sepsis. Oral amoxicillin-clavulanate (45 mg/kg every 12 hours) or clindamycin (15 mg/kg every 8 hours) is used as convalescent therapy. Surgical intervention is indicated if symptoms fail to improve after 24–48 hours of antibiotics or if the abscess exceeds 2–2.5 cm.

Pharyngeal diphtheria requires parenteral penicillin for 14 days along with antitoxin. Three negative cultures at 24-hour intervals are needed to render the patient noninfectious. Bed rest for 2–3 weeks is recommended to prevent cardiac complications.

Treatment for viral pharyngitis is mostly supportive. Warm fluids, gargles, antipyretics for relief of pain and fever, and antihistamines for rhinorrhea may be recommended. Cough suppressants and expectorants are not routinely recommended.

Patients with *IMN* should avoid contact sports for 6–8 weeks due to the risk of splenic rupture.

Individualized approach is essential in the following high-risk patients:

- Severe immunosuppression—long-term steroids, organ and stem cell transplantation, AIDS, neutropenia, other congenital or acquired immune defects
- Severe comorbidities
- Scarlet fever
- Infectious mononucleosis
- Pneumonia, bronchitis, otitis media
- Increased risk of ARF—demographic predilection, past history or family history of ARF

Referral to an ENT specialist is indicated in children with:

- Persistent symptoms >6 weeks,
- Recurrent acute tonsillitis (>6 episodes/year)
- Suspected peritonsillar abscess

Immediate hospitalization is indicated in the following situations:

- Stridor or difficulty in breathing (suspected epiglottitis, IMN)
- Severe systemic disease (e.g., meningitis, diphtheria, KD, Lemierre syndrome)
- Suppurative complications (peritonsillar and para- or retropharyngeal abscess)

MONITORING AND FOLLOW-UP

- *Prognosis is good, as most cases of pharyngitis are typically self-limiting and resolve within 7–10 days.* Streptococcal pharyngitis typically improves within 24–48 hours of treatment. Treatment failures are usually due to antibiotic resistance, poor compliance, and untreated close contacts.
- Patients should be reassessed if symptoms worsen or findings are suggestive of a more serious illness or condition emerges.

KEY LEARNING POINTS

- Most episodes of pharyngitis are self-limiting and require only analgesics and reassurance.
- Irrational use of antibiotics for viral sore throat leads to drug resistance and should be avoided.
- Antibiotics are only prescribed for probable streptococcal infection based on high-risk assessment scores (refer to algorithm); GABHS can be treated effectively with narrow-spectrum antibiotics.
- Importance of hand washing and personal hygiene to prevent spread to household contacts; rest and hydration should be imparted to children and caretakers.
- Nonsuppurative complications of GABHS like ARF and PSGN may not be always preventable by antibiotic treatment of GABHS, particularly PSGN.
- Epiglottitis, peritonsillar abscess, retropharyngeal abscess, and diphtheria may be life-threatening if not treated with appropriate antibiotics.
- A low threshold for initiation of antibiotics is needed for high-risk groups.
- Immunization against flu and diphtheria should be recommended to prevent recurrence.

CLINICAL ALGORITHM ON APPROACH TO SORE THROAT

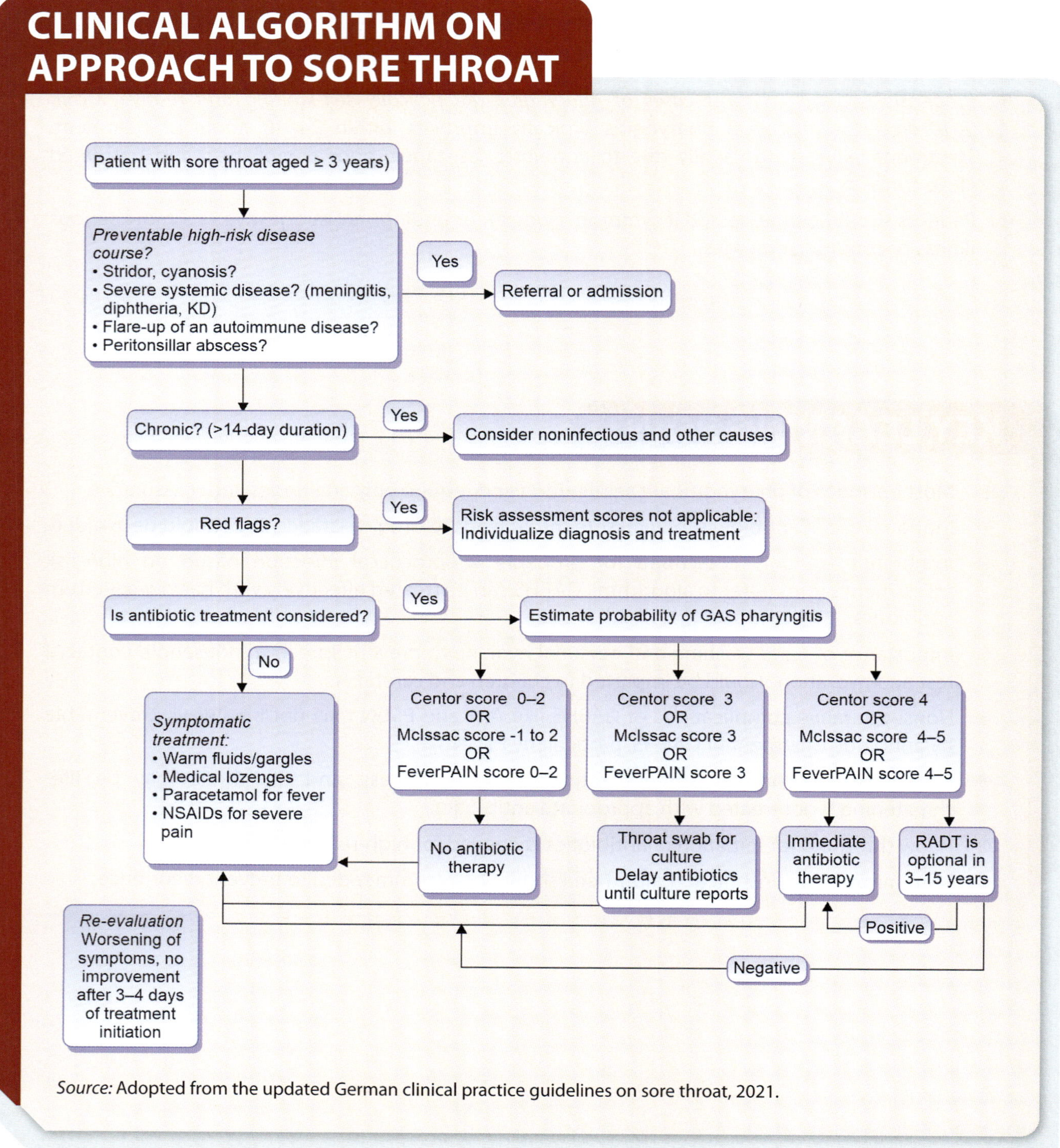

Source: Adopted from the updated German clinical practice guidelines on sore throat, 2021.

SUGGESTED READING

1. Balasubramanian S, Amperayani S, Dhanalakshmi K, Senthilnathan S, Chandramohan V. Rapid antigen diagnostic testing for the diagnosis of group A beta-haemolytic streptococci pharyngitis. Natl Med J India. 2018;31:8-10.
2. Krüger K, Töpfner N, Berner R, Windfuhr J, Oltrogge JH. Clinical practice guideline: Sore throat. Dtsch Arztebl Int. 2021;118:188-94.
3. Marcdante K, Kliegman RM, Schuh AM (Eds). Nelson Essentials of Pediatrics, 9th edition. Philadelphia: Elsevier; 2023.
4. Mustafa Z, Ghaffari M. Diagnostic Methods, Clinical Guidelines, and Antibiotic Treatment for Group A Streptococcal Pharyngitis: A Narrative Review. Front Cell Infect Microbiol. 2020:10:563627.
5. NHS England. (2023). Group A Streptococcus: reinstatement of NICE sore throat guidance for children and young people. [online] Available from https://www.england.nhs.uk/publication/group-a-streptococcus-communications-to-clinicians/ [Last accessed July, 2024]
6. The Royal Children's Hospital Melbourne. (2021). Clinical Practice Guidelines. [online] Available from https://blogs.rch.org.au/clinicalguide/ [Last accessed July, 2024]

7 Stridor

Rohit Bhowmick

INTRODUCTION

- Stridor is an abnormal, harsh monophonic respiratory sound produced by the turbulent air passing through a narrowed airway.
- Stridor indicates a pathology of larger airways, such as obstruction at the level of the supraglottic area, glottis, subglottic airway, or trachea.

TERMINOLOGIES AND DEFINITIONS

A few terminologies and definitions are as follows:

- The supraglottic area includes the nasopharynx, epiglottis, larynx, aryepiglottic folds, and false vocal cords.
- Glottic and subglottic areas are the part of the airway that extends from the vocal cords to the extrathoracic portion of the trachea, just before it enters the thoracic cavity.
- Extrathoracic region includes airways above the thoracic inlet, including supraglottic, glottic, and subglottic areas.
- Intrathoracic airway includes the segment of the trachea that lies within the thoracic cavity and the mainstem bronchi.
- Inspiratory stridor is a high-pitched, harsh sound usually produced due to the involvement of an extrathoracic airway.
- Expiratory stridor generally originates from obstruction in the intrathoracic airway. This sound can be complex to distinguish from wheezing; it can be low-pitched, monophonic, and have a harsh or honking character.
- A biphasic stridor is an inspiratory and expiratory stridor that indicates a fixed central airway obstruction.

ETIOLOGY

Causes of stridor can vary according to the age at presentation **(Table 1)**. Studies found that foreign body aspiration remains one of the leading causes of stridor in Indian children.[1]

TABLE 1: Common causes of stridor with classical features.

Etiology	*Typical age group*	*Type of stridor*	*Fever*	*Typical onset (acute/ subacute/chronic)*	*Salient features*
Viral croup (Laryngo-tracheitis)	3 months–4 years	Inspiratory	+/–	Acute or subacute	Mild upper respiratory infection (URI) or prodrome followed by gradual onset of stridor and barking cough
Bacterial tracheitis	2–6 years	Inspiratory	++	Usually acute or preceded by viral croup (gradual onset)	High-grade fever, toxic appearance, and respiratory distress
Spasmodic croup	6 months–5 years	Inspiratory	–	Subacute	• Mild URI symptoms may precede it • Typically, occurs at night. Intermittent, with abrupt and brief episodes • Recurrences are common
Retropharyngeal abscess	Infant–5 years	Inspiratory	++	Acute	• Starts with a sore throat, then progresses to fever associated with dysphagia • Muffled voice
Peritonsillar abscess	5 years or more	Inspiratory	++	Acute/subacute	• Usually preceded by tonsillitis or pharyngitis (Streptococcal) • Associated with a muffled voice ("hot potato" voice)
Diphtheria	Any age	Inspiratory, expiratory (in severe cases)	+	Subacute	Stridor preceded by swelling over neck (bull neck) and URI, unimmunized child, adherent gray pseudomembrane on throat examination
Anaphylaxis	6 months–any age	Inspiratory, expiratory (in severe cases)	–	Acute	May be associated with itching, urticaria, choking sensation, and/or wheezing
Foreign body aspiration	6 months–5 years	Inspiratory	–	Acute	• History of a witnessed choking episode is common in acute presentation. • Sometimes, classical history may not be available in smaller infants in delayed presentation.

Contd...

Contd...

Etiology	*Typical age group*	*Type of stridor*	*Fever*	*Typical onset (acute/subacute/chronic)*	*Salient features*
Epiglottitis	6 months–14 years	Inspiratory	++	Acute	• Younger patients present with respiratory distress, anxiety, high fever associated with dysphagia, drooling, and muffled speech. Older children may prefer a propped-up or tripod posture • It can rapidly progress to life-threatening airway obstruction
Postextubation	Any age (usually common in infants and smaller children)	Inspiratory	–	–	• Large (improper for age) tube size, multiple reintubations, and inadequate sedation are some critical risk factors • Usually develops within 2–4 hours postextubation but can develop as late as 24 hours postextubation

HISTORY AND PHYSICAL EXAMINATION

History

Factors such as age, symptom, onset, severity, and history of chronic/recurrent stridor are essential in guiding the differential diagnosis. Based on the age, the possible diagnoses that can be considered are given in **Table 2**.

TABLE 2: Age of presentation and differentials of stridor.

Age of onset	*Probable causes*
Neonate	*Congenital abnormalities:* Laryngomalacia, tracheomalacia, subglottic stenosis, and extrinsic compression of trachea by vascular abnormalities
Infants and toddlers	• *Congenital abnormalities:* Bronchogenic and laryngeal clefts • *Acquired:* Croup and foreign body of aspiration
School-age adolescents	Peritonsillar abscess and vocal cord dysfunction
Any age	Bacterial tracheitis, anaphylaxis, and post-trauma/burn

Other Associated Symptoms

Other associated symptoms are as follows:

- *Cough:* The presence of a barking cough is suggestive of croup.
- *Fever:* Fever can be present with croup, bacterial tracheitis, retropharyngeal/peritonsillar abscess, and epiglottitis.[2]
- *Rash:* A history of skin rash and allergies should prompt a rapid evaluation for anaphylaxis.
- *Association with feeding:* Can be seen in swallowing dysfunction, tracheoesophageal fistula, or severe gastroesophageal reflux disease.
- *Drooling:* This is a significant symptom that gives clues to life-threatening etiologies **(Flowchart 1)**.
- *Altered sensorium:* An altered sensorium, particularly when associated with increased work of breathing, can be a warning sign of an impending loss of airway.

Flowchart 1: An algorithmic approach to a child with stridor.

Stridor
- Chronic
- Acute onset → Fever
  - Present → *Evidence of:* • Dysphagia • Drooling • Respiratory distress
    - Yes → *Presence of hoarseness, indicates laryngeal involvement:* • Bacterial tracheitis • Diphtheria • Epiglottitis
    - No → *Presence of muffled voice, indicates pharyngeal involvement:* • Peritonsillar abscess • Retropharyngeal abscess
  - Absent → *History suggestive of:* Choking/foreign body aspiration trauma/burn/caustic injury intubation → • Foreign body-induced stridor • Postinjury stridor • Postextubation stridor

EXAMINATION

- *General physical examination:* Failure to thrive indicates a chronic cause of stridor and associated feeding difficulties.
- *Decubitus:* Patients with epiglottis prefer to sit up in a "tripod" or "sniffing" position.
- *Skin:* Urticarial rash with tongue swelling can be seen in anaphylaxis. A dermal hemangioma can be associated with subglottic hemangioma.
- *Upper airway examination (ear, nose, and throat):* The clinician should be careful when assessing a suspected epiglottitis. Ideally, the local examination should be done in a controlled setting, such as the operating room or pediatric intensive care unit (PICU). Healthcare providers should assess patients' tongue size and pharynx for signs of edema, and membrane or a peritonsillar abscess.
- *Respiratory system examination:* Breathing should be observed during rest and after activity. In the early phase of illness or mild disease, stridor can only be heard during agitation. Cyanosis, retractions, nasal flaring, and the use of accessory muscles can be seen in severe diseases.

INVESTIGATIONS

Relevant investigations are given in **Table 3**.

TABLE 3: Relevant investigations for stridor.

Investigations	*Significance*
Complete blood count	Neutrophilic leukocytosis can be seen in bacterial tracheitis, and peritonsillar and retropharyngeal abscesses
Polymerase chain reactions (PCR) from nasopharyngeal swab	Parainfluenza types 1, 2, and 3 positivity in croup (though rarely indicated)
Radiology	• *Steeple sign:* Seen on anteroposterior (AP) view of the neck in patients of croup (though it is a nonspecific sign) • *X-ray neck lateral view:* Helpful in the diagnosis of epiglottitis and retropharyngeal abscess • X-ray chest can help evaluate for mediastinal lymphadenopathy or masses • *Chest and neck computed tomography (CT) with contrast:* Helpful to diagnose retropharyngeal/peritonsillar abscess, mediastinal mass, and vascular ring
Nasopharyngoscopy	• Useful tool in the diagnosis of laryngomalacia • Detects anatomical defects between the nose and pharynx • Assess vocal cord movement
Bronchoscopy	Essential for management of foreign body aspiration

SEVERITY ASSESSMENT

Westley clinical croup score **(Table 4)** may be used to assess the severity of croup and develop a management plan.[3]

TABLE 4: Westley croup score.	
Components	***Scores***
Level of consciousness	• Normal, including sleep (0 points) • Disoriented (5 points)
Cyanosis	• None (0 points) • With agitation (4 points) • At rest (5 points)
Stridor	• None (0 points) • With agitation (1 point) • At rest (2 points)
Air entry	• Normal (0 points) • Decreased (1 point) • Markedly decreased (2 points)
Retractions	• None (0 points) • Mild (1 point) • Moderate (2 points) • Severe (3 points)

Categories: Mild croup = Score 0–2; Moderate croup = Score 3–5; Severe croup = Score 6–11; and impending respiratory failure = Score 12–17.

MANAGEMENT

Initial Management

The initial management involves the following:

- Patients should be kept in a comfortable position (mother's lap for infants).
- Avoid agitation and postpone cannulation and other painful stimulation.
- *Oxygen therapy:* In a nonthreatening manner to maintain oxygen saturation (SpO_2) >94%.
- Do not insert a tongue depressor and avoid aggressive local oral cavity examination unless indicated and the patient is stable.
- Avoid sedation until the airway is secured.
- Endotracheal intubation or tracheostomy, in severe cases or if medical management fails.

Specific Management

After initial stabilization, patients are to be managed as per the underlying cause (**Table 5**).

The croup should be treated as per the severity:[4]

- Mild croup
  - Oral dexamethasone at 0.6 mg/kg
  - Explain the warning signs (worsening of stridor, altered sensorium, and poor feeding) before discharge
- Moderate-to-severe croup
  - Admit the patient.
  - *Adrenaline nebulization:* Undiluted 1:1,000 adrenaline 0.5 mL/kg is mixed with normal saline (NS) to a maximum dose of 5 mL.[5]

TABLE 5: Specific management plan for different causes of stridor.

Etiology	*Specific management plan*
Bacterial tracheitis	IV antibiotics [Cloxacillin (200 mg/kg in 4 divided doses per day), amikacin (15 mg/kg/day OD dose), and clindamycin (10 mg/kg/dose TID)]
Retropharyngeal abscess	IV antibiotics, and surgical drainage
Angioneurotic edema	Adrenaline (1:1000) intramuscular 0.01 mL/kg (maximum 0.5 mL); Hydrocortisone 10 mg/kg IV and antihistamines
Diphtheria	Antibiotics (crystalline penicillin) and diphtheria antitoxin
Postextubation	IV dexamethasone and adrenaline nebulization
Postburn	Early elective endotracheal intubation

REFERENCES

1. Patnaik S, Zacharias G, Jain MK, Samantaray KK, Surapaneni SP. Etiology, clinical profile, evaluation, and management of stridor in children. Indian J Pediatr. 2021;88(11):1115-20.
2. Casazza G, Graham ME, Nelson D, Chaulk D, Sandweiss D, Meier J. Pediatric bacterial tracheitis–a variable entity: Case series with literature review. Otolaryngol Head Neck Surg. 2019;160(3):546-9.
3. Westley CR, Cotton EK, Brooks JG. Nebulized racemic epinephrine by IPPB for the treatment of croup: A double-blind study. Am J Dis Child. 1978;132(5):484-7.
4. Yang WC, Lee J, Chen CY, Chang YJ, Wu HP. Westley score and clinical factors in predicting the outcome of croup in the pediatric emergency department. Pediatric Pulmonol. 2017;52(10):1329-34.
5. Gelbart B, Parsons S, Sarpal A, Ninova P, Butt W. Intensive care management of children intubated for croup: A retrospective analysis. Anaesth Intensive Care. 2016;44(2):245-50.

8 Croup

Mihir Sarkar, Moumita Samanta

INTRODUCTION

Croup, also known as acute laryngotracheobronchitis, is a common childhood viral respiratory illness. Most cases of croup are mild and self-limiting; however, it may occasionally cause severe airway obstruction and, rarely, death.[1] Among the patients presenting at emergency, 85 % have mild croup, and only 1–8 % need hospital admission.[2]

ETIOPATHOGENESIS

Though usually caused by parainfluenza virus (types 1 and 3), other viruses such as influenza A and B, adenovirus, respiratory syncytial virus, and metapneumovirus are also implicated.[1-4] Inflammation and obstruction of the upper airway, especially the subglottic area, results in sudden-onset barking cough, inspiratory stridor, hoarseness, and respiratory distress.[4] Subglottis is the narrowest part of the pediatric airway. Croup is prevalent during the autumn and winter seasons. Children aged 6 months to 3 years are typically affected, with a predilection toward males.

CLINICAL FEATURES

Following a prodrome of mild upper respiratory tract infection (nonspecific cough, coryza, and low-grade fever), the child may present with sudden-onset seal-like barking cough often associated with inspiratory stridor and hoarseness. A mild wheeze may be present if there is lower airway involvement. The severity of symptoms varies over time and tends to worsen at night.[4]

Risk factors for severe croup include:

- Pre-existing congenital or acquired upper airway narrowing, e.g., Down's syndrome and subglottic stenosis
- Previous admission with severe croup
- Underlying chronic lung disease, congenital heart disease, neuromuscular disease, or immunodeficiency

DIFFERENTIAL DIAGNOSIS

Differentiating croup from other acute illnesses like epiglottitis, bacterial tracheitis, retro- or parapharyngeal abscess, or foreign body can be challenging.[5] Although the incidence of epiglottis has drastically reduced due to widespread vaccination against *Haemophilus influenzae*, it is important to distinguish it from croup because of its potential rapid deteriorating course. **Table 1** describes acute life-threatening differential diagnosis of stridor.

TABLE 1: Differential diagnosis of acute-onset stridor.[4,5]

With high-grade fever	
Clinical condition	***Presentation***
Epiglottitis	Acute onset of dysphagia, drooling, toxic appearance, and muffled voice
Bacterial tracheitis	Barking cough, respiratory distress, and rapid deterioration
Retropharyngeal abscess	Drooling, neck pain or torticollis, dysphagia, and odynophagia
Without fever	
Foreign body	Choking episode, wheezing, hoarseness, biphasic stridor, dyspnea, and decreased air entry
Angioedema	Rapid onset of stridor, wheezing or dysphagia, and possible cutaneous allergic signs such as urticarial rash

Alternative diagnosis must be considered if the following features (red flags) are present:

- Very sudden onset, within minutes
- High-grade fever or toxic appearance
- Biphasic, prolonged, or recurrent stridor
- Prominent wheezing or rales
- Drooling, difficulty swallowing, trismus, and torticollis
- Facial or neck swelling
- Skin rash, erythema, and shock
- Age below 3 months
- Poor response to treatment

ASSESSMENT

Assessment of the severity of airway obstruction can be done by the Westley croup score **(Tables 2 and 3)**. Vital parameters including heart rate, respiratory rate, and oxygen saturation should be recorded and monitored as required. Croup is a disease of the upper airway, and gas exchange in the alveoli is usually unaffected; thus, decreased oxygen saturation or hypoxia is a late sign indicating life-threatening croup. The loudness of stridor is not a good indicator of the severity of obstruction. Soft stridor in the presence of a worsening clinical picture may be a sign of imminent airway obstruction.

TABLE 2: Westley croup score.

Clinical feature	*Level of consciousness*	*Stridor*	*Retraction*	*Air entry*	*Cyanosis*
Assigned score	• Normal including sleep = 0 • Disoriented = 5	• None = 0 • With agitation = 1 • At rest = 2	• None = 0 • Mild = 1 • Moderate = 2 • Severe = 3	• Normal = 0 • Decreased = 1 • Markedly decreased = 2	• None = 0 • With agitation = 4 • At rest = 5

TABLE 3: Classification of severity of croup based on Westley croup score.

Clinical feature	*Mild croup Score ≤ 2*	*Moderate croup Score 3–7*	*Severe croup Score 8–11*	*Impending respiratory failure Score ≥ 12*
Consciousness and activity	• Normal • Occasional barking cough • Able to talk and/or feed	• Mild agitation/ anxiety • Frequent barking cough • Some limitation in talking/feeding	• Increased agitation/ irritability • Frequent barking cough • Breathless to talk or feed	• Depressed level of consciousness/confused/ drowsy • Cough may not be prominent due to fatigue
Stridor	No stridor at rest/ minimal stridor with agitation	Intermittent stridor at rest	Persistent stridor at rest	Persistent stridor at rest or stridor may not be prominent due to fatigue
Respiratory distress/ accessory muscle use	No/minimal retractions	Mild to moderate retractions	Marked retractions + nasal flaring	Severe retractions + nasal flaring + tracheal tug or poor respiratory effort due to fatigue
Air entry	Normal	Decreased	Markedly decreased	Markedly decreased
Cyanosis	None	With agitation	At rest	Cyanosis at rest or pallor

Source: Modified from Bjornson et al. (2013).

INVESTIGATIONS

Croup is essentially a clinical diagnosis, and investigations are rarely of any value. Radiography should not be routinely used to diagnose croup but may be warranted when the diagnosis is uncertain. In croup, a classical steeple sign secondary to glottic and subglottic narrowing may be seen, but sensitivity and specificity are low. During radiography, the patient should be monitored by staff trained in airway management. Nasopharyngeal aspiration should not be undertaken in children with suspected croup. Viral cultures, rapid antigen testing, and blood investigations are not routinely indicated. Complete and differential blood counts and C-reactive protein may help distinguish croup from bacterial causes of stridor where required.[5]

MANAGEMENT

Children with croup should be kept calm, and distressing procedures should be kept to a minimum as agitation may worsen airway obstruction. The treatment is determined by the severity of airway obstruction. The algorithmic management is described in **Flowchart 1**.[3-5]

Flowchart 1: Algorithmic management of croup.

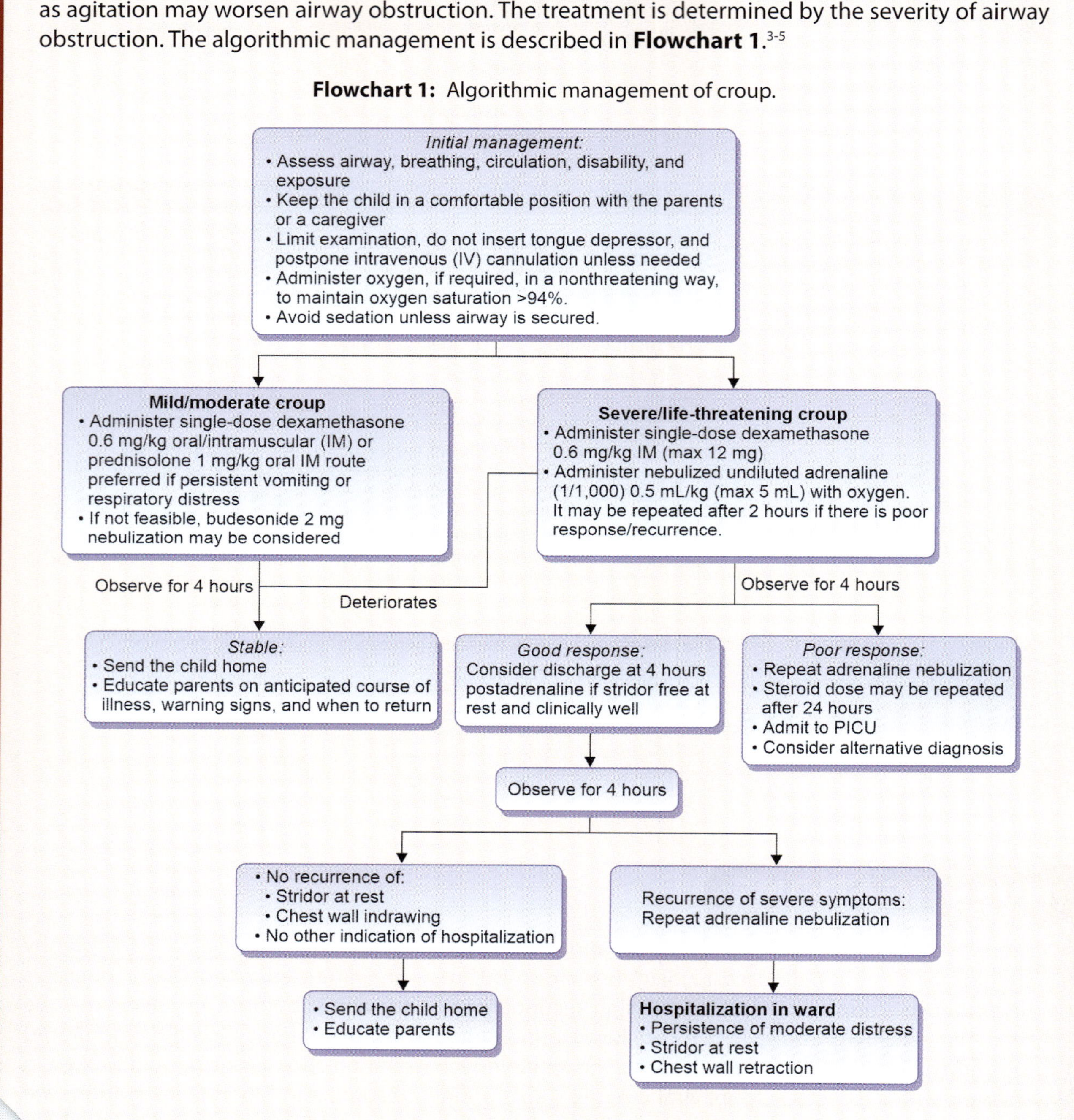

Corticosteroid

- Corticosteroids play a pivotal role in the therapeutic spectrum for croup of all degrees of severity.
- They act by reducing airway inflammation and edema.
- Dexamethasone, in particular, has been the focus of examination in a substantial majority of randomized controlled trials.[6]
- Comparatively, both intramuscular and oral administration of corticosteroids have demonstrated efficacy that is equivalent or superior to that of nebulized form.
- Concomitant use of inhaled budesonide with oral dexamethasone did not yield additional clinical benefit.[7]
- The dosage of dexamethasone employed in the bulk of these clinical investigations was 0.6 mg/kg, administered in a single dose.

Adrenaline Nebulization

- Adrenaline ameliorates manifestations of croup in patients via arteriolar vasoconstriction.
- It is recommended for moderate to severe manifestations of croup.
- It is associated with a reduction in the necessity for both intubation and tracheostomy procedures.[8]
- Adrenaline is administered in synergy with corticosteroids due to its rapid onset yet transient duration of action, in contrast to corticosteroids, which exhibit a more protracted therapeutic effect but maintain an extended half-life.
- Racemic epinephrine is not readily available in India. Nebulized 1:1000 L-epinephrine at a dose of 0.5 mL/kg (max 5 mL) is equally effective.

Supportive Care

- Antipyretic agents are concurrently employed to mitigate pyrexia and alleviate discomfort.
- *There is no role for antibiotics and short-acting $\beta 2$ agonists.*

Indications of Hospitalization or Referral

(If the treating health facility is not equipped to manage)[5-9]

- Severe croup with decreased air entry in chest and altered consciousness
- Persistent or deteriorating work of breathing in the emergency despite treatment with corticosteroid and nebulized epinephrine
- Clinical suspicion of other conditions like epiglottitis, bacterial tracheitis, or retropharyngeal abscess
- Croup in a young infant <6 months of age
- Presence of other comorbid conditions such as severe dehydration or sepsis

Criteria for Discharge from Emergency Department[9,10]

- There is no stridor at rest, tachypnea, or intercostal retractions.
- Normal heart rate and temperature
- The child has been observed in the emergency department for at least 2–4 hours after administering steroid and aerosolized epinephrine.
- No other indications for hospitalization such as poor oral intake or signs of bacterial infection
- In case of deterioration, the child can return to the emergency department promptly.

Life-threatening episodes are rare (<1%) in croup and may warrant urgent measures to secure the airway. It needs prompt attention and intervention to avoid mortality. Severe neurological impairment or cardiorespiratory failure may ensue. Urgent measures like endotracheal intubation may be required.

Indications for intubation or tracheostomy:

- Poor Glasgow Coma Scale (GCS) ≤8 or rapidly deteriorating score
- Rapid desaturation, not improving with oxygen and medical management
- Features of cardiorespiratory failure
- Cyanosed or ashen color

Endotracheal intubation should be done by an experienced intensivist or anesthetist or otorhinolaryngologist, preferably in the operation theater. A smaller size endotracheal tube may be used, and an emergency tracheostomy set must be kept ready.

RECURRENT CROUP

Recurrent croup is most acceptedly defined as two or more episodes per year.[11] Underlying etiologies of recurrent croup are heterogeneous. Glottic, subglottic, or tracheal pathology is typically assumed to be the most common cause of recurrent croup;[12] however, the presence of asthma, allergies, and gastroesophageal reflux disease are also potential causes.[11] Evaluation of such patients is multidisciplinary.

Infants with recurrent croup, and children below the age of 3 years who have a history of endotracheal intubation, warrant an assessment via bronchoscopic examination. Should such an evaluation not disclose any anatomical impediments, a comprehensive triple endoscopy—consisting of bronchoscopy, esophagoscopy, and laryngoscopy—may be deemed necessary. Patients devoid of airway anomalies ought to undergo evaluation for asthma and gastroesophageal reflux disease (GERD), and empirical therapy should be commenced for these conditions.[11]

KEY LEARNING POINTS

- Croup is one of the most common causes of stridor in children and is a clinical diagnosis.
- Management is determined by the severity of airway obstruction.
- Minimize distressing procedures to prevent agitation and worsening airway obstruction.
- Systemic corticosteroids are the mainstay of management. In severe croup, the addition of nebulized epinephrine improves symptoms.
- Recurrent croup is usually associated with airway abnormalities and needs appropriate evaluation.

REFERENCES

1. Bjornson CL, Johnson DW. Croup in children. CMAJ. 2013;185(15):1317-23.
2. Rosychuk RJ, Klassen TP, Metes D, Voaklander DC, Senthilselvan A, Rowe BH. Croup presentations to emergency departments in Alberta, Canada: A large population-based study. Pediatr Pulmonol. 2010; 45(1):83-91.
3. Rajapaksa S, Starr M. Croup-assessment and management. Aust Fam Physician. 2010;39(5):280-2.
4. Ortiz-Alvarez O. Acute management of croup in the emergency department. Paediatr Child Health. 2017; 22(3):166-9.
5. Smith DK, McDermott AJ, Sullivan JF. Croup: Diagnosis and management. AmFam Physician. 2018;97(9): 575-80.
6. Russell KF, Liang Y, O'Gorman K, Johnson DW, Klassen TP. Glucocorticoids for croup. Cochrane Database Syst Rev. 2011;(1):CD001955.
7. Geelhoed GC. Budesonide offers no advantage when added to oral dexamethasone in the treatment of croup. Pediatr Emerg Care. 2005;21(6):359-62.
8. Bjornson C, Russell K, Vandermeer B, Klassen TP, Johnson DW. Nebulized epinephrine for croup in children. Cochrane Database Syst Rev. 2013;10:CD006619
9. Petrocheilou A, Tanou K, Kalampouka E, Malakasioti G, Giannios C, Kaditis AG. Viral croup: Diagnosis and a treatment algorithm. Pediatr Pulmonol. 2014;49(5):421-9.
10. Elder AE, Rao A. Management and outcomes of patients presenting to the emergency department with croup: Can we identify which patients can safely be discharged from the emergency department? J Paediatr Child Health. 2019;55(11):1323-28.
11. Quraishi H, Lee DJ. Recurrent Croup. Pediatr Clin North Am. 2022;69(2):319-28.
12. Hodnett BL, Simons JP, Riera KM, Mehta DK, Maguire RC. Objective endoscopic findings in patients with recurrent croup: 10-year retrospective analysis. Int J Pediatr Otorhinolaryngol. 2015;79(12):2343-7.

Airway Foreign Body in Children

U Vijaya Kumar

INTRODUCTION

- Foreign body aspiration (FBA) is one of the common emergencies in children <3 years of age, however even older children and very elderly people also tend to aspirate foreign body (FB).
- Aspiration of FB could be a life-threatening emergency in children due to their small airways and less functional respiratory reserve in them. Whenever there is a suspicion of FBA, it warrants immediate evaluation with airway evaluation with or without imaging. The exact incidence in our country is not known, due to a lack of reporting and lack of registries.
- In the American population, the incidence of fatal choking among children <5 years is around 0.43 per 100,000.

PREDISPOSING FACTORS IN CHILDREN

The predisposing factors in children include:

- Incompletely developed laryngeal reflexes
- Habit of keeping nonedible things in the mouth
- Talking and crying while eating
- Incomplete developmental of teeth—poor chewing of food

COMMON OBJECTS ASPIRATED

The most commonly aspirated edible items are peanuts and other nuts, seeds, carrots, apples, and inadequately chewed vegetable items. Nonedible items commonly aspirated are pen caps, small whistles, erasers, safety pins, nose pins, needles, etc., It has been reported that 26% of aspiration is due to food, bone pieces, peanuts, and seeds. Nearly about 50% of the times aspiration occurs even if an adult is supervising the children.

CLINICAL FEATURES

Symptoms depend on the foreign object's size, shape, nature, and place of impaction **(Table 1)**:

- Heathy child starts having cough, which is sudden onset, especially during eating or playing with toys having small parts.
- Symptoms can range from persistent cough, stridor, wheezing, respiratory distress, cyanosis, and respiratory arrest.

TABLE 1: Clinical symptoms of foreign body aspiration.

Place of impaction of foreign body	*Symptoms*
Larynx	Severe coughing, choking, hoarseness, and stridor (partial obstruction)
Subglottic/tracheal	Stridor, cough, and dyspnea
Bronchial	Wheezing and persistent pneumonia/collapse (less symptomatic)

Foreign body aspiration should be considered as one of differentials in the nonemergent respiratory conditions such as persistent noisy breathing, chronic cough, difficult asthma, persistent/recurrent pneumonia, persistent collapse, and bronchiectasis.

Bronchial FB can also present with pneumothorax with or without subcutaneous emphysema if it acts like a ball valve in the airway leading to hyperinflation.

INVESTIGATIONS

The investigations done are as follows:

- **Chest X-ray:**
  - Typical finding is unilateral hyperinflation, which may be more evident in expiratory film.
  - Focal hyperinflation is possible when the foreign body is lodged in the segmental bronchus.
  - Unilateral pneumothorax and subcutaneous emphysema can be seen in complicated cases. Collapsed segment or consolidation changes are generally seen in cases of longstanding bronchial FBs.
  - Although chest X-ray may give indirect evidence of FBA, a normal one cannot rule out aspiration.
- **Computed tomography (CT):**
  - CT is superior to chest X-ray in identifying FB by direct demonstration or indirect evidence such as air trapping and atelectasis.
  - CT can also identify the nonradio-opaque FBs, which are often missed by plain radiographs.
  - Hence, CT is useful when plain radiograph fails to demonstrate FB and suspicion is high. It is also helpful to know the exact place of impact, which would help in the removal.
  - Another role of CT is to identify the mimics of FB such as intraluminal obstruction by mass or external compression, where plain radiographs are suggestive of FBA.
- **Virtual bronchoscopy:**
  - It is a noninvasive technology where multidetector CT creates 3D image of the airway using volume and surface rendering techniques.
  - The clinical implications of virtual bronchoscopy are that it helps in planning FB removal, helps to avoid bronchoscopy whether flexible/rigid, and helps to visualize the airway beyond the obstruction.
- **Bronchoscopy:**
  - The gold standard investigation for diagnosing airway FB is direct visualization of it using the flexible/rigid bronchoscopy.
  - Rigid bronchoscopy alone was used for removal of FBs earlier, nowadays the flexible bronchoscopy also serves the therapeutic purpose.

DIFFERENTIAL DIAGNOSES

The differential diagnoses include:

- Mucus plugging
- Large airway infections, for example, tuberculosis (TB) granuloma
- Large airway neoplasms, for example, hamartoma, hemangioma, inflammatory myofibroblastic tumor, and carcinoid tumor
- Tracheobronchomalacia

MANAGEMENT

- The first-line management for any aspirated FB is removal of it by rigid or flexible bronchoscopy. When removal of the FB is planned, the following facts are taken into consideration: Size, shape, material composition and place of impaction, host factors age, approximate diameter of the airways and clinical stability, with respect to equipment the size of the bronchoscope, working channel, and available accessories (raptor forceps, basket, and net). Pediatric anesthesia support is an essential component of procedure, mandatory for rigid bronchoscopy and ensures safety of the child during flexible bronchoscopy. However, experienced interventional pulmonologists may be able to remove under sedation with flexible bronchoscopy.
- Every FBA is different in terms of the object aspirated, the child, and clinical presentation, hence any one equipment or accessory or technique cannot be recommended. It is always good to have discussion on how to proceed, possible methods of removal, and expected complications. The team should consist of interventional pulmonologist, pediatric anesthetist, ENT surgeon, and intensivist. Although no consensus guidelines are available to manage airway FB, **Flowchart 1** depicts overall approach to management of airway FBs in children.

Flowchart 1: Approach to airway foreign body.

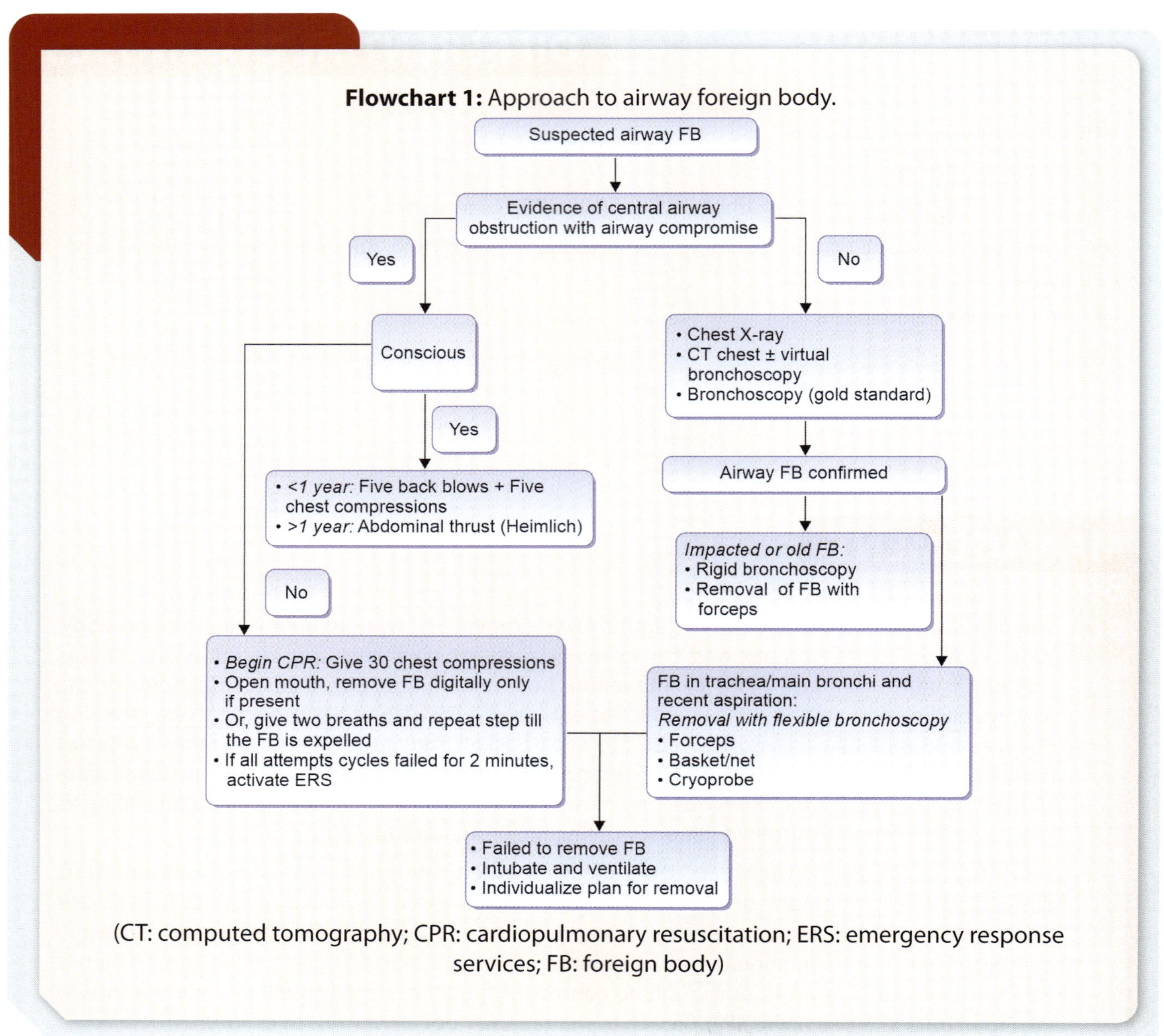

(CT: computed tomography; CPR: cardiopulmonary resuscitation; ERS: emergency response services; FB: foreign body)

ANESTHETIC CONSIDERATIONS

- During induction, the child has to be kept as quiet as possible to avoid dislodgement of FB, which would cause airway compromise. For the FBs that are located proximally (trachea and main bronchi), it is desirable to remove them with flexible bronchoscopy with appropriate accessory under sedation and maintaining spontaneous ventilation. While using flexible bronchoscopy, one would use nasopharyngeal airway or laryngeal mask airway (LMA) for maintaining oxygenation and ventilation.
- If FB is old and impacted or located distally, which needs more controlled airway, then rigid bronchoscopy with inhalational anesthesia should be used. The quantity of inhaled medication would be more as the there will be leakage through the bronchoscope. During the procedure, manual jet ventilation can be used, which would prevent the hypoxemia during the procedure.

BRONCHOSCOPY ACCESSORIES FOR FOREIGN BODY REMOVAL

The following accessories are used for FB removal:

- *Raw-tooth forceps:* These could grasp the plastic and metal FBs and are inserted through a flexible bronchoscope. Food items like peanuts or vegetable pieces cannot be removed using the forceps as it would the FBs leading more worse situation. Biopsy forceps can also be used if raw-tooth forceps are not available. The main disadvantage of the forceps is that the smaller airways would not allow the complete opening of forceps.
- *Baskets and net:* Baskets are used for ureteric stone removal with cystoscopy and can be used for removal of FBs in airway through flexible bronchoscopy. FBs with round margins and organic ones, for example, peanuts, beads, seeds, and vegetable pieces can be removed using baskets. Net is similar to basket and it can fully accommodate the FB and close all around.
- *Cryotherapy:* A cryoprobe can be used to remove the FBs that are impacted more distally. It uses liquid nitrogen to freeze the FB and then it is removed by cryoadhesion. Earlier, only thick cryoprobes were available, now probes as thin as 1.1 mm are available enabling their utility in thin scopes with small working channels. The organic FBs can be best removed by cryo technique.
- *Bronchoscopic balloon:* Impacted FBs can be mobilized using a balloon, which is passed beyond the FB and inflated, which makes the FB move proximally. Mobilized FB can be removed later by using forceps or basket. Balloon is best suited for FB with hole at the center through which a catheter can be passed, and then the balloon is subsequently inflated and removed en bloc.

COMPLICATIONS

The complications include the following:

- *FB-related:*
  - Airway obstruction and respiratory compromise, hypoxemia, and hypoventilation leading to cardiorespiratory arrest
  - Sharp objects would cause injury to the airway leading to bleeding, pneumomediastinum, and pneumothorax.
  - Retained FB can cause recurrent pneumonia and focal bronchiectasis.
- *Procedure-related:*
  - Displacement of FB to central airway from periphery leading to obstruction
  - Airway edema and bleeding
  - Tracheal laceration

SUGGESTED READING

1. Behera G, Tripathy N, Maru YK, et al. Role of virtual bronchoscopy in children with a vegetable foreign body in the tracheobronchial tree. J Laryngol Otol. 2014;128(12):1078-83.
2. Goldfarb S, Piccione J. Diagnostic and Interventional Bronchoscopy in Children. New Jersey: Humana press; 2021. pp. 317-32.
3. Hegde SV, Hui PK, Lee EY. Tracheobronchial foreign
4. Karišik M. Foreign body aspiration and ingestion in children. Acta Clin Croat. 2023;62(Suppl1):105-12.
5. Kendigelen P. The anaesthetic consideration of tracheobronchial foreign body aspiration in children. J Thorac Dis. 2016;8(12):3803-7.
6. Salih AM, Alfaki M, Alam-Elhuda DM. Airway foreign bodies: A critical review for a common pediatric emergency. World J Emerg Med. 2016;7(1):5-12.

10 Epistaxis in Children

Vishnu Mohan PT, Vinitha KA

INTRODUCTION

- Epistaxis is a benign condition of childhood and accounts for about 0.5% of all emergency department visits. Usual age of presentation is between 2 and 10 years of age.
- There is no consensus on the duration or frequency of episodes defining recurrent epistaxis, and in some studies, recurrent epistaxis is defined as five or more episodes per year.

TERMINOLOGIES AND DEFINITIONS

- *Epistaxis* is defined as bleeding from the nostril, nasal cavity, or nasopharynx that is sufficient to warrant medical advice or care.
- *Primary epistaxis:* Idiopathic bleeds without identifiable and precipitating factors
- *Secondary epistaxis:* Bleeding associated with clear and definitive cause

ETIOPATHOLOGY

- Epistaxis may be idiopathic or may have secondary causes.
- Secondary causes are given in **Table 1**.

TABLE 1: Secondary causes of epistaxis.

Trauma	• Digital manipulation (nose picking) • Facial trauma and blunt force • Septal perforation
Inflammation and infection	• Upper respiratory tract infections • Allergic rhinitis/sinusitis • Foreign body • Vasculitis
Neoplasms and masses	• Nasal polyps • Rhabdomyosarcoma of the head and neck • Juvenile nasopharyngeal angiofibroma (JNA)
Hematologic conditions and coagulopathies	• Hemophilia • von Willebrand disease • Leukemia • Platelet dysfunction/disorder • Liver disease
Medications	• Anticoagulants • Nasal steroid sprays • Illicit drug inhalation • Natural medications

SITES OF BLEEDING

Fig. 1: Sites of bleeding.

The sites of bleeding are as follows **(Fig. 1)**:

- *Superficial portion of anterior nasal septum due to network of small blood vessels:* Kiesselbach's plexus
- Lateral nasal wall, particularly the branches of the sphenopalatine artery
- Posteriorly, bleeding can arise from posterior branches of the sphenopalatine artery, Woodruff plexus, and venous sources.

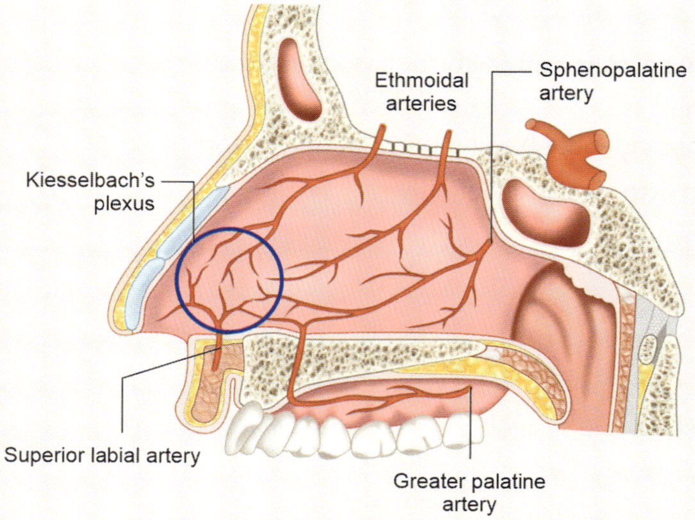

CLINICAL FEATURES

The clinical features of epistaxis are given in **Table 2**.

TABLE 2: Signs, symptoms, and etiology of epistaxis.

S.No	*Symptoms*	*Signs*	*Etiology*
1	Unilateral epistaxis accompanied by foul-smelling nasal discharge in a young child		Foreign body
2	Nasal itch and blockage, watery rhinorrhea, and sneezing	• Transverse nasal skin crease (allergic salute) and periorbital markers such as "allergic shiners" and "Dennie–Morgan lines" • Pale or bluish nasal mucosa and turbinates	Allergic rhinitis
3	*Adolescent males presenting with:* Dramatic bleeding, difficult to control and facial swelling		Juvenile nasopharyngeal angiofibroma (JNA)
4	• Young children presenting with severe intermittent epistaxis • Nasal obstruction with or without mucopurulent or bloody nasal discharge • Pain and cranial neuropathy	Eustachian tube dysfunction such as unilateral middle ear effusion	Rhabdomyosarcoma
5	Neck mass with neck pain	Distortion of nasal anatomy, intranasal mass, polyps, or cervical lymphadenopathy	Nasopharyngeal carcinoma
6	• Family history of bleeding disorders • Recurrent or extremely refractory epistaxis • Bleeding from other anatomical sites or a history of easy bruising	Pallor, jaundice	Primary and acquired coagulopathies
7	Nosebleeds present at a mean age of 12 years and progressively worsen with age	Gastrointestinal bleeding, pulmonary arteriovenous malformations and mucocutaneous telangiectasias	Hereditary hemorrhagic telangiectasia (HHT)
8	Adolescent epistaxis with fever, arthralgia, and weight loss		Granulomatosis with polyangiitis (Wegener's granulomatosis)

BLEEDING POINT IDENTIFICATION

The bleeding point identification is done as follows:

- Examine for visible bleeding points with a nasal speculum.
- Place cotton into the posterior nasal cavity to prevent blood from running down the pharynx.
- If bleeding point is not identified, refer to an otolaryngologist for detailed examination using a flexible/rigid endoscope.
- When the patient is seated, the blood flows from top to bottom, hence the search for a bleeding point with an endoscope is performed in the following order: Upper olfactory cleft, upper middle meatus, lower olfactory cleft, lower middle meatus, common meatus, inferior meatus.
- *Rigid nasal endoscopy* is not tolerated well by children.
- For posterior view of the nasal cavity and nasopharynx, fine 2.2 mm flexible nasal endoscope can be used after application of topical anesthetic and vasoconstricting agent.
- If an adequate view cannot be obtained or in case of a noncooperative child, examination under general anesthesia may be required.

INVESTIGATIONS

- Routine blood testing is not needed.
- Laboratory tests should be considered for children with:
  - Prolonged (i.e., more than 30 minutes) or severe bleeding despite appropriate application of pressure
  - Age <2 years and when the history and physical findings are suggestive of a bleeding disorder, malignancy, liver or other systemic disease.

Laboratory Tests

The following laboratory tests are done:

- Full blood count (FBC) with differential white cell count and platelet count
- Coagulation screen comprising prothrombin time (PT) and activated partial thromboplastin time (APTT)
- International normalized ratio (INR)
- Factor assays and von Willebrand factor
- Platelet function assays (hematologist option, if any abnormalities)
- Computed tomography (CT)/magnetic resonance imaging (MRI)/selective digital subtraction angiography (DSA) [for suspected neoplasm/juvenile nasopharyngeal angiofibroma (JNA)]

MANAGEMENT

The stepwise management of epistaxis is as follows:

- In an acute episode, stabilize child's *airway, breathing, and circulation.*
- Direct pressure over the soft cartilaginous part of the nose (alae nasi) for 10–15 minutes (*the Hippocratic method)is applied with the* child seated, head tilted slightly forward, and mouth open to prevent airway obstruction and swallowing of blood.
- As blood clots are a source of fibrinolytic enzymes, chance of persistent bleeding after 5–10 minutes is there; therefore, the nose should be gently blown to evacuate any clots.
- If bleeding is not controlled, gently place *cotton pledgets soaked in vasoconstrictor and local anesthetic* such as co-phenylcaine (lignocaine hydrochloride 5% with phenylephrine hydrochloride 0.5%) or oxymetazoline is applied in the anterior nasal cavity, followed by further digital pressure for 5 minutes.
- If bleeding continues, proceed with *chemical cautery with silver nitrate.* If a bleeding point can be seen anteriorly and the child can tolerate the procedure, 75% silver nitrate is applied to the bleeding point for up to 5 seconds until a grey-white eschar develops. Avoid applying on both sides as it can cause septal perforation.
- *Anterior nasal packing* under direct vision may be required if the bleeding continues. Absorbable packs are preferred in children over nonabsorbable packs because their removal can cause further trauma to the anterior nasal septum. Admit the child for observation.
- Examination under anesthesia may be required if bleeding continues, or if a young child is unable to tolerate/cooperate for intervention.
- Posterior bleeding in children is much less common but more severe, rarely, *posterior nasal packing or balloon* inflation under general anesthesia is needed.
- The child with persistent anterior or posterior epistaxis refractory to these measures in the absence of a correctable bleeding disorder may require consideration of either *arterial ligation or radiological selective arterial embolization.* Transnasal endoscopic sphenopalatine artery ligation (TESPAL) is routinely performed.

Management of Recurrent Episodes of Bleeding

If the child or underlying cause for recurrent epistaxis is not high risk, treatment options should be discussed and include:

- Mucosal hydration with saline drops or spray
- Emollients, for example, petroleum jelly
- Topical antiseptic cream
- Bipolar electrocautery

The algorithmic approach to the management of epistaxis is given in **Flowchart 1**.

Flowchart 1: The algorithmic approach to the management of epistaxis.

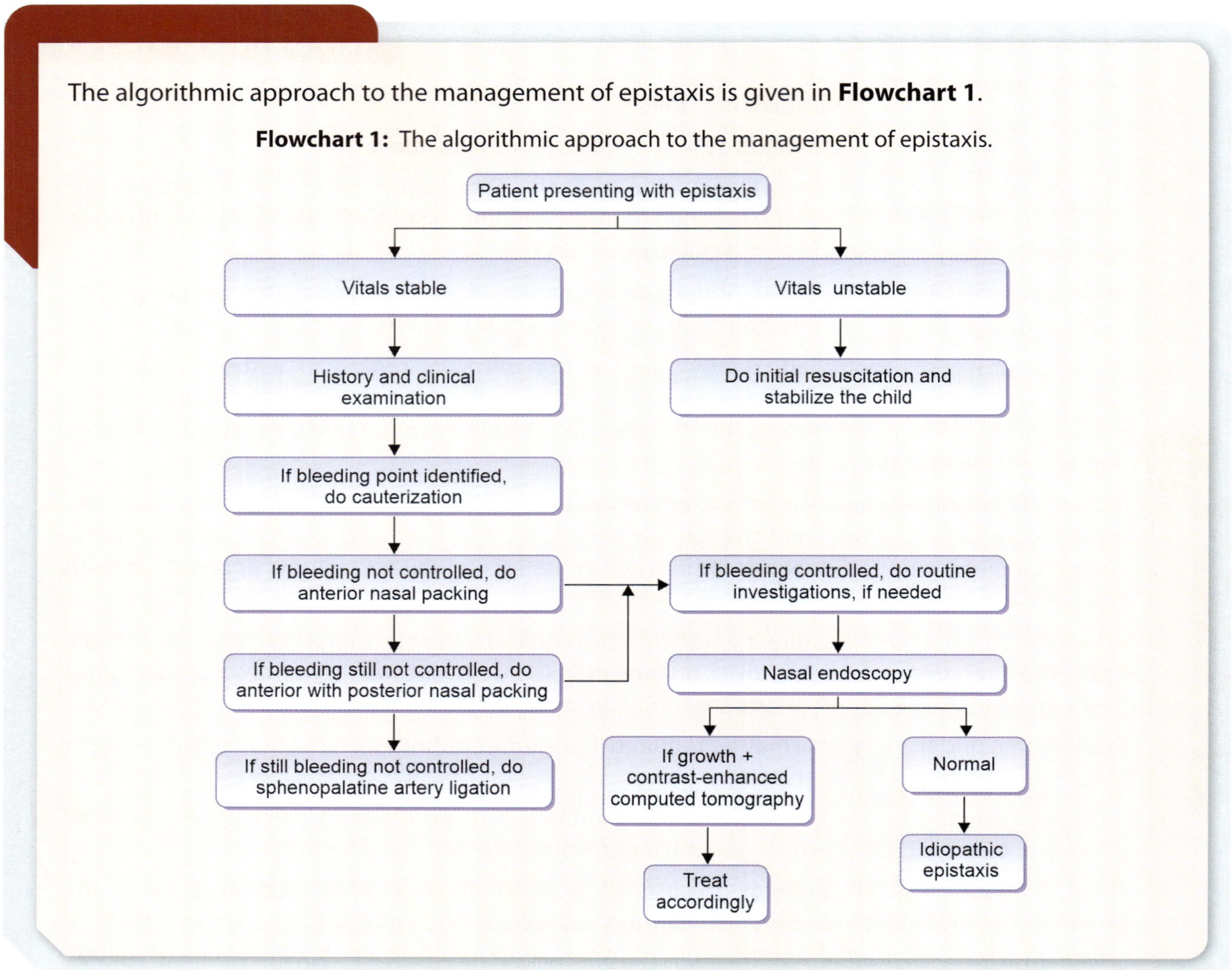

PREVENTION

- Educate the correct first-aid management in the event of recurrence.
- Keep fingernails trimmed and clean.
- Manage suspected or proven allergic rhinitis.
- Teach parents how to apply child's nasal steroid spray correctly.

KEY LEARNING POINTS

- Anterior bleeds are the most common type of epistaxis. They originate from Little's area on the anterior nasal septum either from Kiesselbach's plexus or from retrocolumellar veins.
- No laboratory investigations are required unless an underlying cause is suspected.
- If a bleeding point is visible, do chemical cautery with silver nitrate.

SUGGESTED READING

1. Kucik CJ, Clenney T. Management of epistaxis. Am Fam Physician. 2005;71(2):305-11.
2. Send T, Bertlich M, Eichhorn KW, Ganschow R, Schafigh D, Horlbeck F, et al. Etiology, management, and outcome of pediatric epistaxis. Pediatr Emer Care. 2021;37(9):466-70.
3. Svider P, Arianpour K, Mutchnick S. Management of epistaxis in children and adolescents: Avoiding a chaotic approach. Pediatr Clin N Am. 2018;65(3):607-21.
4. Tunkel DE, Anne S, Payne SC, Ishman SL, Rosenfeld RM, Abramson PJ, et al. Clinical practice guideline: Nosebleed (Epistaxis). Otolaryngol Head Neck Surg. 2020;162(1_suppl):S1-38.
5. Watkinson JC, Clarke RW (Eds). Scott-Brown's otorhinolaryngology, head and neck surgery, eighth edition. Boca Raton, Florida: CRC Press; 2018.

11 Management of Acute Viral Bronchiolitis

Karthik Narayanan

INTRODUCTION

Acute viral bronchiolitis (AVB) is the most common cause of respiratory distress in children <24 months of age. It usually happens during winter, and wheezing is the most common presentation. Many viruses are implicated to cause AVB out of which respiratory syncytial virus (RSV) contributes to 30–80% in various studies.[1,2] Other viruses include human metapneumovirus, Bocavirus, parainfluenza virus, adenovirus, and rhinovirus.

PATHOPHYSIOLOGY

Acute viral bronchiolitis is characterized by inflammation of the bronchioles leading to edema, accumulation of necrotic debris of epithelial cells, bronchospasm, and increased mucous production leading to obstruction of small airways, air trapping, and atelectasis.

HISTORY AND PHYSICAL EXAMINATION

Most infants present with an acute history of symptoms of viral prodrome like low-grade fever, running nose, nose block, reduced feeding, and cough for the initial 3 days. As the disease progresses, the infant develops tachypnea, nasal flaring, and use of accessory muscles of respiration resulting in chest retractions and wheezing. Auscultation can reveal both wheeze and crepitations. The infant becomes more irritable due to difficulty breathing. Later, hypoxia and respiratory failure occur and the child becomes drowsy. Young infants <3 months of age can also have episodes of apnea as a manifestation of severe bronchiolitis. Disseminated viral infection can lead to myocarditis (gallop, murmur), hepatitis (hepatomegaly), rhabdomyolysis (oliguria), encephalopathy, and cytokine storm leading to multiorgan dysfunction.[2]

EVALUATION

Acute viral bronchiolitis is a clinical diagnosis. Laboratory investigations and chest radiography are not warranted in all patients and are not recommended as a routine.[3,4]

In children with associated comorbid conditions and children in impending respiratory failure requiring ventilation where the incidence of associated sepsis/secondary bacterial infection is high, investigations may be performed. Risk factors for serious illness include:

- Prematurity
- Congenital heart disease
- Chronic neurological conditions with hypotonia and pharyngeal incoordination
- Immunocompromised children
- Chromosomal abnormalities like trisomy 21
- Chronic lung disease

Identification of causative virus using antigen detection testing for RSV from nasopharyngeal aspirate by direct immunofluorescence or enzyme-linked immunosorbent assay (ELISA) technique or multiplex polymerase chain reaction (PCR) can help in preventing indiscriminate use of antibiotics in these children, isolation, and cohort cases.[4,5]

Chest radiographs may provide information about the baseline lung condition and help to rule out other lung conditions like congenital lung malformations, foreign body, and pneumonia when such diagnoses are suspected based on clinical history.

Other investigations include total and differential WBC counts, C-reactive protein, serum procalcitonin, and blood culture which should be done as a part of sepsis workup to decide on initiation or continuation of antibiotics.

Investigations to evaluate organ functions like liver function tests, renal function tests, cardiac biomarkers, and neuroimaging can be performed based on the clinical situation.

ASSESSMENT OF SEVERITY

There have been many severity scoring systems developed for assessment in AVB, but none of them has been extensively validated. Almost all of these have emphasized on the following clinical examination findings for moderate-to-severe bronchiolitis:

- Respiratory rate >2 SD for age
- Use of accessory muscles (chest retractions)
- Nasal flaring
- Saturation <92% in room air (hypoxia)

Children with severe bronchiolitis require respiratory support more than supplemental oxygen to decrease the work of breathing and improve oxygenation.

MANAGEMENT OF ACUTE VIRAL BRONCHIOLITIS

Acute viral bronchiolitis is a mild and self-limiting illness that is managed conservatively at home in most children with saline nasal drops to clear nasal blocks and oral hydration. Reporting to health care facilities for hospitalization in otherwise normal children with no risk factors is advised in case of signs of worsening (poor feeding, labored breathing, lethargy, and excessive irritability).

Children with a high risk for severe disease are hospitalized if they have chest auscultatory findings and are monitored for worsening. In hospitalized children, the cornerstone of treatment is supportive care with continuous monitoring for the progression of diseases, appropriate respiratory support to deliver heated humidified oxygen to ensure normoxia and reduce work of breathing, hydration using oral/nasogastric or intravenous fluids, and fever management.

Respiratory Support in Acute Viral Bronchiolitis

- *Supplemental oxygen:*
  - Supplemental oxygen should be initiated in all children with moderate bronchiolitis with increased work of breathing or room air SpO_2 <92%.[3,4]
  - Ensure that oxygen is heated and humidified.
  - Oxygen support can be discontinued if there is no respiratory distress and room air SpO_2 >92%.
- *Heated humidified high-flow nasal cannula (HHHFNC):*
  - Start in children with severe bronchiolitis—increased work of breathing or hypoxia (saturation <92% at 40% FiO_2) in spite of providing adequate supplemental oxygen for 2 hours.
  - Closely monitor the child for deterioration—worsening heart rate, respiratory rate, sensorium, and SpO_2/FiO_2 ratio.
  - Start with a flow of 2 L/kg/min and 60% FiO_2.
  - Choose the appropriate size nasal interface (the diameter of the interface should not be more than 50% of the diameter of the nostril size).
  - Use intravenous sedation only if the baby is irritable and does not settle down with pacifiers and mild oral sedatives like chloral hydrate.
- *Continuous positive airway pressure (CPAP):*
  - Start in severe bronchiolitis if HHHFNC is not available.
  - Ensure appropriate interface (nasal pillow, nasal mask, face mask depending upon infant's comfort).
  - Do not start in infants with an inability to handle oral secretions, hemodynamic instability requiring inotropes, and uncooperative child.
  - Use intravenous sedation only if the baby is irritable and does not settle down with pacifiers and mild oral sedatives like Triclofos.

- *Noninvasive positive-pressure ventilation (NPPV):*
  - Use of NPPV is limited as most children recover either with HHHFNC or with CPAP.
  - It has been observed that NPPV delays intubation in impending respiratory failure with no additional benefit in AVB.
  - NPPV requires high-level unit expertize to maintain the interface, titrate pressure, and ensure synchrony.
- *Intubation and invasive mechanical ventilation:*
  - Indications of mechanical ventilation include:
    - Hypoxia (SpO_2/FiO_2 <150 in spite of adequate CPAP/HHHFNC support for at least 2 hours)
    - Hypercarbia ($paCO_2$ >60 mm Hg and pH <7.2)
    - Impending cardiorespiratory failure [impaired neurological status, recurrent apnea, poor perfusion, Glasgow Coma Score (GCS) < 8, poor respiratory efforts, and bradycardia]
  - Lung-protective ventilation should be done.
  - Auto-positive end-expiratory pressure (PEEP) should be avoided by providing adequate expiratory time.
  - Appropriate sedation and analgesia should be provided to prevent asynchrony.

Aerosol Therapy in Acute Viral Bronchiolitis

Aerosol therapy that has been studied in AVB includes the following:

- Hypertonic saline (3%)
- Nebulized epinephrine
- Nebulized bronchodilators
- Nebulized corticosteroids

There is no significant available evidence on the above therapies to demonstrate a reduction in pediatric intensive care unit (PICU) admission or the need for respiratory support in acute viral bronchiolitis. However, they have been found to reduce the work of breathing and offer symptomatic relief when used. Hence, they are not routinely recommended as part of care in children with AVB.

In children with a clinical history of atopy, a trial of bronchodilator nebulization can be given in the emergency room to assess response. Nebulized bronchodilators can be continued if there is a good response to bronchodilators in these children.

The following has no role in the treatment of bronchiolitis and should not be used routinely unless indicated:

- Systemic corticosteroids
- Macrolides and other antibiotics
- Antivirals
- Caffeine for apnea

- Routine use of aerosolized bronchodilators and epinephrine
- Hypertonic saline
- Oral cough syrups containing mucolytics
- Nebulized n-acetyl cysteine
- Chest physiotherapy

Hydration

- Oral feeding is preferred in children with mild-to-moderate bronchiolitis. This will help the child to be calm and settled. Use nasal saline drops and do gentle nasal suctioning to clear nasal secretions before oral feeding.
- Nasogastric feeding is reserved for children with CPAP or HHHFNC therapy. Nasogastric feeding is preferable to intravenous fluids for hydration unless contraindicated.
- Intravenous fluid is reserved for children who do not tolerate nasogastric feeding or in circumstances where nasogastric feeding is not possible.
- It is recommended to start hydration at two-thirds of maintenance due to the risk of SIADH (syndrome of inappropriate antidiuretic hormone secretion).

Weaning of Respiratory Support

- Target SpO_2 between 94 and 97%.
- Taper FiO_2 if $SpO_2 > 97\%$.
- Trial off supplemental nasal oxygen can be given every 6 hours to assess SpO_2.[5]
- If $SpO_2 < 92\%$ or work of breathing increases, restart supplemental oxygen.
- If a child is on HHHFNC/CPAP, titrate FiO_2 to maintain SpO_2 between 92 and 97%.
- Trial off HHHFNC to supplemental low-flow nasal oxygen can be given if FiO_2 <40% to maintain $SpO_2 > 92\%$.
- Restart HHHFNC/CPAP if there is a fall in $SpO_2 < 92\%$ or if there is an increase in work of breathing.

Indications for Pediatric Intensive Care Unit/High Dependency Unit Admission

- Requirement of supplemental oxygen with FiO_2 >50% to maintain SpO_2 >92%
- Requirement of HHHFNC/CPAP/NPPV
- Children with comorbidities with moderate bronchiolitis requiring supplemental oxygen
- Children with complications of viral infection—myocarditis, encephalopathy, hepatitis, cytokine storm, and acute kidney injury

Criteria for Discharge

- Normal respiratory rate and heart rate
- Room air SpO_2 >94%

- Adequate oral intake
- Absence of respiratory distress

Algorithmic Approach to Acute Viral Bronchiolitis

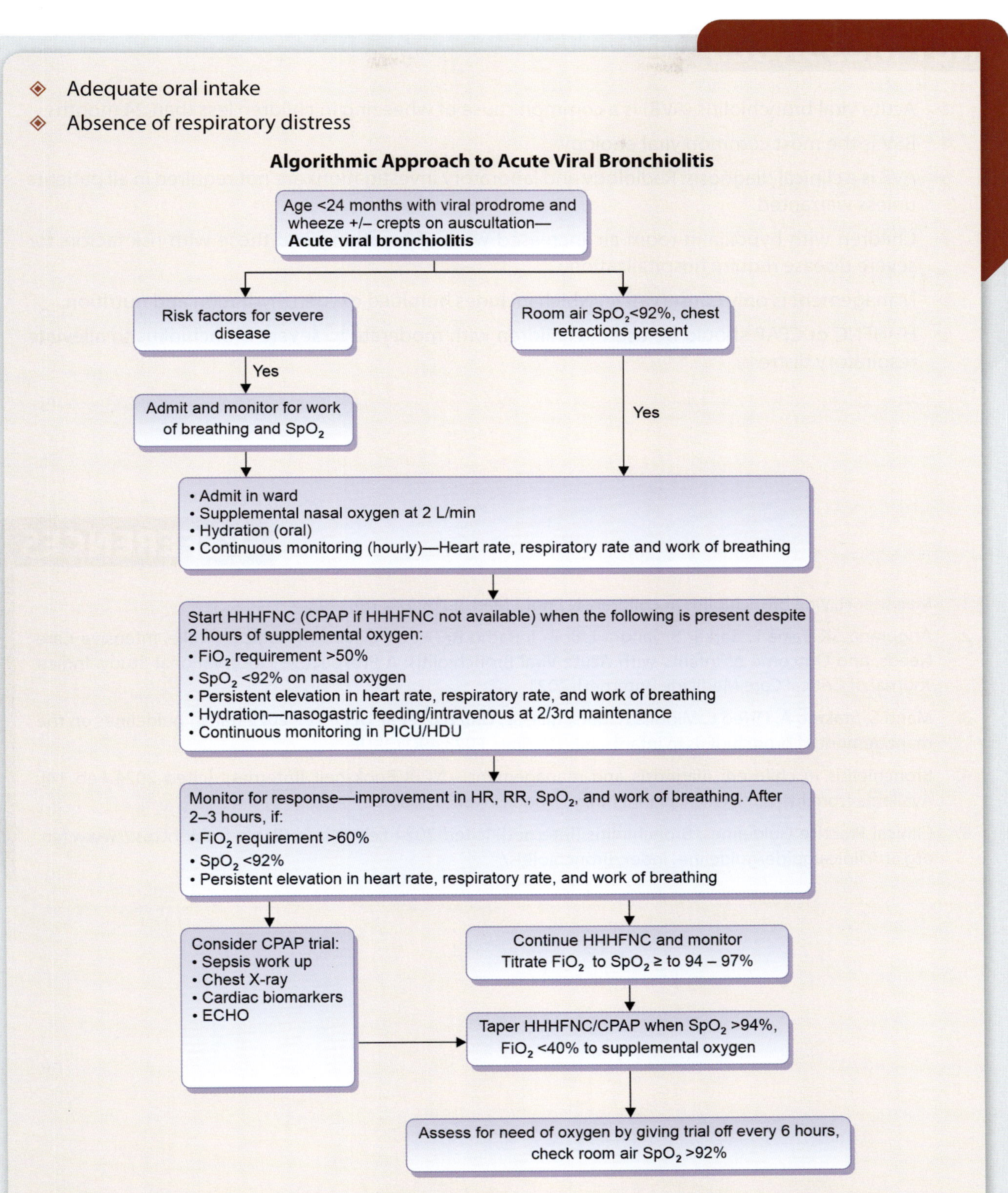

(CPAP: continuous positive airway pressure; HDU: high dependency unit; HHHFNC: heated humidified high-flow nasal cannula; HR: heart rate; PICU: pediatric intensive care unit; RR: respiratory rate)

KEY MESSAGES

- Acute viral bronchiolitis (AVB) is a common cause of wheezing in children less than 24 months.
- RSV is the most common viral etiology.
- AVB is a clinical diagnosis. Radiology and laboratory investigations are not required in all patients unless warranted.
- Children with hypoxia in room air, increased work of breathing and those with risk factors for severe disease require hospitalization.
- Management is only conservative, which includes humified oxygen, hydration and nutrition.
- HHHFNC or CPAP should be used in children with moderate to severe bronchiolitis to alleviate respiratory distress.

REFERENCES

1. Meissner H. Viral bronchiolitis in children. N Engl J Med. 2016;374(18):1793-4.
2. Angurana SK, Takia L, Sarkar S, Jangra I, Bora I, Ratho RK, et al. Clinico-virological Profile, Intensive Care Needs, and Outcome of Infants with Acute Viral Bronchiolitis: A Prospective Observational Study. Indian Journal of Critical Care Medicine [Internet]. 2021
3. Manti S, Staiano A, Orfeo L, Midulla F, Marseglia GL, Ghizzi C, et al. UPDATE - 2022 Italian guidelines on the management of bronchiolitis in infants. Ital J Pediatr. 2023;49(1):1-18.
4. Bronchiolitis in children: diagnosis and management - NCBI Bookshelf [Internet]. [cited 2024 Feb 14]. Available from:https://www.ncbi.nlm.nih.gov/books/NBK573086/
5. Clinical Practice Guidelines: Bronchiolitis [Internet]. [cited 2024 Feb 14]. Available from: https://www.rch.org.au/clinicalguide/guideline_index/Bronchiolitis/

12 Pneumonia in Children

Mullai Baalaaji AR

INTRODUCTION

Pneumonia refers to acute infection of lung parenchyma caused by a wide variety of viruses, bacteria, and other atypical organisms. It is a leading cause of morbidity and mortality in children and accounts for 22% of all deaths in children aged between 1 and 5 years.[1] Lower respiratory tract infection represents a broad variety of conditions, namely bronchitis, bronchiolitis, pneumonia, or a combination of the three.

COMMUNITY-ACQUIRED PNEUMONIA

Community-acquired pneumonia (CAP) is defined as a clinical diagnosis of pneumonia caused by a community-acquired pathogen in a previously healthy child **(Table 1)**.

TABLE 1: Etiologic agents for community-acquired pneumonia (CAP) in children.

Age	*Microbial agent*
1–3 months	• *Chlamydia trachomatis* • *Mycoplasma hominis* • *Ureaplasma urealyticum* • *Treponema pallidum* • *Streptococcus pneumoniae*
Children <5 years	• *Viruses:* Respiratory syncytial virus, influenza A and B, human metapneumovirus, parainfluenza viruses 1, 2, and 3, coronaviruses, adenovirus, rhinovirus, and bocavirus • *Streptococcus pneumoniae* • *Streptococcus pyogenes* • *Staphylococcus aureus*
Children ≥5 years	• Viruses • *Chlamydia pneumoniae* • *Mycoplasma pneumoniae*
Aspiration pneumonia	Anaerobic oral flora such as anaerobic streptococci (*Peptostreptococcus*), *Fusobacterium*, *Bacteroides*, and *Prevotella melaninogenica*

CLINICAL FEATURES

Clinical symptoms can be subtle, especially in infants and young children, who present with fever, feeding difficulty, and restlessness. Fever may be a sign of occult pneumonia in young children. Cough may not be an initial feature since alveoli have few cough receptors unlike airways and may appear later when there is airway irritation due to the alveolar exudates. Older children may complain of pleuritic chest pain or abdominal pain, due to referred pain from the lower lobes.

Tachypnea and signs of increased work of breathing are more specific for lower respiratory tract involvement. Presence of retractions, grunting, nasal flaring, and hypoxemia (oxygen saturations less than 94% in room air) are predictive of lower respiratory tract involvement. Lung auscultation would reveal the presence of crepitations, decreased breath sounds, and bronchial breath sounds over the involved lung fields. Wheeze may be present in atypical/viral pneumonia. Markedly diminished breath sounds and stony dullness to percussion indicate complications such as pleural effusion.

There may be findings in general systemic examination that may point toward the etiology such as conjunctivitis (*Chlamydia trachomatis* and adenovirus), impetigo (*Staphylococcus*), vesicles (varicella), postmeasles desquamation, and maculopapular rash (*Mycoplasma*) **(Table 2)**.

TABLE 2: Clinical clues to differentiate different etiological agents of pneumonia.

Viral etiology	*Bacterial etiology*	*Atypical bacterial etiology*
Usually, children <5 years	Children all ages	Most common in children >5 years
Upper respiratory symptoms/ signs	Abrupt onset and ill appearance	Abrupt onset and constitutional findings—malaise, rash, and conjunctivitis
Bilateral findings and wheeze	Focal auscultatory findings	Wheeze
Nontoxic appearance	Neutrophilia and elevated acute phase reactants	Extrapulmonary manifestations (rash and hepatitis)
Interstitial infiltrates, bronchiolitis, and hyperinflation	Lobar/segmental consolidation	Lobar/parahilar infiltrates, patchy reticulonodular infiltrates

INDICATIONS FOR HOSPITALIZATION

The need to hospitalize a child with CAP depends upon a variety of factors such as age, severity of illness, and underlying medical problems. The following criteria may be considered for hospitalization:[2]

- Infants younger than 3–6 months of age
- Inability to maintain hydration orally
- Increased work of breathing
- Hypoxemia
- Underlying conditions that predispose to severe course (e.g., immunocompromised host, cardiopulmonary disorders, neurological disorders, genetic syndromes)
- Complications of pneumonia (pleural effusion/empyema, necrotizing pneumonia, and lung abscess)
- Failure of outpatient treatment (no response/worsening) in 48–72 hours

DIAGNOSIS

Laboratory Evaluation

Community-acquired pneumonia is a clinical diagnosis and may not require any investigation in an outpatient setting. Complete blood count cannot reliably differentiate bacterial from viral etiologies. Neutropenia may be seen in severely ill patients or might indicate an underlying immunocompromised status. Acute phase reactants such as C-reactive protein (CRP) or procalcitonin may help to distinguish bacterial from viral etiologies when taken together with the clinical picture. A negative procalcitonin has a better predictive value to identify children at a lower risk for bacterial pneumonia.[3]

Serum electrolyte abnormalities, especially dysnatremias, are commonly observed and need monitoring. Dehydration and syndrome of inappropriate antidiuresis (SIAD) are the common reasons for sodium imbalances.

Chest radiograph is indicated in children who need hospitalization, those with risk factors, where diagnosis is unclear, and when we suspect complications due to pneumonia. Routine chest radiographs are not necessary in children who appear well enough to be treated on an outpatient basis and these are not sensitive enough to differentiate viral from bacterial etiologies.[4] Ultrasonogram (USG) chest is evolving as a bedside investigative modality to diagnose pneumonia and is comparable to radiograph with no radiation. Pleural-based pathologies such as effusion and empyema are better detected using USG.[5]

DIFFERENTIAL DIAGNOSIS

There are many noninfectious conditions that might mimic pneumonia in children **(Table 3)**.

TABLE 3: Differential diagnosis of pneumonia in children.

Conditions	*Examples*
Anatomical causes	• Pulmonary sequestration • Congenital lobar emphysema • Vascular rings • Bronchogenic cysts
Aspiration	• Neuromuscular disorders • Gastroesophageal reflux • Tracheoesophageal fistula
Chronic lung disorders	• Asthma • Cystic fibrosis • Bronchiectasis • Bronchopulmonary dysplasia • Primary ciliary dyskinesia • Alpha-1 antitrypsin deficiency • Pulmonary hemosiderosis

Contd...

Contd...

Conditions	*Examples*
Cardiac disorders	• Congestive cardiac failure due to structural heart diseases • Myocarditis
Others	• Foreign body aspiration • Mucus plugging and atelectasis • Inhalation lung injury (smoke) • Chemical pneumonitis (hydrocarbon) • Lipoid pneumonia • Graft versus host disease

EMERGENCY CARE

Presence of red flag signs such as inability to drink, persistent vomiting, lethargy, altered consciousness, and stridor would indicate a severe disease. According to pediatric advanced life support (PALS) guidelines, respiratory rate, work of breathing, cyanosis, level of consciousness, and oxygen saturations are used to categorize children into various severity groups at presentation **(Table 4)**.

TABLE 4: Clinical findings to categorize severity of illness.

Clinical parameter	*Mild illness*	*Severe illness*
Respiratory rate (RR)	Normal-to-mild tachypnea	Tachypnea (RR > 70/min for infants, RR > 50/min for older children), and bradypnea
Work of breathing	Mild or no retractions	Moderate/severe retractions, grunting, and nasal flaring
Color	Normal	Cyanosis
SpO_2	Normal	Hypoxemia
Sensorium	Normal	Altered
Feeding	Normal	Not feeding or vomiting, and signs of dehydration
Heart rate	Normal	Tachycardia
Capillary refill	<2 seconds	≥2 seconds

SUPPORTIVE CARE

Supportive care includes fluid therapy, respiratory support, chest physiotherapy, and adjunctive medications:

- *Fluid therapy:* Inability to drink/feed and vomiting could result in dehydration. Children who are not able to feed enterally due to risk of aspiration and respiratory fatigue require intravenous fluids. Isotonic fluids are recommended, and monitoring of electrolytes is warranted.
- *Respiratory support:* Children who are hypoxemic and in respiratory distress need supplemental oxygen to maintain oxygen saturation ≥94%. Children with significant tachypnea and increased work of breathing would need initiation of respiratory support in the form of high-flow nasal cannula (HFNC) or continuous positive airway pressure (CPAP). Close monitoring is essential to identify failure of noninvasive support and appropriate timely escalation to invasive ventilation.
- *Chest physiotherapy:* It is not beneficial in children with CAP and is not recommended in routine uncomplicated patients. It has a role in persistent lung collapse and in conditions such as cystic fibrosis.
- *Adjunctive steroids:* Steroids have shown to be harmful, resulting in treatment failure, and hence not recommended in childhood CAP.

INDICATIONS FOR PEDIATRIC INTENSIVE CARE UNIT TRANSFER

- Increased work of breathing and tachypnea [respiratory rate (RR) >70/min for infants and RR >50/min for older children]
- Signs of impending respiratory failure such as bradypnea/apnea or irregular respirations, altered mental status, and respiratory fatigue
- Shock/hypotension
- Need for ventilatory support—noninvasive, invasive, failure to maintain blood oxygen saturation (SpO_2) >92% with fraction of inspired oxygen (FiO_2) >50%
- *Comorbidities:* Malnutrition, immunocompromised such as nephrotic syndrome, malignancies, immunodeficiency disorders, etc.
- Worsening oxygenation parameters (arterial partial pressure of oxygen:inspired oxygen fraction <250)

SPECIFIC THERAPY

Empiric antimicrobial therapy is determined by the age of the child, suspected pathogens and their antimicrobial susceptibility, and severity of involvement. **Tables 5** and **6** give broad guidelines on the empirical treatment in children. It is a common practice to switch from parenteral therapy to oral therapy once the child is afebrile for 24–48 hours and has no emesis. A total treatment duration of 5–7 days is effective in uncomplicated cases. In children with complications such as empyema, treatment duration is determined by the clinical response. Generally, prolonged therapy for 3–4 weeks is usually practiced.[3,6]

TABLE 5: Empirical antimicrobial therapy for inpatient treatment of pneumonia in children.

Age group and pathogens	*Antimicrobial agent*	*Comments*
	1–3 months	
Bacterial	Cefotaxime/Ceftriaxone	Add vancomycin when *Staphylococcus aureus* is suspected
Chlamydia trachomatis	Azithromycin	
	3 months–5 years	
Bacterial	Ampicillin/Amoxicillin–Clavulanate/Cefotaxime/Ceftriaxone	Children unimmunized/incompletely immunized against *Streptococcus pneumoniae* should receive Cefotaxime/Ceftriaxone
Mycoplasma pneumoniae or *Chlamydia pneumoniae*	Azithromycin/Erythromycin/Levofloxacin	
	>5 years	
Bacterial/Atypical bacterial	Ampicillin/Amoxicillin–Clavulanate/Cefotaxime/Ceftriaxone/Azithromycin	
	Any age	
Complicated pneumonia (effusion/empyema/necrotizing pneumonia/lung abscess)	Ceftriaxone/Cefotaxime + Clindamycin/Vancomycin	
Severe pneumonia requiring PICU admission	Ceftriaxone/Cefotaxime + Vancomycin	*Antiviral:* Oseltamivir during influenza season

(PICU: pediatric intensive care unit)

TABLE 6: Empirical antimicrobial therapy for outpatient treatment of pneumonia in children.

Age group	*Antimicrobial agent*
<3 months	Needs hospitalization
3 months to 5 years, typical bacterial	High-dose Amoxicillin or Amoxicillin–Clavulanate or Cefpodoxime/Cefuroxime
≥5 years, typical bacterial	High-dose Amoxicillin or Amoxicillin–Clavulanate
≥5 years, *Mycoplasma pneumoniae* or *Chlamydia pneumoniae*	Azithromycin/ Clarithromycin/ Levofloxacin/Doxycycline
≥5 years, aspiration pneumonia	Amoxicillin–Clavulanate

FOLLOW-UP

Clinical recovery is marked by resolution of fever, toxic appearance, work of breathing, and hypoxemia. Cough may persist for several weeks, following viral pneumonia or pertussis.[7] Follow-up radiographs are usually not necessary in asymptomatic children. X-ray chest may be helpful when there are diagnostic dilemmas or when there are coincident conditions in children with recurrent pneumonia or persistent symptoms.

KEY LEARNING POINTS

- Pneumonia is a common reason for hospitalization in children.
- Clinical features help to categorize the severity of illness at presentation and should be used to decide on need for hospitalization and PICU transfer.
- No laboratory investigation is needed to diagnose pneumonia in outpatient setting.
- Empirical therapy depends on age of child, immunization status, and suspected etiologies.

REFERENCES

1. World Health Organization, (2022). Pneumonia in children. [online] Available from https://www.who.int/news-room/fact-sheets/detail/pneumonia [Last accessed February, 2024].
2. Bradley JS, Byington CL, Shah SS, Alverson B, Carter ER, Harrison C, et al. The management of community-acquired pneumonia in infants and children older than 3 months of age: Clinical practice guidelines by the Pediatric Infectious Diseases Society and the Infectious Diseases Society of America. Clin Infect Dis. 2011;53(7):e25-76.
3. Harris M, Clark J, Coote N, Fletcher P, Harnden A, McKean M, et al. British Thoracic Society guidelines for the management of community acquired pneumonia in children: Update 2011. Thorax. 2011;66(Suppl 2):ii1-23.
4. Andronikou S, Lambert E, Halton J, Hilder L, Crumley I, Lyttle MD, et al. Guidelines for the use of chest radiographs in community-acquired pneumonia in children and adolescents. Pediatr Radiol. 2017;47(11): 1405-11.
5. Orso D, Guglielmo N, Copetti R. Lung ultrasound in diagnosing pneumonia in the emergency department: A systematic review and meta-analysis. Eur J Emerg Med. 2018;25(5):312-21.
6. World Health Organization. (2014). Revised WHO classification and treatment of childhood pneumonia at health facilities. Evidence Summaries. Available from https://iris.who.int/bitstream/handle/10665/137319/9789241507813_eng.pdf?sequence=1 [Last accessed February, 2024].
7. Gaston B. Pneumonia. Pediatric Rev 2002;23(4):132-40.

13 Pertussis

Kavitha TK, Krishna Mohan R

INTRODUCTION

Pertussis (whooping cough) cases have been reported from various parts of the globe lately. Reemergence of this vaccine-preventable disease is a global concern because of its high morbidity and mortality, especially among infants. Infantile age group has predilection for severe forms of the disease like critical pertussis or malignant pertussis. Disease transmission in the community is attributed to weaning vaccine immunity among adolescents and adults. In 2014, global data showed 24.1 million pertussis cases and 160,700 deaths in <5 years of age. India reported 46706 pertussis cases in 2014. Pertussis outbreaks occur periodically in every 3–5 years, and in 2022 India reported only 4362 cases.

DEFINITION

For surveillance purpose, the Centers for Disease Control and Prevention (CDC) recommends pertussis case definition as confirmed or probable based on the criteria given in **Box 1**.

BOX 1: Criteria to determine a pertussis case for surveillance.

Clinical criteria: In the absence of an alternative diagnosis, cough illness lasting ≥2 weeks, at least one of the following:
- Paroxysms of coughing, *or*
- Inspiratory whoop, *or*
- Post-tussive vomiting, *or*
- Apnea (with or without cyanosis)

Laboratory criteria:
- *Bordetella pertussis* isolation from clinical specimen
- Positive polymerase chain reaction (PCR) for *Bordetella pertussis*

Confirmed Pertussis Case

Any cough illness of any duration with isolation of *Bordetella* from clinical specimen or positive polymerase chain reaction (PCR) for *Bordetella*

Probable Pertussis Case

- Any case meeting the clinical criteria in the absence of an alternative diagnosis
- Any cough illness of any duration with least 1 symptom or sign of clinical criteria and contact with a laboratory confirmed case

Critical Pertussis

It refers to pertussis cases requiring intensive care unit admissions and/or resulting in death.

Malignant Pertussis

It is a severe form of pertussis resulting in acute respiratory distress syndrome, severe pulmonary artery hypertension (PAH), or multiorgan failure.

ETIOPATHOGENESIS

The causative agent is a gram-negative bacterium, *Bordetella pertussis*, and in minority of cases *Bordetella parapertussis*. The mode of infection is aerosols through which bacteria invade ciliated epithelium of the respiratory tract. Bacterial toxins induce inflammation of the respiratory tract and extrapulmonary systemic effects. Various virulence factors have been identified which include filamentous hemagglutinin (*Fha*), fimbria (*Fim*), and adenylate cyclase toxin (*Act*). Fim and Fha are adherence factors. Local immunosuppression by Fha aids in reducing host response to initial infection leading to persistence of bacteria in the respiratory tract. Adenylate cyclase toxin (Act or Cya-A) has antiphagocytic and neutrophil oxidative burst inhibition actions, which help bacteria to escape the host defense. The pathogenesis of the disease is mainly toxin mediated. Major toxins are pertussis toxin (Ptx), tracheal cytotoxin (TCT), and adenylate cyclase toxin-hemolysin. Ptx helps in bacterial colonization by immunomodulatory effect and mediates leukocytosis which is a major predictor of mortality. It also affects cardiac function and has shown to cause PAH in mouse models. Ptx has a proinflammatory effect on the respiratory tract. In an infant, Ptx is known to cause the lethal infection predominantly due to its extrapulmonary effects. Act, another immunomodulatory agent along with promoting bacterial colonization, induces apoptosis of bronchial and pulmonary cells adding to respiratory dysfunction. TCT induces nitric oxide production and cell death. It also promotes IL-1α-mediated inflammation in the respiratory system and immunosuppression in the host by preventing neutrophil chemotaxis. Ptx-induced leukocytosis and systemic inflammation lead to stasis in microcirculation and organ damage, ensuing PAH, cerebral infarcts, and other systemic features.

CLINICAL FEATURES

The incubation period is usually 7–10 days and it ranges from 4 days to 3 weeks. Pertussis classically presents with three stages: Initial catarrhal phase, followed by paroxysmal phase and convalescence.

The *catarrhal phase* may last for 1–2 weeks where it presents similar to any respiratory tract infection with symptoms of mild fever, runny nose, or conjunctival injection. At the end of this phase, patients would develop cough which gradually might increase in severity.

It proceeds to *paroxysmal phase* in which the patient develops paroxysms of repeated coughing bouts with increasing intensity which might end in classical whooping (prolonged inspiratory efforts with difficulty in drawing air inside resulting in whoop sound). The paroxysmal phase may last for 1–6 weeks. This phase also results in post-tussive vomiting, apnea, or cyanosis during paroxysmal cough bouts. Infants may present only with apnea. Paroxysms of cough may increase in the first 2 weeks of paroxysmal stage and remain in the same intensity for 1–3 weeks and then gradually improves.

The disease then moves to the *convalescent phase* where paroxysmal cough improves to nonparoxysmal cough and might take weeks or months to resolve fully.

In infants, the disease takes a lethal course. Critical pertussis is seen predominantly in < 3 months of age, with a median age of 45 days to 3.5 months. It affects infants even before completion of their primary vaccination series making them much vulnerable to disease. Lower maternal antibodies and their transfer are another reason for susceptibility. Mothers and siblings are the usual source of infection.

Critical pertussis often presents with rapid breathing, typical paroxysmal cough, or apnea. Fever is a less common symptom. Encephalopathy and seizures are also other common presentations. Most of the cases may present with hypoxemia at admission. The disease can progress to developing refractory hypoxemia, PAH, cerebral infarcts, acute kidney injury, and shock. The mortality rate in critical pertussis ranges from 4.8 to 34%. Female gender, hyperleukocytosis, PAH, need for vasoactive support, and encephalopathy are predictors of mortality.

INVESTIGATIONS

Laboratory evaluation would show hyperleukocytosis or thrombocytosis. In patients with hyperleukocytosis, the total leukocyte count ranges from 27,000 to 64,000, although higher counts more than 1 lakhs are also reported in few cases. For laboratory confirmation, nasopharyngeal swab or aspirate can be sent for pertussis PCR. Dry nasopharyngeal swab is preferred for PCR in view of potential contamination during handling of liquid medium. Culture of nasopharyngeal swab or aspirate for *B. pertussis* is considered to be gold standard, but it has poor sensitivity. In vaccinated children, IgM response to infection is very negligible; hence, serological testing for IgG antibody against specific pertussis antigen is regarded as another sensitive marker for pertussis diagnosis. IgA elevation is less seen after vaccination; hence, it is also used to differentiate recent infection and recent vaccination.

MANAGEMENT

Management strategies focusses on initial stabilization, early initiation of macrolide antibiotics, leukodepletion measures, and organ support measures.

- *Initial stabilization:* At admission, all children with pertussis should undergo airway stabilization, initiation of oxygen support as per scenario, hemodynamic stabilization, and proper hydration initiation.
- Early initiation of macrolide antibiotics in the catarrhal phase would clear the bacteria from the airways and might reduce the disease severity. The preferred agent in children >1 month of age is erythromycin 40–50 mg/kg/day in four divided doses for 14 days. Alternative agents are azithromycin 10 mg/kg/day for 5 days in all age groups or clarithromycin 15 mg/kg/day in two divided doses for 7 days in infants and children more than 1 month of age. In possible macrolide allergy, sulfamethoxazole–trimethoprim combination may be tried.
- Hyperleukocytosis increases mortality risk in critical pertussis. It can be managed with hyperhydration and leukodepletion measures which include leukocytapheresis or exchange transfusion. Exchange transfusion in pertussis-related hyperleukocytosis has been found to have mortality benefit in few case series. Hydroxyurea was successfully tried in hyperleukocytosis in pertussis in one to two case reports.
- Since hypoxemic respiratory failure is a common complication, oxygen support in the form of nasal prongs or high-flow nasal cannula (HFNC) in mild cases and noninvasive ventilation or advanced mechanical ventilation in severe cases are the most common intensive care needs. Infants may develop refractive hypoxemia complicated by PAH.
- Vasoactive support and renal replacement therapy for acute kidney injury should be started as per requirement on a case-to-case basis.
- The extracorporeal membrane oxygenation (ECMO) trial in critical pertussis has showed only marginal survival benefits with 26% survival.
- In PAH, leukodepletion or ECMO might help marginally.

PREVENTION

Pentavalent vaccination which includes DPT (diphtheria, pertussis, tetanus) at 6, 10, 14 weeks and booster doses at 16–24 months and 5–6 years of age are recommended by the national immunization schedule. Maternal Tdap (tetanus, diphtheria, and acellular pertussis) has been found to reduce infantile pertussis in various countries. Weaning immunity in adolescents helps in disease persistence in community. The IAP ACIP (Indian Academy of Pediatrics (IAP) Advisory Committee on Vaccines and Immunization Practices) recommends additional TdaP for adolescents 10–12 years of age and pregnant women 27–36 weeks of gestation.

CONCLUSION

Pertussis is reemerging in various countries. Critical pertussis or malignant pertussis is lethal, especially in infants. Initiation of macrolide antibiotics, adequate organ support measures and tackling of hyperleukocytosis are the cornerstones of pertussis management. Macrolides and organ support leukodepletion measures are the cornerstones in disease treatment. High susceptibility and subsequent mortality in infants can be reduced by Tdap vaccination in pregnancy and single booster dose in adolescents.

SUGGESTED READING

1. Berger JT, Carcillo JA, Shanley TP, Wessel DL, Clark A, Holubkov R, et al. Critical pertussis illness in children: a multicenter prospective cohort study. Pediatr Crit Care Med. 2013;14(4):356-65.
2. Brousseau N, Skowronski DM, Bellemare D, Amini R, Joffres Y, Clarke Q, et al. Impact of the adolescent pertussis booster dose on the incidence of pertussis in British Columbia and Quebec, Canada. Vaccine. 2020;38:427-32.
3. Carbonetti NH. Bordetella pertussis: new concepts in pathogenesis and treatment. Curr Opin Infect Dis. 2016;29:287-94.
4. Carrasquilla G, Porras A, Martinez S, DeAntonio R, Devadiga R, Caceres DC, et al. Incidence and mortality of pertussis disease in infants <12 months of age following introduction of pertussis maternal universal mass vaccination in Bogotá, Colombia. Vaccine. 2020;38:7384-92.
5. Domico M, Ridout D, MacLaren G, Barbaro R, Annich G, Schlapbach LJ, et al. Extracorporeal membrane oxygenation for pertussis: Predictors of outcome including pulmonary hypertension and leukodepletion. Pediatr Crit Care Med. 2018;19:254-61.
6. Jackson DW, Rohani P. Perplexities of pertussis: recent global epidemiological trends and their potential causes. Epidemiol Infect. 2014;142:672-84.
7. Kasi SG, Shivananda S, Marathe S, Chatterjee K, Agarwalla S, Dhir SK, et al. Indian Academy of Pediatrics (IAP) Advisory Committee on Vaccines and Immunization Practices (ACVIP): Recommended Immunization Schedule (2020-21) and Update on Immunization for Children Aged 0 Through 18 Years. Indian Pediatr. 2021;58(1):44-53.
8. Kavitha TK, Samprathi M, Jayashree M, Gautam V, Sangal L. Clinical profile of critical pertussis in children at a pediatric intensive care unit in Northern India. Indian Pediatr. 2020;57:228-31.
9. Kazantzi MS, Prezerakou A, Kalamitsou SN, Ilia S, Kalabalikis PK, Papadatos J, et al. Characteristics of Bordetella pertussis infection among infants and children admitted to paediatric intensive care units in Greece: A multicentre, 11-year study. J Paediatr Child Health. 2017;53(3):25762.
10. Maitre G, Schaffner D, Natterer J, Longchamp D, Ferry T, Diezi M, et al. Leukemoid reaction in infant pertussis: Is there a place for hydroxyurea? A case report. Front Pediatr. 2018;6:261.
11. Nunes A, Abreu A, Furtado B, Soares da Silva A, Coelho EB, de Barros EN. Epidemiology of pertussis among adolescents, adults, and older adults in selected countries of Latin American: a systematic review. Human Vaccines Immunother. 2021;17:1733-46.
12. Son PT, Reda A, Viet DC, Quynh NXT, Hung DT, Tung TH, et al. Exchange transfusion in the management of critical pertussis in young infants: a case series. Vox Sang. 2021;116(9):976-82.

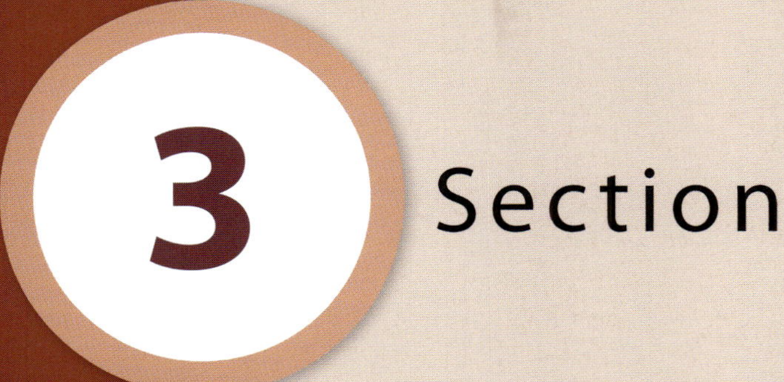

Cardiovascular System

14 Heart Failure

Bharat Choudhary, Ashwini Chityala

INTRODUCTION

Pediatric heart failure is associated with considerable morbidity, mortality, and financial burden. Therefore, early recognition in emergency settings is important to prevent mortality.[1] Heart failure results from structural or functional cardiac conditions that hamper the ability of ventricles to fill with and/or to eject the blood.

TERMINOLOGIES AND DEFINITIONS

Heart failure, a syndrome with clinical and pathophysiological implications, occurs when the heart is unable to meet the metabolic demands of the body. It leads to respiratory distress, feeding issues, and poor growth along with circulatory, neurohormonal, and molecular abnormalities.[2]

ETIOPATHOLOGY

The etiology of heart failure is physiologically categorized, which aids in comprehending the underlying pathology and clinical presentations, thereby directing management strategies. The cardiac causes of ventricular dysfunction in children are divided into structurally normal heart with ventricular dysfunction and congenital heart disease with ventricular dysfunction **(Flowchart 1)**.[3,4]

Flowchart 1: Categorization based on physiology.

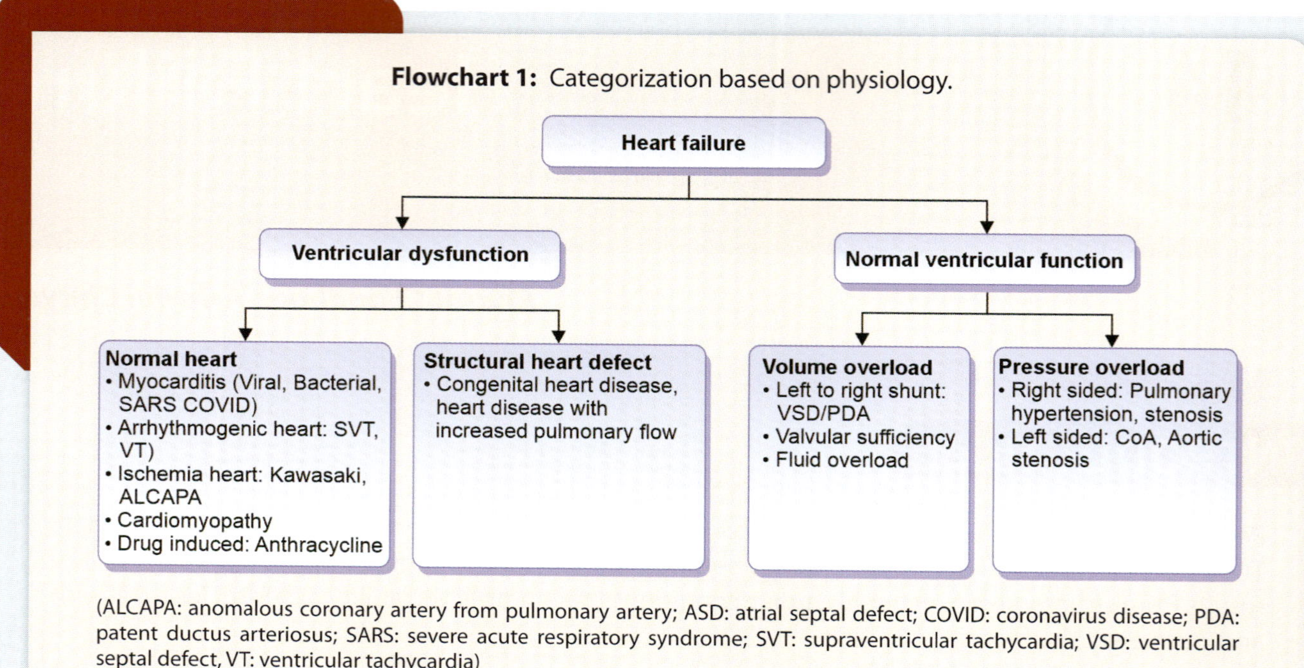

(ALCAPA: anomalous coronary artery from pulmonary artery; ASD: atrial septal defect; COVID: coronavirus disease; PDA: patent ductus arteriosus; SARS: severe acute respiratory syndrome; SVT: supraventricular tachycardia; VSD: ventricular septal defect, VT: ventricular tachycardia)

Clinical Features

Symptoms and signs arise due to reduced cardiac output and/or fluid overload. It may also vary with the age.

- *Infants*: The most common presentation is tachypnea, irritability, and feeding difficulty which ranges from prolonged feeding (>20 minutes), feeding diaphoresis (suggestive of effort intolerance), and failure to thrive.
- *Children:* They may present with easy fatigability, cough, dyspnea and syncope, chest pain, and abdominal complaints.

EVALUATION

History

Careful history of abovementioned symptoms should be taken. In addition, for ruling of a specific underlying cause, history of fever, rash, joint pain, abnormal movement (acute rheumatic fever/ rheumatic heart disease), scorpion sting, and poisoning/ingestion (aluminum phosphide) should be asked.

Physical Examination

Children may have tachypnea, disproportionate tachycardia, and poor perfusion with or without gallop rhythm on auscultation. Underlying congenital heart disease or valvular disease may have disease-specific murmurs. They also show signs of systemic congestion like raised jugular venous pressure (JVP), edema, hepatomegaly, ascites, and basal crepitations in lungs. Severity of the heart failure can be assessed as per modified Ross classification **(Table 1)**. Investigations include point-of-care tests and specific tests as mentioned in **Table 2**.

TABLE 1: Modified Ross heart failure classification for children.[3]

Class I	Asymptomatic
Class II	Mild tachypnea or diaphoresis with feeding in infants, dyspnea on exertion in older children
Class III	Marked tachypnea or diaphoresis with feeding in infants, with marked dyspnea on exertion, prolonged feeding with growth failure
Class IV	Symptoms such as tachypnea, retractions, grunting, or diaphoresis at rest

TABLE 2: Diagnostic evaluation of children with heart failure in emergency.

Tests	*Findings*
Blood gas	Hypercapnia, hypoxia, lactic acidosis, electrolytes
CBC	Anemia, evidence of infection
ECG	Arrythmia, myocarditis, specific conditions like ALCAPA, ARF
Chest X-ray	Cardiomegaly, pulmonary plethora, specific heart shapes of CHD
CRP/PCT	Sepsis, ARF, KD
ESR	ARF, KD
KFT	AKI, CKD
LFT	Congestive hepatopathy
Cardiac markers	Evidence of myocarditis, heart failure (troponin I, CKMB, pro-BNP)
Point-of-care ultrasound (POCUS)	Evidence of fluid overload: Confluent B lines, distended IVC, cardiac contractility (ejection fraction and cardiac index)
Echocardiogram	Definitive CHD diagnosis

(AKI: acute kidney injury; ALCAPA: anomalous left coronary artery from pulmonary artery; ARF: acute rheumatic fever; CBC: complete hemogram; CHD: congenital heart disease; ECG: electrocardiogram; IVC: inferior vena cava; KD: Kawasaki disease)

DIFFERENTIALS

As respiratory distress is a common presenting symptom of heart failure in children in an emergency, other conditions that are more common which have similar presentation create dilemmas for clinicians. These are bronchiolitis, pneumonia, and other fluid overload conditions such as severe anemia, and renal and hepatic failure patients. Careful history, examination, and relevant point-of-care tests help in differentiating the cause of respiratory distress.

MANAGEMENT IN THE EMERGENCY ROOM[5]

The key goals of managing heart failure in the emergency room are to stabilize the patient, identify the cause, assess the severity, and implement appropriate interventions to optimize the heart function, reduce the complications, and improve the quality of life **(Flowchart 2)**.

Airway, Breathing, Circulation (ABC) Stabilization

In children with heart failure, the airway should be stabilized promptly and oxygen should be supplemented in case children have respiratory failure. If there is no improvement by general measures, intubation and positive-pressure ventilation may be required. Postintubation, higher positive end-expiratory pressure (PEEP) is helpful to decongest the alveoli and decrease the afterload and improve the cardiac output.[6] Children may require frequent airway clearance through suctioning in case of frank pulmonary edema.

These children may be in shock at presentation. In case of feeble pulses, a small aliquot bolus of 5–10 mL/kg can be given slowly over 1 hour to restore the perfusion, but a large amount and rapid bolus should be avoided. POCUS (Point-of-Care Ultrasound) should be utilized to guide further fluid therapy and ionotropic support. If cardiac contractility is poor on POCUS, early inotropes (dobutamine/adrenaline/milrinone) help in improving the perfusion. Beta-blockers should be avoided in children with decompensated heart failure.[7]

If the patient is not in shock and cardiac contractility is good, then diuretics are used to decongest the accumulated fluids and maintenance fluids should be restricted to 50–60%.[4]

General Measures

Fluid and Electrolyte Management

Most of these children have fluid overload or are at risk of fluid overload. Fluid restriction goals should be individualized based on age, severity of heart failure, urine output, amount of fluid overload, and response to treatment which can be guided using POCUS. The potassium level should be carefully monitored (target 4–5 mEq/L) as both hypokalemia and hyperkalemia have adverse effects on the failing heart.

Flowchart 2: Approach to heart failure management in emergency.

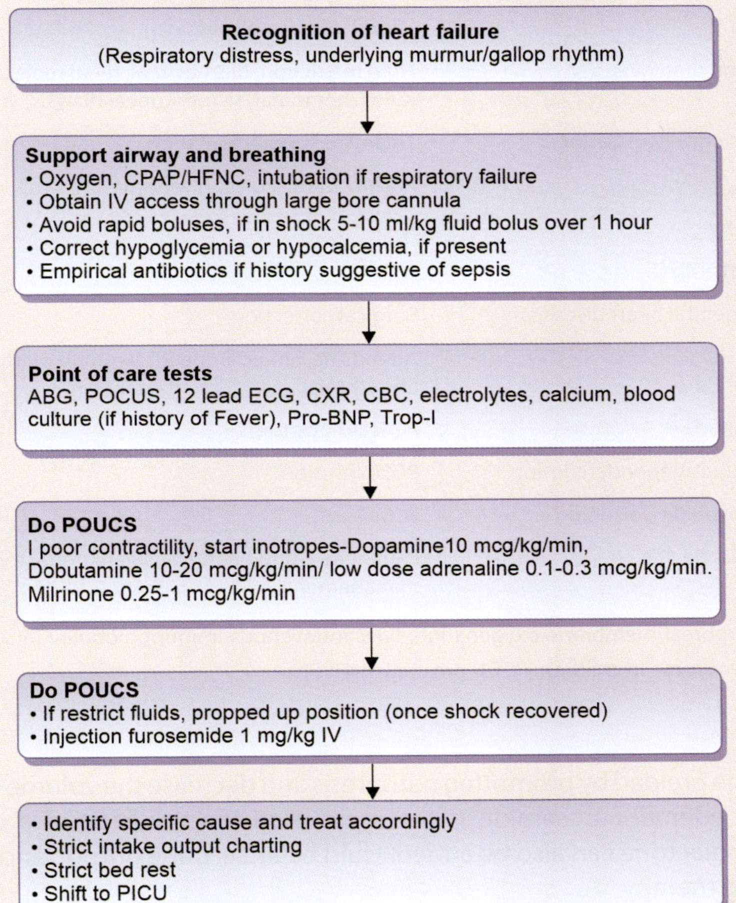

(ABG: arterial blood gas; BNP: brain natriuretic peptide; CPAP: continuous positive airway pressure; CXR: chest X-ray; HFNC: high-flow nasal cannula; PICU: pediatric intensive care unit)

Specific Treatment

Heart failure in children may be due to underlying secondary causes. Addressing and treating the reversible causes help clinicians halt or even reverse the progression of disease, thereby improving the outcome **(Table 3)**.

TABLE 3: Secondary causes of heart failure and their treatment.

Secondary causes of heart failure	*Specific treatment*
Hypertensive emergency	Control of hypertension (Labetalol or sodium nitroprusside infusion)
Severe anemia	Packed RBC (small aliquots)
Renal failure and fluid overload	Fluid restriction, diuretic trial, renal replacement therapy (CRRT/hemodialysis/peritoneal dialysis)
Thiamine deficiency (wet beriberi)	Thiamine supplementation
Scorpion sting	Prazosin, antiscorpion venom
Kawasaki disease	IVIG
Viral myocarditis/MISC	IVIG
Structural congenital heart diseases	Surgical correction
Arrhythmias	Adenosine, amiodarone (depending on the type of arrhythmia)
Cardiac tamponade	Pericardiocentesis
Neonate with duct-dependent lesion	PGE1 infusion
Aluminum phosphide poisoning	ECMO
Ventricular assist device	Patient awaiting heart transplant, refractory to medical management[8]

(ECMO: extracorporeal membrane oxygenation; IVIG: intravenous immunoglobulin; MISC: multisystem inflammatory syndrome in children; PGE1: prostaglandin E)

Diuretics

Diuretics decrease the preload by promoting natriuresis and decrease the volume overload symptoms such as pulmonary edema. Furosemide is the most used loop diuretic at a dose of 1–2 mg/kg q6–12 hourly. Spironolactone can also be added. Fluid balance, urine output, and electrolytes should be monitored during therapy.

Angiotensin-converting Enzyme Inhibitors

Heart failure leads to activation of the renin–angiotensin–aldosterone system and increased sympathetic tone. Enalapril at a dose of 0.1–0.5 mg/kg/day in three divided doses can be used. Side effects like cough and renal failure should be monitored.

MONITORING

All children with heart failure require close continuous monitoring to assess improvement or worsening following treatment and for timely intervention.

- Heart rate and rhythm should be continuously monitored as this child is at risk of arrhythmia. Improvement in heart rate indicates a response to treatment, whereas persistent/worsening tachycardia indicates a failure to the given treatment and indicates further assessment.
- Signs of perfusion like capillary refilling time (CRT) and pulse volume for monitoring of shock
- *Clinical:* JVP, bilateral crepitation, and hepatomegaly
- Strict intake–output charting for fluid balance
- Electrolytes monitoring every 6–12 hourly (sodium and potassium monitoring)
- POCUS for inferior vena cava (IVC) diameter and cardiac contractility

KEY LEARNING POINTS

- In all children, especially infants presenting with respiratory distress in the emergency room, heart failure should be suspected and ruled out.
- Heart failure may present with or without a murmur.
- Airway, Breathing, Circulation, and Disability (ABCD) stabilization is a priority in children with heart failure.
- POCUS is an important tool in the management of heart failure in an emergency.
- Strict fluid charting and electrolyte monitoring are required.
- Secondary causes should be identified and treated.

REFERENCES

1. Mejia EJ, O'Connor MJ, Lin KY, Song L, Griffis H, Mascio CE, et al. Characteristics and Outcomes of Pediatric Heart Failure-Related Emergency Department Visits in the United States: A Population-Based Study. J Pediatr. 2018;193:114-8.e3.
2. Kirk R, Dipchand AI, Rosenthal DN, Addonizio L, Burch M, Chrisant M, et al. The International Society for Heart and Lung Transplantation Guidelines for the management of pediatric heart failure: Executive summary. J Heart Lung Transplant. 2014;33:888-909.
3. Hsu DT, Pearson GD. Heart failure in children: part I: history, etiology, and pathophysiology. Circ Heart Fail. 2009;2(1):63-70.
4. Hsu DT, Pearson GD. Heart failure in children: part II: diagnosis, treatment, and future directions. Circ Heart Fail. 2009;2:490.
5. Masarone D, Valente F, Rubino M, Vastarella R, Gravino R, Rea A, et al. Pediatric Heart Failure: A Practical Guide to Diagnosis and Management. Pediatr Neonatol. 2017;58:303-12.
6. Kovacikova L, Skrak P, Dobos D, Zahorec M. Noninvasive positive pressure ventilation in critically ill children with cardiac disease. Pediatr Cardiol. 2014;35:676.
7. Frobel AK, Hulpke-Wette M, Schmidt KG, Läer S. Beta-blockers for congestive heart failure in children. Cochrane Database Syst Rev. 2009(1):CD007037.
8. Adachi I, Khan MS, Guzmán-Pruneda FA, Fraser 3rd CD, Mery CM, et al. Evolution and impact of ventricular assist device program on children awaiting heart transplantation. Ann Thorac Surg. 2015;99:635.

Arrhythmias

Kaustabh Chaudhuri, Debdatta Mukhopadhyay

INTRODUCTION

Arrhythmias are relatively common in pediatric ER, PICU, and pediatric cardiac ICUs. Prompt diagnosis and appropriate early management can potentially prevent life-threatening events.

CLASSIFICATION

Arrhythmias can be classified into the following:

- *Primary arrhythmias:*
  - With or without structural heart disease or in channelopathies
  - Without secondary causes
- *Secondary arrhythmias:*
  - Electrolyte and acid–base imbalance
  - Vasoactive drugs
  - Postcardiac surgical repair and long cardiopulmonary bypass times
  - Inflammation/carditis seen in myocarditis, Kawasaki disease, and rheumatic fever
  - Ventricular volume overloading, valvular regurgitation, and congestive heart failure
  - Pulmonary hypertension

CLINICAL ASSESSMENT

- *History:*
  - Family history of heart disease, death at a young age, sudden death, history of syncope, palpitations, seizures, exercise intolerance, and feeding intolerance
  - Past history of any diagnostic investigations, previous surgical repair, and postsurgical anatomy.
  - It is important to inquire about events preceding rhythm disturbance.
- *On examination:* Nonspecific features like irritability, feeding intolerance, sudden pallor, sweating, respiratory distress, tachycardia/bradycardia for age, irregular heart rate/pulse, prolonged capillary refill time, lethargy, congestive heart failure, syncope, and absent pulses/cardiac arrest.
- *Heart rate and rhythm:* Sinus tachycardia is the most frequently seen arrhythmia, with supraventricular tachycardia (SVT) being the next most common, followed by sinus bradycardia.
- *Cardiac assessment* includes auscultation of heart sounds for murmurs, any abnormal heart sounds, abnormal blood pressure, and assessment of vital signs including pulse oximetry is essential.
- *Cardiac surgeries* that involve the conduction tissue around the membranous septum and atrioventricular (AV) node such as repair of ventricular septal defect (VSD) and atrioventricular septal defects (AVSD) can be at increased risk of junctional ectopic tachycardia (JET), and heart block. VSD closure and intracardiac repair (ICR) for tetralogy of Fallot are at increased risk of ventricular arrhythmias.
- Arrhythmias in the early *postoperative period* like premature atrial contractions (PACs) and premature ventricular beats (bigeminy) are usually transient and well tolerated. Others like JET and atrial flutter may cause significant hemodynamic instability and even sudden cardiac death.
- *Neonates* with structurally normal hearts commonly have PACs, atrial flutter, and atrioventricular reentry tachycardia (AVRT). Congenital heart block is associated with maternal autoimmune diseases like systemic lupus.
- *Acute hemodynamic* state of the child is the key to determining the course of management. Treatment focuses on termination of the arrhythmia and prevention of future recurrences. The combination of pharmacotherapy, electrical therapies, antibradycardia devices (pacemakers), antitachycardic pacing, antiarrhythmic devices, surgical or interventional catheterization/electrophysiological studies, and radiofrequency ablation are the treatments that are used in managing patients with cardiac arrhythmias.

Normal heart rates in children:

- *Newborn:* 110–150 bpm
- *2 years:* 85–125 bpm
- *4 years:* 75–115 bpm
- *6 years+:* 60–100 bpm

TACHYARRHYTHMIAS

- Tachyarrhythmia may be sinus tachycardia, SVT, or ventricular tachycardia (VT)/ventricular fibrillation.
- SVT is a narrow complex tachyarrhythmia and most common symptomatic arrhythmias in children.

Classification of Supraventricular Tachycardia by Site of Origin and Regularity

The classification of SVT is as follows:

- Regular atrial
  - Sinus tachycardia
  - Atrial tachycardia
  - Atrial flutter
  - Sinus nodal reentry tachycardia (SNRT)
- Irregular atrial
  - Atrial fibrillation
  - Atrial flutter (variable block)
  - Multifocal atrial tachycardia (MAT)
- Regular atrioventricular
  - Atrioventricular reentry tachycardia (AVRT)
  - Atrioventricular nodal reentry tachycardia (AVNRT)
  - Junctional ectopic tachycardia

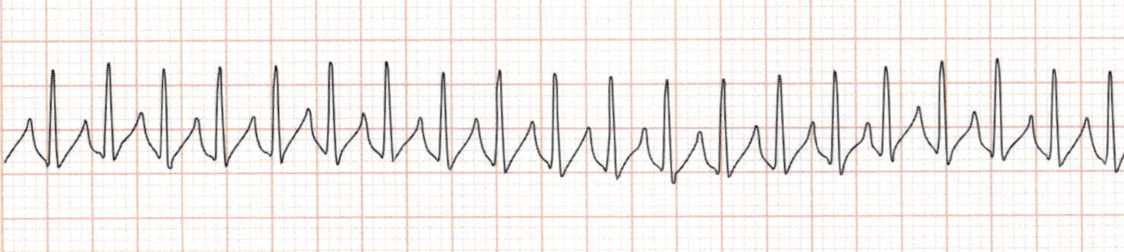

SUPRAVENTRICULAR TACHYCARDIA

Management of Supraventricular Tachycardia

A 12-lead electrocardiogram (ECG) in SVT and postconversion is essential. Monitoring with a rhythm strip during maneuvers in SVT and postconversion allows later assessment of underlying rhythm.

Acute Treatment

- Vagal maneuvers
  - *Infants:* Ice plus water in a plastic bag placed on face for up to 10 seconds—often effective. (avoid pressure on the eyeballs)
  - *Older children:* Carotid sinus massage, Valsalva maneuver (30–60 seconds), deep inspiration/ cough/gag reflex, and headstand.
- Adenosine (1 mL = 3 mg)
  - *Half-life* <10 seconds and side effects, including flushing, nausea, dyspnea, and bronchospasm, are short-lived.
  - *0.1 mg/kg* into a large vein *(rapid bolus/2 syringes flush technique)*; repeat after 2 minutes with 0.2 mg/kg
  - Maximum total dose = 12 mg
  - Transient AV nodal block as well as sinus node block, negative chronotrope, and ionotope.
- *Cardioversion:* If hemodynamically unstable, synchronized cardioversion is indicated 0.5–2 J/kg.

Chronic Treatment

Either medical (beta blockers—propanolol and nadolol) or surgical/catheter pathway ablation is done in older children.

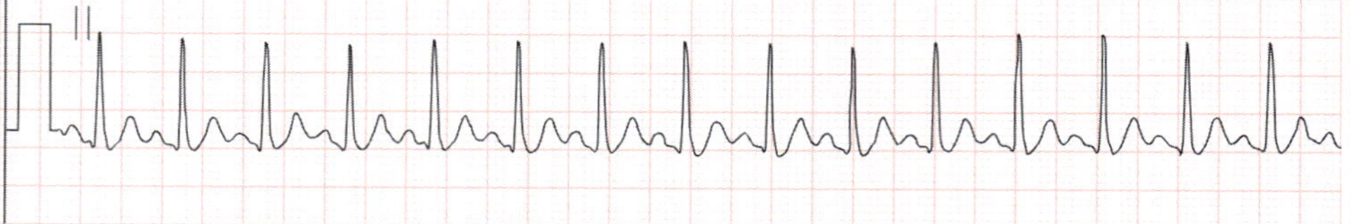

Sinus Tachycardia

- With very fast heart rates the P waves may be hidden in the preceding T wave.
- Each R wave is preceded by a P wave of the same morphology and PR intervals are constant and normal for age.

Cause (physiological/nonpharmacological): Exercise, pain, anxiety, hypoxia, hypercarbia, acidemia, sepsis, pyrexia, hyperthyroidism, and drugs (adrenaline, isoprenaline, salbutamol, etc.)

An algorithmic approach to the management of sinus tachycardia and supraventricular tachycardia is given in **Flowchart 1**.

Flowchart 1: Algorithmic approach to the management of sinus tachycardia and supraventricular tachycardia.

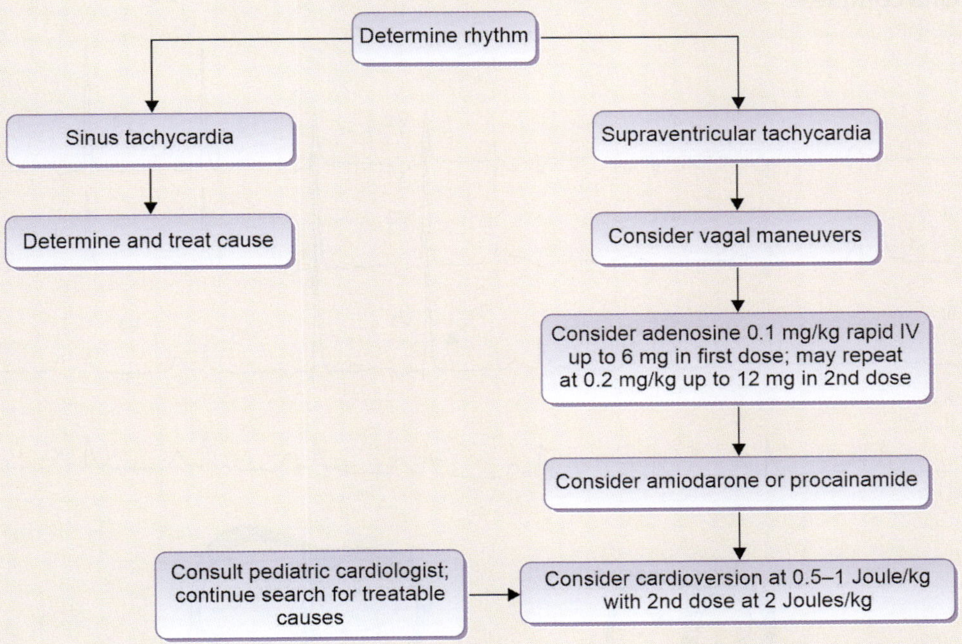

A comparison of ECG features of supraventricular tachycardia versus sinus tachycardia is given in **Table 1**.

TABLE 1: Supraventricular tachycardia versus sinus tachycardia.

	Sinus tachycardia	*Supraventricular tachycardia*
P wave preceding QRS complex	Present	Absent/retrograde
Beat-to-beat variability	Present	Absent
Rate >180 bpm in children and >220 bpm in infants	Unusual	Present

Wolff–Parkinson–White Syndrome

The Wolff–Parkinson–White (WPW) syndrome is a combination of the presence of a congenital accessory pathways that can conduct impulses *anterograde*, toward the ventricle; *retrograde*, away from the ventricle, or in both directions causing episodes of tachyarrhythmia.

The *ECG features of WPW in sinus rhythm:*

- PR interval <120 ms
- *Delta wave:* Slurring slow rise of the initial portion of the QRS
- QRS prolongation >110 ms
- ST segment and T-wave discordant changes, i.e., in the opposite direction to the major component of the QRS complex

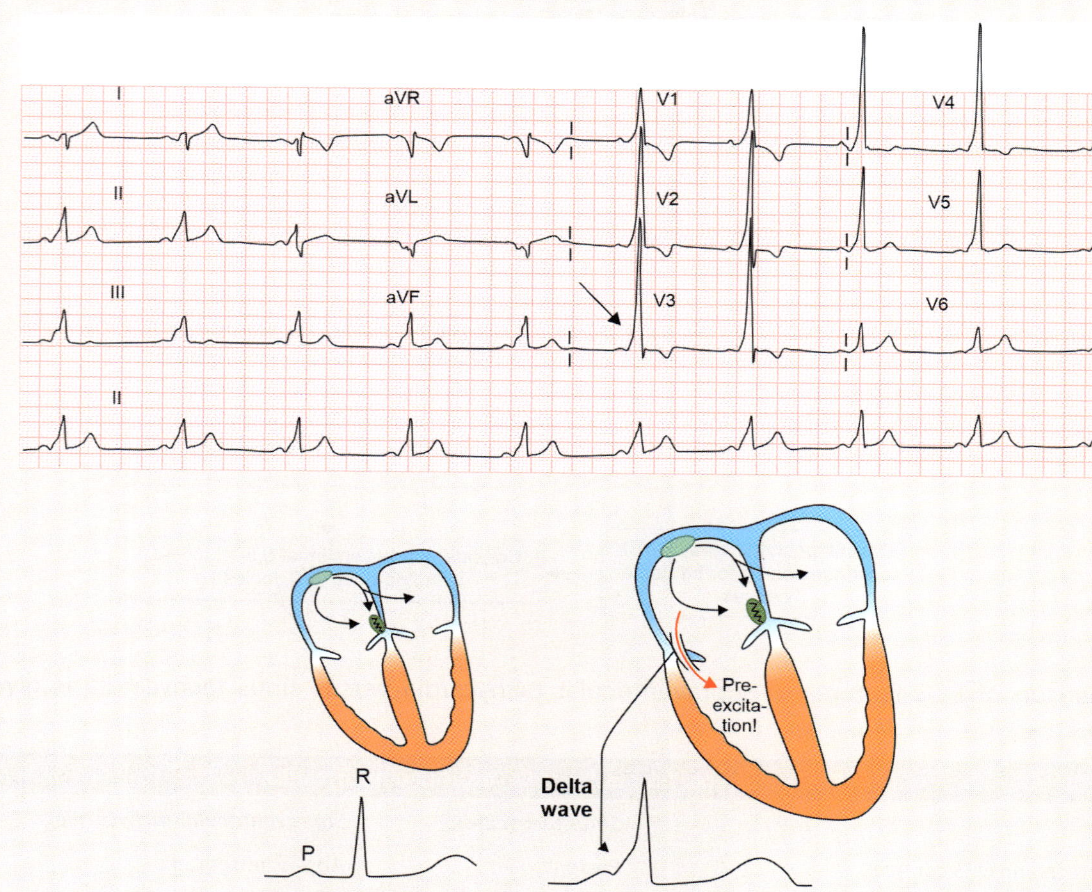

Fig. 1: Normal atrioventricular (AV) transmission and pre-excitation.

Atrioventricular Reentry Tachycardia (AVRT)

Atrioventricular reentry tachycardia is a form of paroxysmal SVT. A reentry circuit is formed by the normal conduction system and the accessory pathway resulting, in circus movement **(Fig. 1)**.

The AVRT is often triggered by premature atrial or premature ventricular beats. AVRTs are further divided into *orthodromic* (anterograde conduction occurs via the AV node) or *antidromic* (retrograde conduction via the AV node).

The ECG features of AVRT with orthodromic conduction are:

- Rate usually 200–300 bpm
- P waves may be buried in QRS complex or retrograde
- Narrow QRS

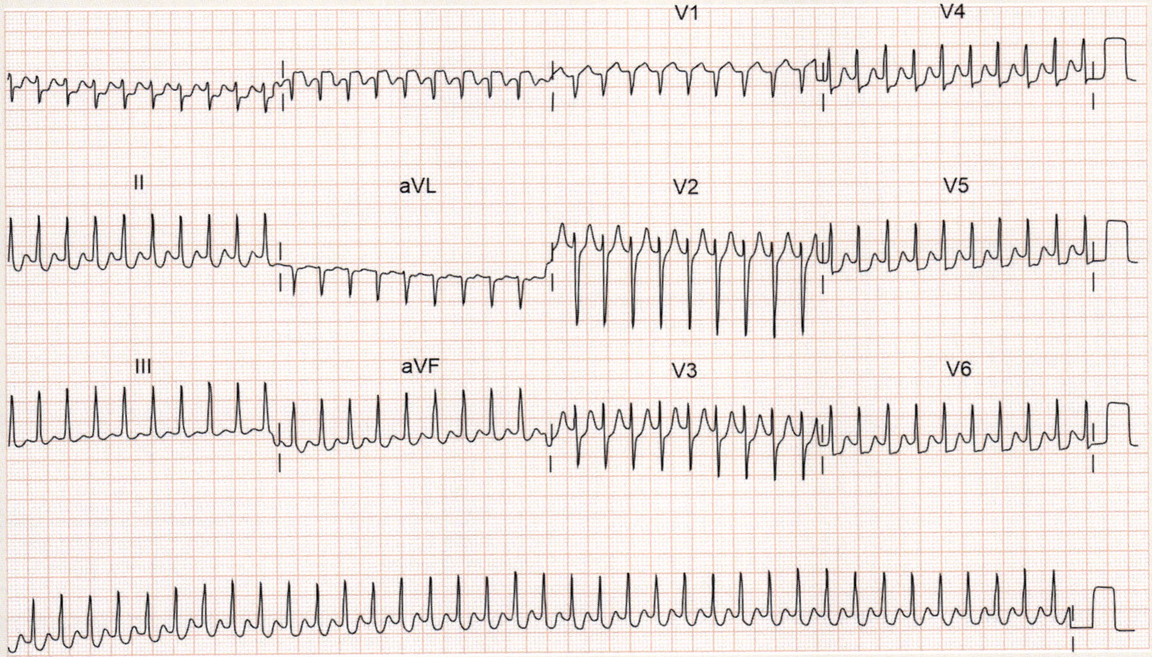

The approach to the management of tachyarrhythmias is given in **Flowchart 2**.

Flowchart 2: Approach to the management of tachyarrhythmias.

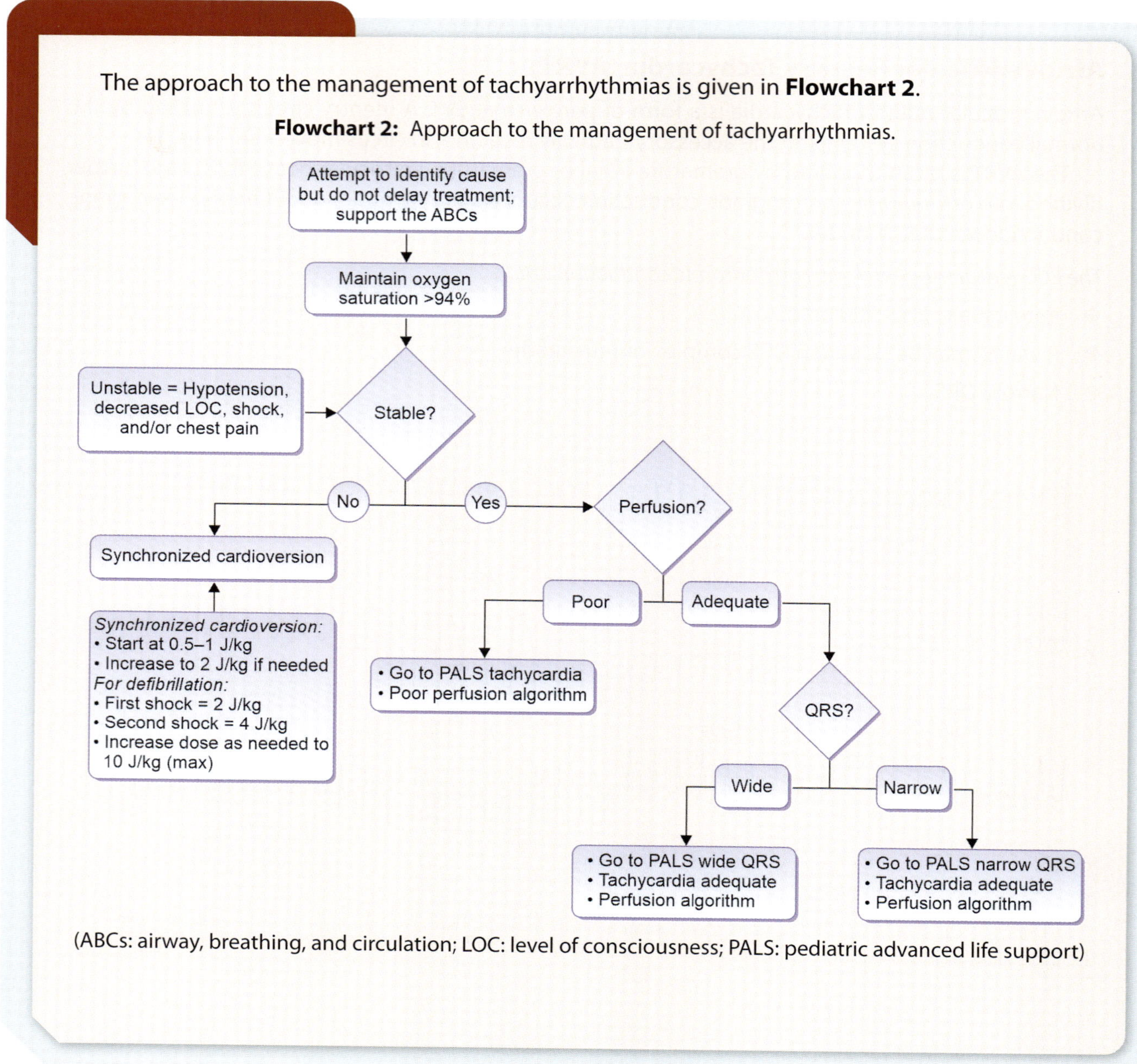

(ABCs: airway, breathing, and circulation; LOC: level of consciousness; PALS: pediatric advanced life support)

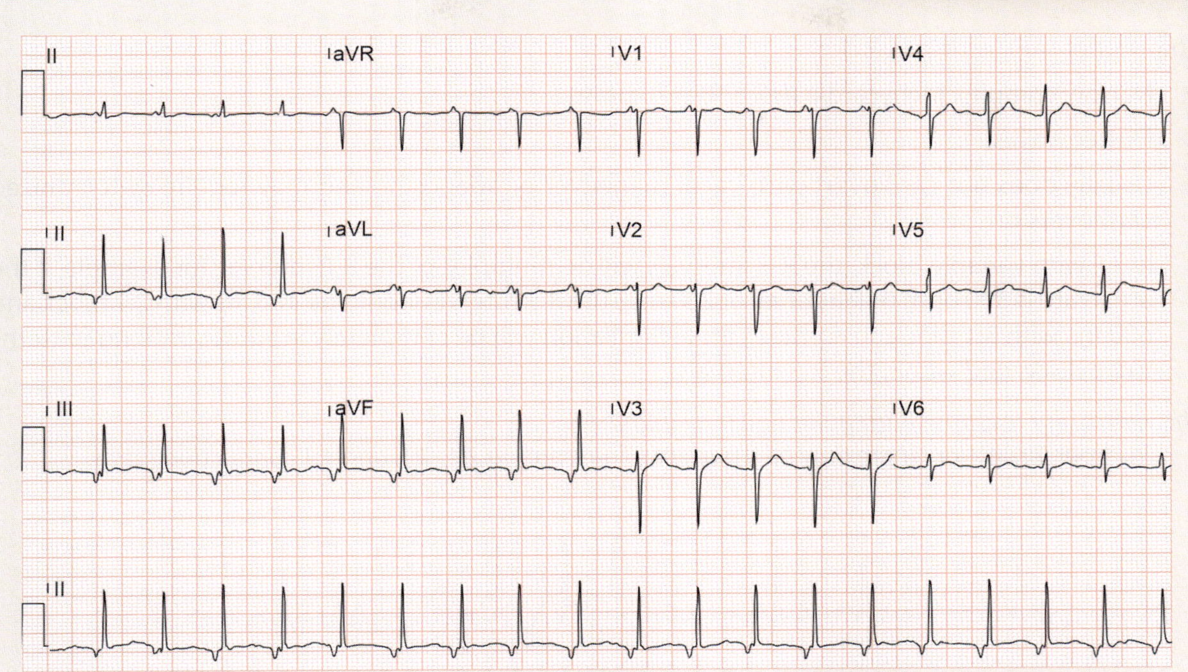

Junctional Ectopic Tachycardia

- Narrow complex tachycardia
- *Retrograde P waves:* Inverted in II, III, and aVF; upright in V1 and aVR).
- Short PR interval (<120 ms) indicates a junctional rather than atrial focus

Heart rate (HR) >170 bpm with either atrioventricular dissociation or 1:1 ventriculoatrial conduction.

It is the most common tachyarrhythmia in postoperative period. Long cardiopulmonary bypass (CPB) time, inotrope use, and repair of conotruncal defects are associated with increased incidence of JET.

This is conventionally treated with cooling, correction of electrolyte imbalance, moderate inotrope therapy, pain relief, and amiodarone.

The addition of magnesium during the rewarming phase of CPB, and use of dexmedetomidine and ivabradine are beneficial in controlling JET.

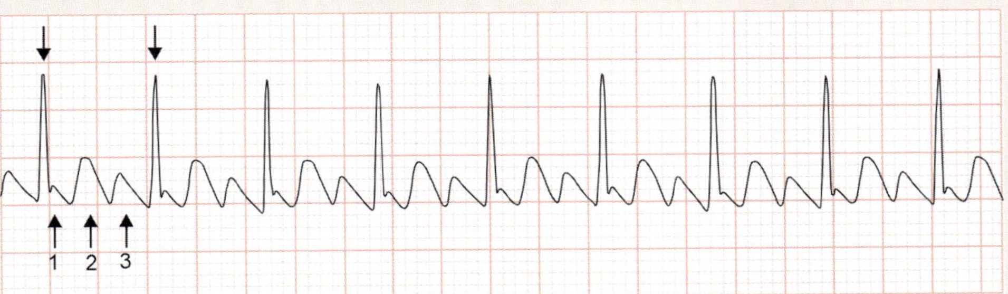

Atrial flutter (AF) *(with 3:1 block)*:

- Narrow complex tachycardia (*HR:* 130–170 bpm)
- Flutter waves
- Usually does not cardiovert with vagal maneuver or adenosine and may require synchronized cardioversion
- In AF with variable block, the R-R intervals will be multiples of the P-P interval; for example, if the atrial rate is 300 bpm (P-P interval of 200 ms), the R-R interval would be 400 ms with 2:1 block and 600 ms with 3:1 block. In contrast, atrial fibrillation will be completely irregular, with no patterns to be discerned within the R-R intervals.

The ventricular response is irregular and may mimic AF.

On closer inspection, there may be a pattern of alternating 2:1, 3:1, and 4:1 conduction ratios.

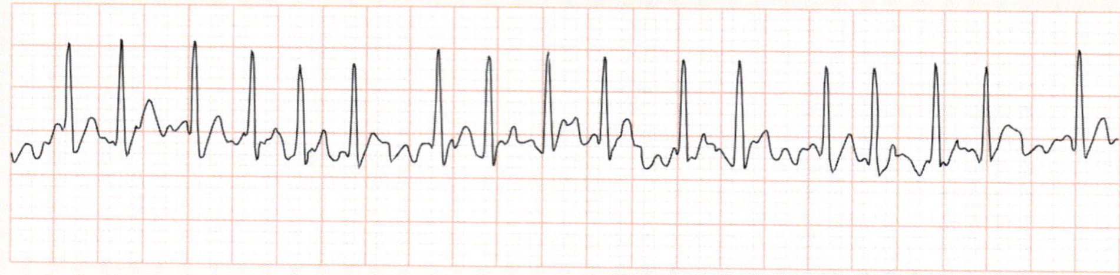

Atrial Fibrillation

- Irregularly irregular rhythm
- No P waves; fibrillatory waves may mimic P waves leading to misdiagnosis
- Variable ventricular rate
- QRS complexes are usually <120 ms unless preexisting bundle branch block, accessory pathway, or rate-related aberrant conduction.
- Fibrillatory waves may be present and can be either fine (amplitude < 0.5 mm) or coarse (amplitude > 0.5 mm).

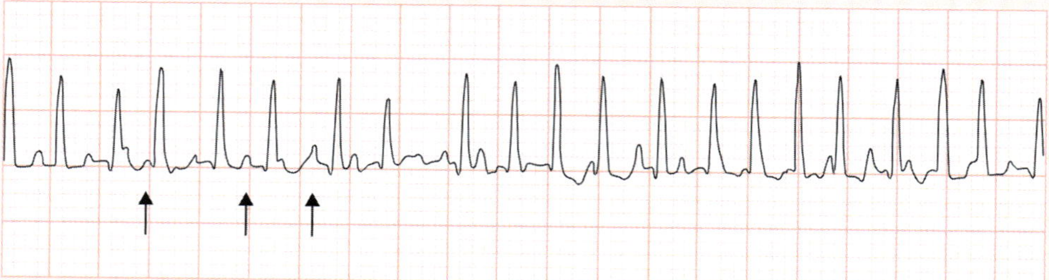

Multifocal Atrial Tachycardia

The features of multifocal atrial tachycardia (MAT) are as follows:

- Heart rate >100 bpm (usually, 100–150 bpm; may be as high as 250 bpm)
- Irregularly irregular rhythm with varying PP, PR, and RR intervals
- At least three distinct P-wave morphologies in the same lead
- Isoelectric baseline between P-waves (i.e., no flutter waves)
- Absence of a single dominant atrial pacemaker (i.e., not just sinus rhythm with frequent PACs)
- Rate controlled by beta blockers and treatment of the underlying disorder
- The development of MAT during an acute illness is a poor prognostic sign, associated with a 60% inhospital mortality.

Wide Complex Tachycardia (QRS > 0.9 ms)

Examples of wide complex tachycardia are as follows:

- Ventricular tachycardia
- SVT with aberrant conduction due to bundle branch block
- SVT with aberrant conduction due to the WPF syndrome
- Paced beats

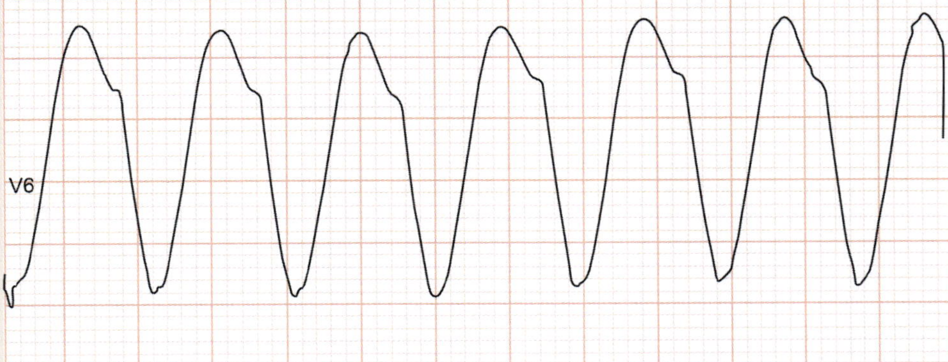

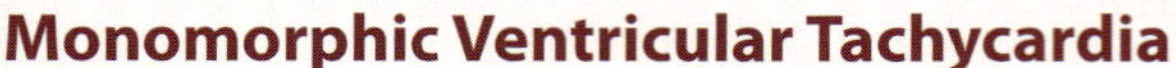

Monomorphic Ventricular Tachycardia

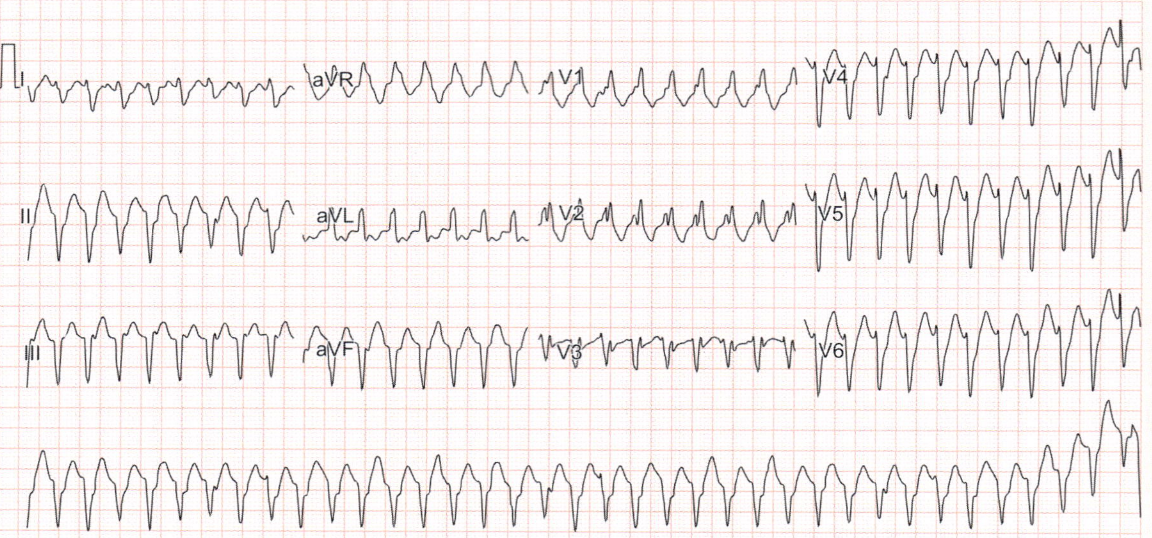

The features and treatment of VT are given in **Table 2**.

TABLE 2: Ventricular tachycardia (VT).

Features	*Causes*	*Treatment*
• More than three premature ventricular contractions (PVCs) in a row at a rate faster than 120 bpm (If slower, can be considered an accelerated ventricular rhythm) • Atrioventricular (AV) dissociation with more QRS complexes than P waves • Wide QRS, usually monomorphic, but can be polymorphic • Usually, abrupt onset	• Cardiomyopathies, RVOT VT (benign variant), idiopathic left VT (benign variant), and myocarditis • Long QT syndrome, catecholamine-sensitive polymorphic VT (CPVT), medication toxicity, arrhythmogenic right ventricular cardiomyopathy (ARVC), coronary artery abnormalities, and post-surgical abnormalities	• VT/VF –PALS algorithm • Primary prevention in patients with channelopathies or cardiomyopathies • *Asymptomatic:* Beta blockers • *Deceased function:* Can consider ablation • *Sustained or hemodynamically unstable:* ICD placement

(ICD: implantable cardioverter-defibrillator; RVOT: right ventricular outflow tract; VT: ventricular tachycardia; VF: ventricular fibrillation)

Polymorphic VT/Torsade de pointes:

- Occurs in long QT syndrome and with some drugs
- Causes syncope if self-terminating or cardiac arrest if prolonged [i.e., degenerates to ventricular fibrillation (VF)]

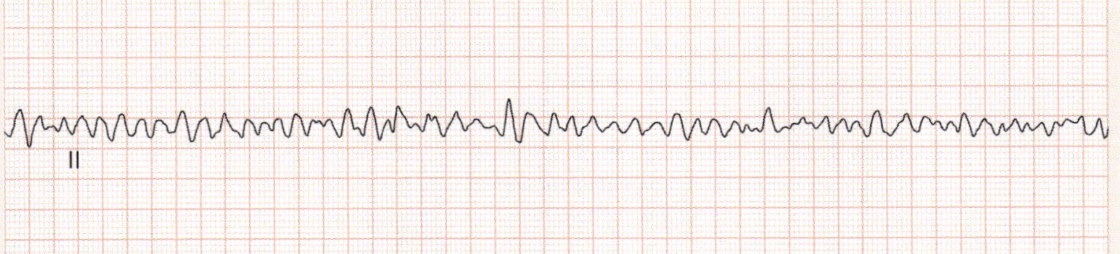

Ventricular fibrillation (VF): Extremely rare in children and associated with congenital cardiac abnormalities/postcardiac surgery. Treatment is defibrillation at 2 J/kg (max 10 J/Kg) and cardiopulmonary resuscitation

BRADYARRHYTHMIAS

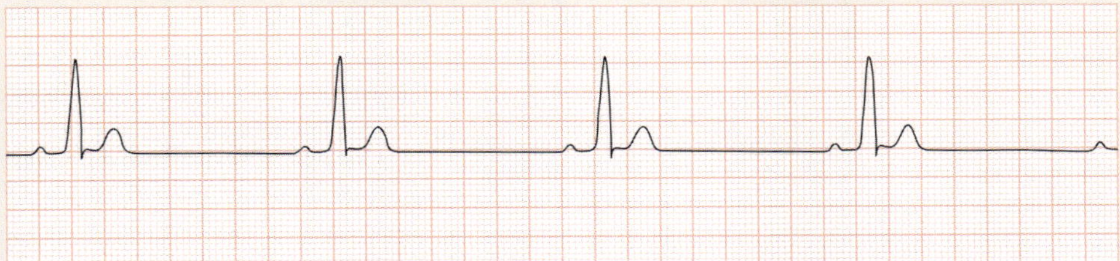

Sinus Bradycardia

- Increased vagal tone (e.g., athletes, sinus node disease, hypothyroidism, hypothermia, and anorexia nervosa)
- *Electrolyte abnormalities:* Hyperkalemia and hypermagnesemia
- Brainstem herniation (the Cushing reflex) and myocarditis
- *Drug:* Amiodarone, beta-blockers, calcium channel blockers (CCB), digoxin, and organophosphate poisoning

Algorithmic approach to the management of bradycardia is illustrated in **Flowchart 3**.

Flowchart 3: Algorithmic approach to the management of bradycardia.

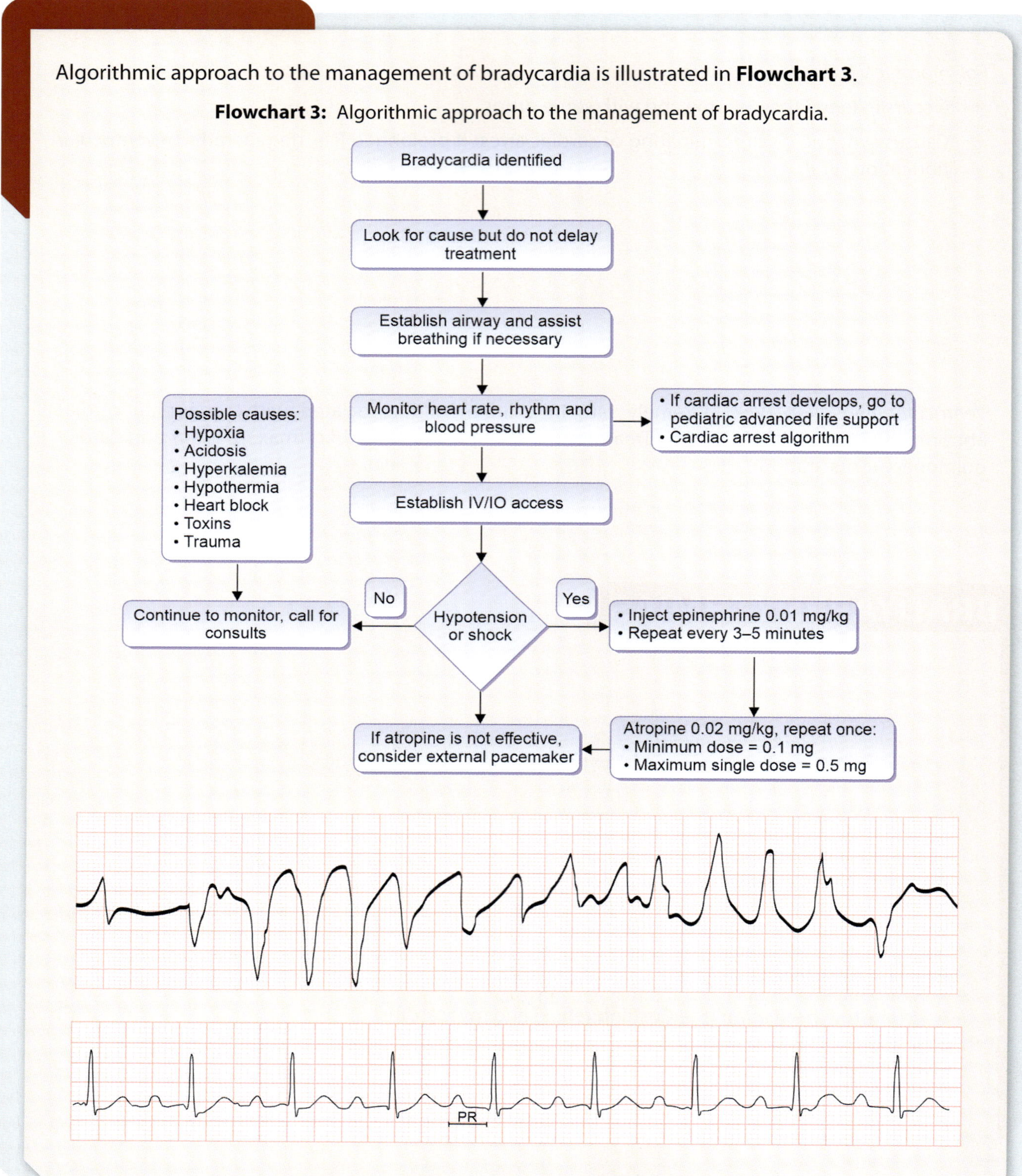

- *First-degree heart block:*
  - PR interval >120 ms (<3 years) and >200 ms (adolescents/adults)
  - *Cause:* Increased vagal tone, myocarditis, atrial septal defect (ASD), structural heart disease, Ebstein's anomaly, rheumatic fever, drugs (digitalis, beta blockers, CCB, and hyperkalemia)
  - Does not cause hemodynamic disturbance and no specific treatment is required.

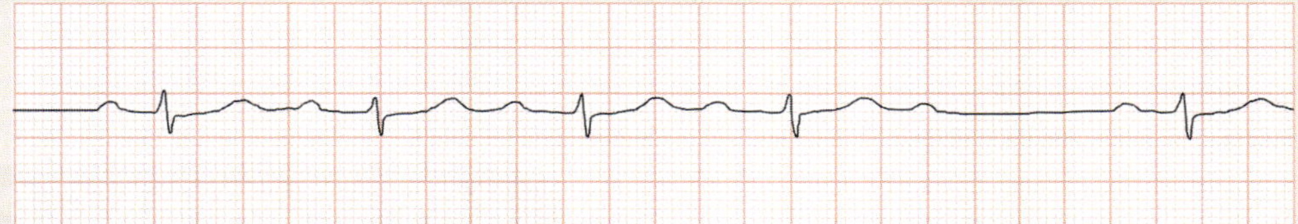

- *Second-degree AV block, Mobitz I (Wenckebach phenomenon):*
  - Progressive prolongation of the PR interval culminating in a nonconducted P wave
  - The PR interval is longest immediately before the dropped beat.
  - The PR interval is shortest immediately after the dropped beat.

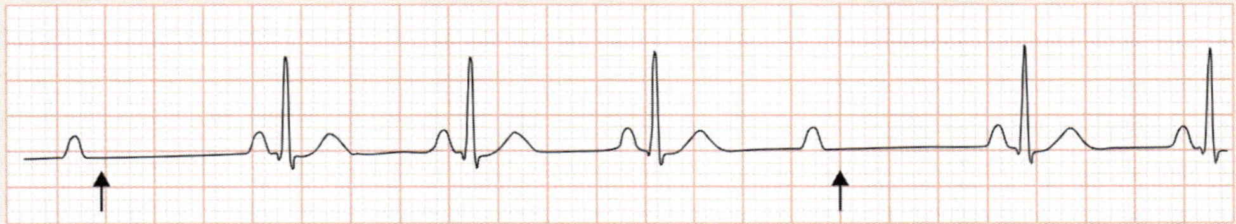

- Arrows indicate "*dropped*" QRS complexes (i.e., nonconducted P waves)

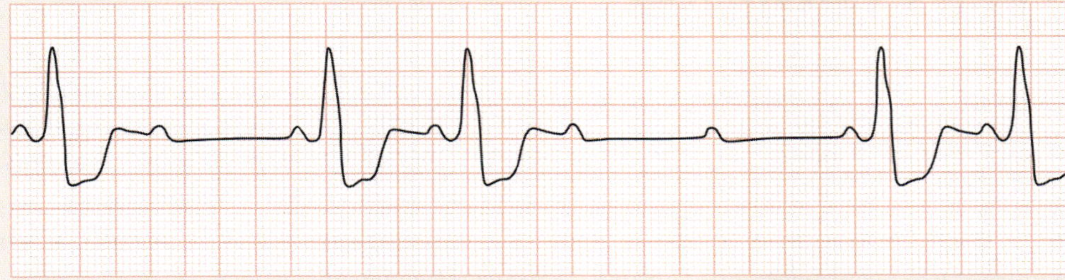

- *Second-degree AV block, Mobitz II*: Intermittent nonconducted P waves without progressive prolongation of the PR interval (PR interval in the conducted beats remains constant).

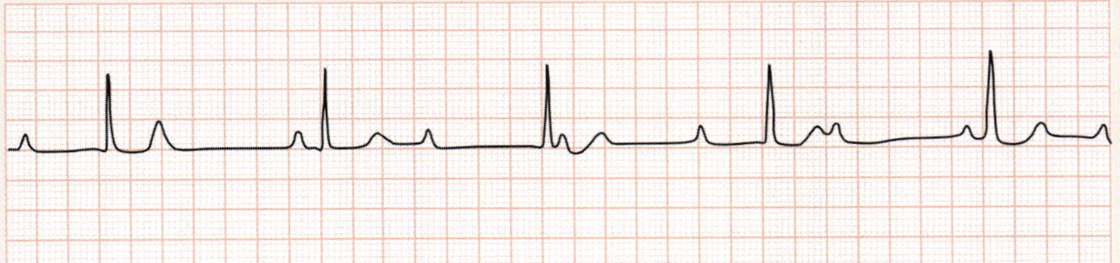

- *Severe bradycardia with independent atrial and ventricular rates, i.e., AV dissociation. Complete heart block (Third-degree heart block):* In a complete heart block, there is complete absence of AV conduction of the supraventricular impulses. Perfusing rhythm is maintained by a junctional or ventricular escape rhythm. Alternatively, the patient may suffer ventricular standstill leading to syncope (if self-terminating) or sudden cardiac death (if prolonged).

KEY LEARNING POINTS

- Arrhythmias are relatively common in the pediatric cardiac intensive care unit.
- Arrhythmia with acute hemodynamic instability is an acute emergency
- Prompt diagnosis and appropriate early management can potentially prevent life-threatening events.
- Always look for reversible factors (H's and T's) if life-threatening arrhythmia is not responding.

SUGGESTED READING

1. Al-Khatib SM, Stevenson WG, Ackerman MJ, Bryant WJ, Callans DJ, Curtis AB, et al. 2017 AHA/ACC/HRS Guideline for Management of patients with ventricular arrhythmias and the prevention of sudden cardiac death: A Report of the American College of Cardiology/American Heart Association Task Force on Clinical Practice Guidelines and the Heart Rhythm Society. Circulation. 2018;138(13):e210-71.
2. Chandar JS, Wolff GS, Garson A Jr, Bell TJ, Beder SD, Bink-Boelkens M, et al. Ventricular arrhythmias in postoperative tetralogy of Fallot. Am J Cardiol. 1990;65(9):655-61.
3. Doniger SJ, Sharieff GQ. Pediatric dysrhythmias. Pediatr Clin North Am. 2006;53(1):85-105.
4. Kaltman J, Shah M. Evaluation of the child with an arrhythmia. Pediatr Clin North Am 2004; 51(6):1537-51.
5. Wisten A, Messner T. Symptoms preceding sudden cardiac death in the young are common but often misinterpreted. Scand Cardiovasc J. 2005;39(3):143-9.
6. Woods WA, McCulloch MA. Cardiovascular emergencies in the pediatric patient. Emerg Med Clin North Am. 2005;23(4):1233-49.

Hypertensive Emergencies

Nitesh Upadhyay, Chirag Sethi

INTRODUCTION

- The incidence of primary hypertension in pediatric population is on rise and its prevalence is estimated to be around 3.5%.[1]
- As per a systematic review, it was observed that considerable proportions (7%) of school-going children are hypertensive in India.[2] Prevalence was higher in urban and overweight children.
- As per the National Health and Nutrition Examination Survey (NHANES), the morbidity of hypertensive crisis was found to be between 1% and 4% in preadolescent and adolescents.[3]

TERMINOLOGIES AND DEFINITIONS

- *Hypertensive crisis* is defined as an acute episode of severely elevated blood pressure (BP) with potential for end-organ damage, often exceeding the limits known for stage II hypertension.
- Hypertensive crisis can be subcategorized as *hypertensive urgency* or *acute severe hypertension*, in which there are no signs of end-organ damage, and *hypertensive emergency*, in which signs of end-organ damage are present.
- The BP classification in children and adolescents is given in **Table 1**.

TABLE 1: Blood pressure classification in children and adolescents.		
	Children 1–13 years	*Age >13–17 years*
Normal blood pressure	<90th centile	<120/<80 mm Hg
Elevated blood pressure	≥90–<95th centile or 120/80 mm Hg to <95th centile (whichever is lower)	120/<80–129/<80 mm Hg
Stage 1: Hypertension	≥95th centile to <95th centile + 12 mm Hg or 130/80–139/89 mm Hg (whichever is lower)	130/80–139/89 mm Hg
Stage 2: Hypertension	≥95th centile + 12 mm Hg, or ≥140/90 mm Hg (whichever is lower)	≥140/90 mm Hg
	Hypertensive Crisis	
Hypertensive urgency	>95th centile + 30 mm Hg without target end-organ damage	>180/120 mm Hg without target end-organ damage
Hypertensive emergency	>95th centile + 30 mm Hg associated with target end-organ damage	>180/120 mm Hg associated with target end-organ damage

ETIOPATHOLOGY

70–80% of the cases of hypertension crisis in children are due to secondary causes. Among the secondary causes of hypertensive crisis, renal parenchymal diseases and coarctation of aorta are the most common.[4,5] Other causes may include renal artery stenosis or thrombosis, glomerular disease, obstructive uropathy, hemolytic uremic syndrome (HUS), pheochromocytoma, and endocrine disorders **(Table 2)**.

TABLE 2: Common causes of hypertensive emergency and urgency in children.	
Age group	*Etiology*
Newborn–1 year	• Renal artery or venous thrombosis • Renal artery stenosis • Congenital renal abnormalities (polycystic kidneys) • Coarctation of aorta • Bronchopulmonary dysplasia • Renovascular disease • Renal parenchymal disease • Iatrogenic tumor • Tumor • Theophylline/caffeine overdose

Contd…

Contd...

Age group	*Etiology*
1–12 years	• Renal parenchymal disease • Polycystic kidneys • Renovascular disease • Tumor • Endocrine causes • Coarctation of aorta
13–18 years	• Essential hypertension • Metabolic syndrome • Renal parenchymal disease • Iatrogenic • Anabolic steroid • Substance abuse • Renovascular disease • Coarctation of aorta • Endocrine causes

Source: Patel et al. (2012).

CLINICAL FEATURES

Of the known presentations of hypertensive emergencies, acute neurological signs are most common. Hypertensive urgency has a greater propensity to present with nonspecific symptoms, such as irritability and poor feeding in infants and headache, nausea, fatigue, and dizziness in children and adolescents.

A severe neurological complication of hypertensive emergency in children is posterior reversible encephalopathy syndrome (PRES), which principally involves damage to the occipitoparietal white matter and may spread to the basal ganglia, cerebellum, and brainstem. Presentation of PRES can vary, ranging from minor symptoms such as headache and nausea to major symptoms, such as altered mentation, seizures, focal neurologic deficit, or blindness. Hypertensive emergency may also affect retina, heart, and kidneys. Retinal changes due to hypertensive emergency may present as vision loss, papilledema, and retinal hemorrhage. Cardiac morbidities like left ventricular hypertrophy, congestive cardiac failure, and cardiogenic shock may be present. Renal symptoms may also be seen such as flank pain, hematuria, and oliguria **(Table 3)**.

TABLE 3: Clinical presentation of hypertensive emergencies in children.

Nonspecific symptoms	• Irritability • Poor feeding
Neurological symptoms	• Headache • Fatigue • Dizziness • Nausea/vomiting • Altered consciousness • Seizures • Focal neurological deficit • Posterior reversible encephalopathy syndrome
Visual symptom	• Acute ischemic optic neuropathy • Retinal hemorrhage • Blindness
Cardiac symptoms	• Left ventricular failure • Cardiogenic shock
Renal symptoms	• Hematuria • Proteinuria • Flank pain • Oliguria • Hyponatremic hypertensive syndrome (renal artery stenosis)

EVALUATION (PHYSICAL EXAMINATION AND INVESTIGATIONS)

Detailed history and physical examination are the cornerstones of evaluation of hypertension emergencies and must include history related to urinary complaints including hematuria, oliguria, or past medical history of urinary tract infection or NICU stay (especially, umbilical artery catheterization), or any drug intake. Physical evaluation must stress on palpation of all peripheral pulses, auscultatory BP measurement of all four limbs, presence of tachycardia, S3 or S4 sounds, location of apex beats, complete neurological examination, and fundus examination. Presence of renal bruit may point toward renovascular hypertension.

Initial investigation battery should include urinalysis, complete blood count, renal function tests, electrocardiography (ECG), chest radiograph, echocardiography, and ultrasonography of abdomen. MRI brain may help diagnose PRES, infarct, or hemorrhage. In selective cases, renal angiography, urinary vanillylmandelic acid (VMA), renal captopril scan, and endocrinological evaluation may be required.

DIFFERENTIALS

Posterior reversible encephalopathy syndrome may mimic acute encephalitis syndrome, intracranial space occupying lesion (ICSOL), or meningitis. Circulatory system involvement may be confused with congenital cardiac shunt [ventricular septal defect (VSD) or patent ductus arteriosus (PDA)] during infancy and ischemic heart disease in older children. Renal damage may mimic glomerulonephritis or acute kidney injury.

EMERGENCY CARE

Emergency-setting management includes initial stabilization of airway, breathing, and circulation along with control of life-threatening conditions like abortion of seizures and control of congestive cardiac failure (CCF), shock, and respiratory failure, if present. High-flow oxygen with nonrebreather mask (NRBM), urinary catheterization, and setting up of intravenous access are required in all cases admitted in the pediatric intensive care unit (PICU) setting **(Flowchart 1)**.

Flowchart 1: Algorithm for management of hypertensive crisis.

Repeated BP reading suggestive of hypertensive crisis on auscultatory BP
Concern of target end-organ damage/red flag?
Yes
No
Hypertensive emergency
Hypertensive urgency
• Stabilize ABC
• Establish IV access
• Draw samples
• Monitor arterial BP
• Start treatment
• Oral medicine + NiBP monitoring + Treat cause
BP <90th centile
Plan discharge and follow up
Concern of life threatening event
No
Yes
Control seizure/CCF/ respiratory failure
Identification of the underlying cause?
Yes
No
CCF or Pulmonary edema?
CNS Pathology? (Consider MRI Brain)
No
Treat secondary cause + Control BP with IV medicine*
Signs of fluid overload?
Yes
Yes
Yes
No
2D echocardiography and cardiology opinion
Neurology and neurosurgery opinion
Consider IV diuretic
Control BP by IV medicine*

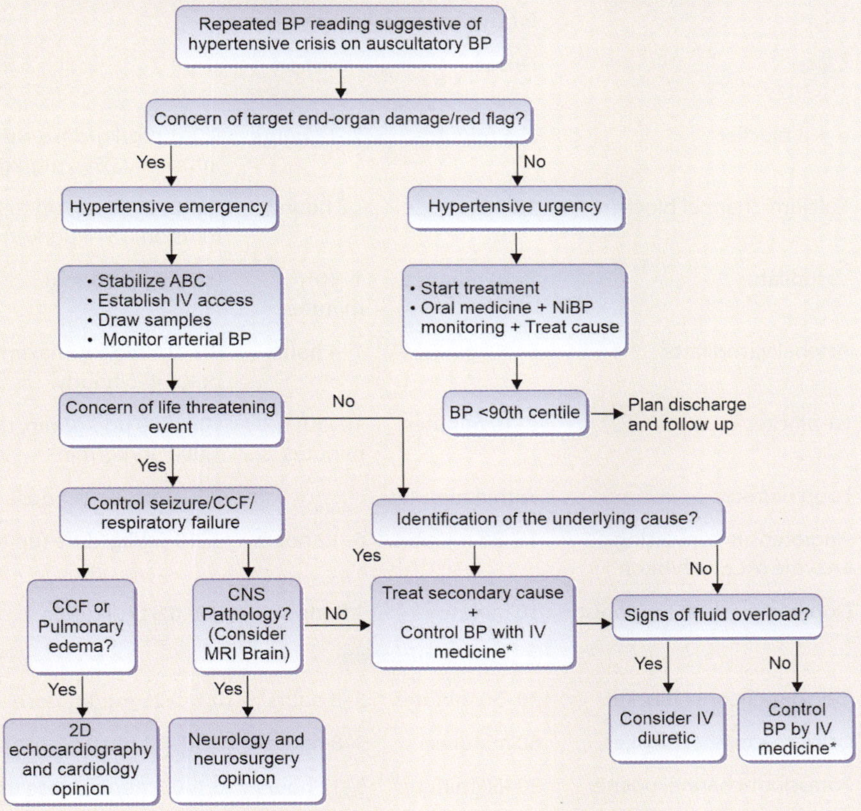

*Target for BP on IV medicine is to achieve 25% reduction in initial 8 hours complete control till 90th centile by 48 hours of ICU admission. After BP control, switch to oral medicine.

(ABC: airway, breathing, circulation; BP: blood pressure; CCF: congestive cardiac failure; CNS: central nervous system; IV: intravenous; MRI: magnetic resonance imaging; NiBP: noninvasive blood pressure)

SPECIFIC MANAGEMENT

In children and adolescents diagnosed with hypertensive crisis, the treatment goal is to achieve reduction in systolic blood pressure (SBP) and diastolic blood pressure (DBP) to <90th percentile and <130/80 mm Hg in adolescents ≥13 years of age.[6-8] The rate of BP reduction should be 25% over a period of 6–8 hours, and then gradually, reduction to the target BP over 24–72 hours is achieved. Sudden and drastic reductions in BP can itself contribute to organ damage secondary to ischemia.

Parenteral therapy is crucial to the management of hypertensive emergencies, while cases of hypertensive urgency can be managed with either intravenous (IV) or rapid-acting oral antihypertensives. Most commonly used first-line IV agent is *labetalol,* a combined alpha and beta blocker, which acts both by reducing peripheral vascular resistance and through its negative chronotropic effect.[9] Labetalol, when used alone or as an add-on drug, is more efficacious than IV nitroprusside/nitroglycerine in children with hypertensive crisis.[10] Other options used are *esmolol, nicardipine, sodium nitroprusside, hydralazine,* or *fenoldopam* (**Table 4**). Some drugs, such as *enalaprilat, phenoxybenzamine, doxazosin, and furosemide*, are used only in specific situations. Oral therapy may be tried in hypertensive urgency with *nifedipine, isradipine,* and *minoxidil.*

TABLE 4: Characteristics of the medications used in management of hypertensive crisis.

Name of Medication	*Class*	*Onset*	*Duration*	*Dose*
Intravenous medications				
Labetalol	α + β blocker	2–5 minutes	2–12 hours	0.2–1 mg/kg/dose, up to 40 mg/dose; infusion 0.25–3 mg/kg/hour
Nicardipine	Calcium-channel blocker	10 minutes	<8 hours	Bolus: 30 µg/kg up to 2 mg/dose; infusion 0.5–4 µg/kg/min
Sodium Nitroprusside	Vasodilator	2–10 minutes	1–10 minutes	0.5–10 µg/kg/min
Hydralazine	Arterial vasodilator	5–10 minutes	1–4 hours	0.2–0.6 mg/kg, maximum 20 mg; repeat bolus 4–6 hourly
Esmolol	β1 blocker	2–10 minutes	10–30 minutes	100–500 µg/kg/min, up to 1,000 µg/kg/min
Furosemide	Loop diuretic	Within minutes		0.5–5 mg/kg per dose
Enalapril	Angiotensin-converting enzyme (ACE) inhibitor	15–30 minutes	6–12 hours	5–10 µg/kg/dose (up to 1.2 mg)
Fenoldopam	Dopamine receptor agonist	10 minutes	1 hour	0.2–0.8 µg/kg/min
Oral medications				
Nifedipine	Calcium-channel blocker	20–30 minutes	3–8 hours	0.1–0.25 mg/kg/dose
Isradipine	Calcium-channel blocker	60 minutes	3–8 hours	0.05–0.1 mg/kg/dose (maximum 5 mg)
Minoxidil	Potassium-channel opener	30–60 minutes	8–12 hours	0.1–0.2 mg/kg/dose (maximum 10 mg)
Clonidine	Central alpha agonist	15–30 minutes	6–8 hours	0.05–0.1 mg/kg/dose, may be repeated up to 0.8 mg total

MONITORING

Continuous intra-arterial BP monitoring is required to make sure gradual reduction of BP is achieved. Along with BP measurement, vital monitoring including heart rate, ECG, respiratory rate, oxygen saturation, mental status, and urinary output with close monitoring of input/output balance is required.

KEY LEARNING POINTS

- Hypertensive crisis is an acute life-threatening emergency, which may mimic neurological or cardiovascular or in rare cases, renal or ocular diseases.
- Goal of treatment in hypertensive emergency is to achieve initial rapid control of 25% reduction over 8 hours followed by gradual reduction in BP over 24–48 hours.
- In hypertensive urgency, oral medicines may be tried but in hypertensive emergency IV medicines are the mainstay of treatment with close monitoring of BP.

REFERENCES

1. McNiece KL, Poffenbarger TS, Turner JL, Franco KD, Sorof JM, Portman RJ. Prevalence of hypertension and pre-hypertension among adolescents. J Pediatr. 2007;150(6):640-4.
2. Meena J, Singh M, Agarwal A, Chauhan A, Jaiswal N. Prevalence of hypertension among children and adolescents in India: A systematic review and meta-analysis. Indian J Pediatr. 2021;88(11):1107-14.
3. Din-Dzietham R, Liu Y, Bielo MV, Shamsa F. High blood pressure trends in children and adolescents in national surveys, 1963 to 2002. Circulation. 2007;116(13):1488-96.
4. Viera AJ, Neutze DM. Diagnosis of secondary hypertension: An age-based approach. Am Fam Physician. 2010;82(12):1471-8.
5. Patel NH, Romero SK, Kaelber DC. Evaluation and management of pediatric hypertensive crises: Hypertensive urgency and hypertensive emergencies. Open Access Emergency Med. 2012;5(4):85-92.
6. Raina R, Mahajan Z, Sharma A, Chakraborty R, Mahajan S, Sethi SK, et al. Hypertensive crisis in pediatric patients: An overview. Front Pediatr. 2020;8:588911
7. Flynn JT, Tullus K. Severe hypertension in children and adolescents: Pathophysiology and treatment. Pediatric Nephrol. 2009;24:1101-12.
8. Flynn JT, Kaelber DC, Baker-Smith CM, Blowey D, Carroll AE, Daniels SR, et al.; Subcommittee on Screening and Management of High Blood Pressure in Children. Clinical practice guideline for screening and management of high blood pressure in children and adolescents. Pediatrics. 2017;140(3):e20171904.
9. Awad L, Sethuraman U. Evaluation and Management of Elevated BP in Children in the ED. Curr Hypertens Rep. 2024;26(3):99-105.
10. Lad S, Patil M, Jayashree M, Bansal A, Baranwal A, Nallasamy K, et al. Efficacy and safety of intravenous labetalol in acute hypertensive crisis in children. Indian J Pediatr. 2022;89(1):7-12.

Central Nervous System

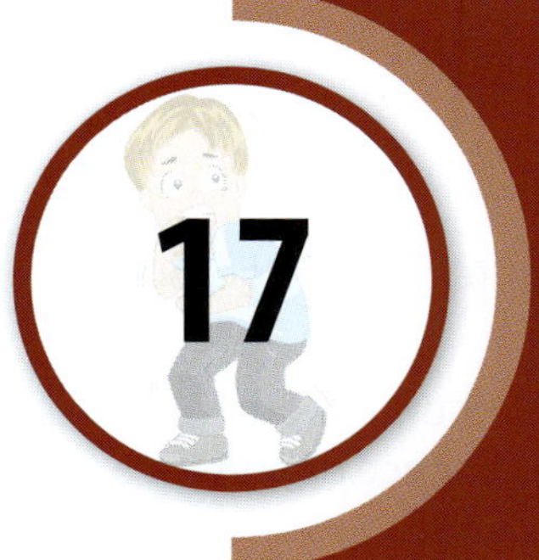

17

Approach to Altered Sensorium

Sasmita Devi Agrawal, Lokesh Lingappa

DEFINITION

- Sensorium is the ability of the brain to receive and interpret sensory stimuli.
  - Wakefulness = Arousal and Alertness
  - Good sensorium = Wakefulness + Awareness
- Altered sensorium is not a disease. It is a symptom.
- Its causes could be varied from easily reversible (hypoglycemia) to permanent (stroke) and from relatively benign (electrolyte imbalance) to life-threatening (meningitis or encephalitis).

PRESENTATION OF PATIENT WITH ALTERED SENSORIUM

Altered sensorium may have varying degrees of severity starting from excessive irritability, drowsiness, delirium, and finally coma.

TERMS USED IN ALTERED SENSORIUM

The following terms are used in altered sensorium:

- *Drowsiness:* State of apparent sleep with brief arousal on oral command
- *Lethargic:* This state resembles sleepiness but patient does not become fully alert; there is slow verbal response and patient is inattentive. Patient is unable to adequately perform simple concentration tasks.
- *Somnolent:* There is easy arousal by voice or touch; patient awakens and follows commands; stimulation is required to maintain arousal.

- *Stupor:* There is unresponsiveness from which the child can be aroused intermittently by vigorous, repeated stimulation.
- *Coma:* An altered state of consciousness in which the child is unarousable and unresponsive to various external stimuli and the only response to repeated stimuli may be the presence of primitive avoidance reflexes.
- *Confusion:* There is impaired attention and concentration; the child manifests disorientation in time, place, and person. There is impersistent thinking, speech, performance, reduced comprehension, and capacity to reason.
- *Delirium:* In this state, the child experiences confusion and associated agitation, hallucination, convulsion, and tremor

STATES OF ALTERED SENSORIUM

Table 1 shows newer terms used for altered sensorium.

TABLE 1: Newer terms used for altered sensorium.

Sensorium	*Wakefulness*	*Awareness*	*Brainstem function*
Conscious	Preserved	Preserved	Normal
Minimally conscious state	Preserved	Suboptimal	Normal
Vegetative state	Preserved	Absent	Preserved
Coma	Absent	Absent	Normal

Altered sensorium can be determined by evaluating level of consciousness by using pediatric Glasgow Coma Scale (PGCS) as shown in **Table 2**.

TABLE 2: Evaluating level of consciousness by pediatric Glasgow Coma Scale (PGCS).

Category	*Score*	*Response <1 year old*	*Response >1 year old*
Eye-opening	4	Spontaneous	Spontaneous
	3	To shouting	To speech
	2	To pain	To pain
	1	None	None
Best motor response	6	Normal movement and obeys command	
	5	Localizes pain	Localizes pain
	4	Flexion withdrawal	Flexion withdrawal
	3	Abnormal decorticate	Abnormal decorticate

Contd...

Contd...

Category	*Score*	*Response <1-year-old*	*Response >1-year-old*
	2	Decerebrate	Decerebrate
	1	None	none
Best verbal response	0–23 months	2–5 years	>5 years
Score: 5	Smiles/coos appropriately	Appropriate words/phrases	Oriented
4	Cries and is consolable	Inappropriate words	Disoriented/confused
3	Persistent inappropriate crying and or screaming	Persistent cries and screams	Inappropriate words
2	Grunts, agitated, and restless	Grunts	Incomprehensible sounds
1	No response	No response	No response

The broad approach is based on how rapidly the encephalopathy has evolved, what structures are likely involved and what is the likely etiopathogenesis.

Identify in the emergency room (ER) all the easily treatable disorders. Check blood pressure (BP), blood sugar, and electrolytes. Stabilize airway, breathing, and circulation. Assess neurology while taking history simultaneously. In infants with cardiogenic shock, administer thiamine:

- The degree of the state of altered sensorium is graded by Glasgow Coma Scale (GCS).
- The lowest score is 3 and the highest score is 15.
- Endotracheal intubation is required if the GCS score is 7 or less. Also, if there are clear feature of raised intracranial pressure (ICP) or systemic complications requiring respiratory support or shock.
- *Total score:* Eye-opening + motor response + verbal response
- In the context of intracranial infections such as acute viral encephalitis or head trauma, a GCS of *8 or less* suggests severe cerebral dysfunction. Serial monitoring is vital as a rapid decline in GCS warrants reevaluation and imaging for sinusoidal obstruction syndrome (SOS).
- *GCS—9–12:* Moderate cerebral dysfunction
- *GCS—13–15:* Minor cerebral dysfunction
- A score of 8 or less suggests greater mortality, and hence, a poor prognosis. Also, it depends on the etiology, extent of changes in MRI Brain. For example, a child with hepatic encephalopathy and poor sensorium can improve well once the liver function improves rapidly, child with sepsis-associated encephalopathy also can improve very well once the systemic complications improve.
- Scores *of 3–5:* If accompanied by fixed pupils or absent oculovestibular response, it is potentially fatal.

- Other scoring systems like AVPU and FOUR scores can also be used to assess the level of consciousness **(Tables 3 and 4)**.

TABLE 3: AVPU score.

A	Alert	Alert and conscious
V	Verbal	Response to verbal stimulus
P	Pain	Respond to painful stimuli
U	Unresponsive	Unresponsive to any form of stimuli

TABLE 4: FOUR score.

Category and response	***Score***
Eye response	
• Eyelid open, tracking or blinking to command	4
• Eyelid open but not tracking	3
• Eye closed but open to loud voice, not tracking	2
• Eye closed, open to pain not tracking	1
• Eye closed with pain	0
Motor response	
• Thumbs up, fist, or peace sign to command	4
• Localizing to pain	3
• Flexion response to pain	2
• Extensor posturing	1
• No response to pain, generalized myoclonus status	0
Brainstem reflexes	
• Pupil and corneal reflex present	4
• One pupil wide and fixed	3
• Pupil or corneal reflex absent	2
• Pupil and corneal reflex absent	1
• Absent pupil, corneal, and cough reflex	0
Respiration	
• Not intubated, regular breathing pattern	4
• Not intubated and Cheyne–Stokes breathing	3
• Not intubated and irregular breathing	2
• Breathes higher than ventilator rate	1
• Breathes at ventilator rate, apnea	0

ETIOLOGY OF ALTERED SENSORIUM AND COMA

Infectious or Inflammatory

- *Infectious:*
  - Bacterial meningitis
  - Viral encephalitis/meningoencephalitis
  - Rickettsial infections
  - Helminthic infestation
  - Protozoan infection
  - Fungal infection
- *Inflammatory:*
  - Sepsis-associated encephalopathy
  - Acute disseminated encephalomyelitis (ADEM)
  - Demyelination
  - Vasculitis
  - Collagen vascular diseases

Structural

- *Traumatic:* Varying degree of severity can be seen in this situation, care has to be closely coordinated with intensivist, radiologist, neurologist, and neurosurgeon. Emergent intervention is advised in epidural hematoma and subdural hematoma:
  - Cerebral contusion
  - Concussion
  - Epidural hematoma
  - Intracerebral hematoma
  - Diffuse axonal injury
  - Abusive head trauma
- *Vascular:* A rapid and emergent neuroimaging in children with abrupt-to-acute onset altered sensorium evolving over minutes to hours with or without hemiparesis is imperative:
  - *Cerebral infarction:* Anterior or posterior circulation arterial ischemic stroke or cerebral venous sinus thrombosis (CVST)
  - *Cerebral hemorrhage:* Subarachnoid hemorrhage, arteriovenous (AV) malformation, and aneurysm
  - Trauma to carotid/vertebral artery
- *Neoplasm*
- *Brain* abscess and cerebritis
- Hydrocephalus

Metabolic, Toxic, and Nutritional

- Metabolic
  - Hypoglycemia, fluid, and electrolyte imbalance always need to be ruled out in all children presenting to emergency with encephalopathy.
  - *With acidosis:* Diabetic ketoacidosis (DKA), organic acidemia, aminoacidopathies (the latter two conditions are common in <1–2 years of age, especially with consanguineous parents.)
  - *With hyperammonemia:* Urea cycle disorder and hepatic encephalopathy
  - *Others:* Uremia, mitochondrial disorder, and Leigh's syndrome
- *Nutritional:* Vitamin deficiencies (thiamine, niacin, pyridoxin dependency, folate, and B_{12})
- *Hypoxic–ischemic encephalopathy*
  - Shock
  - Cardiac/pulmonary failure
  - Near drowning
  - Carbon monoxide (CO) poisoning and strangulation.

Others

- Hypertensive encephalopathy
- Burn encephalopathy
- Alcohol intoxication (predominantly in certain communities in younger children or generally in adolescents)
- Illegal drugs

HISTORY AND EXAMINATION

A careful history will help to identify the etiology and associated complications and determine the prognosis:

- Identification of the cause (primary and secondary) of altered sensorium
- Consideration of all potentially treatable causes that can be completely reversed
- Detection of complications such as raised intracranial complications, cerebral edema, seizures, etc.

Onset of altered sensorium can give a clue:

- *Sudden onset:* Intracranial hemorrhage or a convulsion
- *Acute onset:* In normal child—ingestion of drug, toxin, and poison
- *Gradual onset:* Infectious process and metabolic derangement
- *Intermittent episode:* Ingestion, drug overdose, and inborn errors of metabolism (IEM).
- *Recurrent episode:* Use of ophthalmic drops brimonidine can cause coma in 1-month child, epilepsy, and IEM.

ASSOCIATED SYMPTOMS

- *Fever:* Infections
- *Headache, vomiting, and diplopia:* Increased ICP of any etiology
- *Neck stiffness:* Meningitis and subarachnoid hemorrhage (SAH)
- *Rash:* Dengue, Rickettsial infection, and enteroviral infections
- *History of excess cry, irritability, enlarging head in infants:* Meningitis and SAH
- *Retinal hemorrhage, metaphyseal, rib, subdural hemorrhage, bleeding from ear/nose:* Traumatic brain injury.
- *Seizures:* Intracerebral hemorrhage (ICH), intracranial space-occupying lesion (ICSOL), epilepsy, and postictal
- *History of infectious disease:* Mumps (recently, there has been resurgence of neurological complications associated with mumps as the National Immunization schedule does not include mumps), measles, tuberculosis (TB), malaria, and dengue
- Failure to thrive, vomiting, peculiar skin and urine odor

METABOLIC CAUSES

- *Hepatic encephalopathy:* Jaundice, abdominal distension, hematemesis, melena, and bleeding
- *Uremic encephalopathy:* Decreased urine output, swelling, periorbital puffiness, nausea, vomiting, and loss of appetite
- *CO poisoning:* History of use of stove/heater
- *History of loose stools:* Hemolytic uremic syndrome (HUS), hypovolemia, ingestion of toxins/poisons, and medications
- *History of diabetes:* Hypoglycemia/ketoacidosis
- *History of congenital heart disease*: Brain abscess/infarction
- *History of immunocompromised state*: Malignancy
- History of birth asphyxia and family history of TB, migraine, epilepsy

PHYSICAL AND NEUROLOGICAL EXAMINATION

Vital Signs

- *Temperature:*
  - *Fever:* Meningitis, encephalitis, intracranial abscess, sepsis, and pneumonia
  - *Hypothermia:* Sepsis (especially in infants), shock, barbiturate poisoning, and hypoglycemia
  - Very high fever and dry skin indicate heat stroke (with global warming, this phenomenon is going to be recognized increasingly during the summer times, especially in developing countries)
- *Heart rate:*
  - *Bradycardia*: Increased ICP, myocardial injury due to hypoxia, and sepsis
  - *Tachycardia:* Shock, infections, fever, heart failure (young infant with cardiac failure and encephalopathy, in rice-eating communities, consider acquired thiamine deficiency)
  - *Irregular:* Arrhythmias and myocardial stunning can also happen with rhombencephalitis.
- *Respiratory rate:* Most common abnormal breathing pattern is neurogenic hyperventilation, which is seen with diffuse cortical involvement.
  - *Bradypnea/apnea:* Drug intoxication and septicemia
  - *Tachypnea:* Metabolic acidosis, pneumonia, asthma, pulmonary embolism, and brainstem lesion
  - *Cheyne–Stokes breathing:* B/L cortical damage with intact brainstem
  - *Irregular/ataxic breathing:* Medullary involvement
  - *Hyperventilation:* Low midbrain or pontine lesion
  - *Apneustic:* Lateral tegmentum or lower pontine lesion
  - *Slow periodic:* Raised ICP
- *Blood pressure*:
  - *Hypertension (HTN):* Increased ICP or stroke, HTN encephalopathy, early acute cerebral visual impairment in association with encephalopathy is a clue towards this etiology (detailed evaluation of cause of hypertension is essential, most common pathology being renal in origin).
  - *Hypotension:* Shock, sepsis, drug ingestion, myocardial injury/failure, and adrenal insufficiency
- SPO_2 monitoring

NEUROLOGICAL ASSESSMENT

- Level of consciousness
- Pupillary responses
- Brainstem function
- Motor response
- Other neurological findings
- Herniation syndrome
- The level of consciousness must be recorded in the form of an objective scale.

Eye findings: Careful eye movement examination provides wealth of information to localize the disease and also in estimating the severity of encephalopathy **(Table 5)**.

Eye findings and their common causes are given in **Table 5**.

TABLE 5: Eye findings and their common causes.

Finding	*Common causes*
Position	
Eyes and head deviated to one side	Hemispheric lesion on that side or pontine lesion on opposite side—typically associated with hemiparesis
Ocular fundoscopy	
Papilledema	Increased intracranial pressure
Exudates, hemorrhages, and vessel-crossing changes	Hypertensive encephalopathy
Subhyaloid hemorrhage	Subarachnoid hemorrhage

Size and reactivity of pupil ***(Table 6)****:* All this information is readily available in standard textbooks.

TABLE 6: Pupil findings and causes.

Pupils	*Cause*
Symmetrically reactive round	Usually excludes midbrain damage; if extraocular movements and corneal reflexes are absent, it suggests metabolic disorder or drug toxicity
Mid position—fixed or irregular	Midbrain lesion
Pinpoint	Pons, opiates, and cholinergic intoxication
Unilateral, dilated, and fixed	Uncal herniation
Bilateral, dilated, and fixed	Severe midbrain damage
Skew deviation (one up and one down)	Brainstem lesion
Forced downward deviation	Thalamic hemorrhage
Findings	Cause
Oculocephalic or doll's eye reflex	Full and conjugate eye movements rule out brainstem lesion; if suspected cervical spine injury, do oculovestibular reflex testing instead

Contd…

Contd...

Pupils	*Cause*
Ocular bobbing (brisk downward and slow upward movement with loss of horizontal movements)	Bilateral pontine damage
Ocular dipping (slower arrhythmic downward and faster upward movements with normal horizontal gaze)	Diffuse anoxic damage to cerebral cortex
Oculovestibular reflex	Bilateral deviation toward nystagmus away from the stimulated side excludes a structural brainstem lesion; abnormal slow phase in one or both directions suggests brainstem damage; abnormal fast phases in either direction with normal slow phases suggest bilateral cerebral hemisphere disorder

BRAINSTEM FUNCTION

- Pupillary light reflex
- Oculocephalic reflex (doll's eye reflex)
- Corneal reflex
- Oculovestibular reflex (caloric reflex)
- Gag and cough reflex

MOTOR RESPONSE

- *Decorticate posturing:* Flexion of the upper extremities and extension of the lower extremities suggest involvement of the cerebral cortex and preservation of brainstem function.
- *Decerebrate posturing:* Rigid extension of the arms and legs is indicative of cortical and brainstem damage.
- *Flaccid response:* No response to painful stimuli has the worst prognosis with injury to deep brainstem lesions.

INITIAL INVESTIGATIONS

- Blood sugars, sodium, potassium, magnesium, calcium
- *Blood counts:* Hemoglobin, blood counts, platelets, peripheral smear study, and coagulation profile
- Liver function test (LFT), renal function test (RFT) (end-organ dysfunction)
- Urine analysis, sugar, albumin, casts, reducing sugars, ketones, bile pigments, etc.
- Microbiological workup, blood, and cerebrospinal fluid (CSF) culture and serological studies for bacteria, mycobacteria, virus, fungus, *Leptospira*, and protozoa
- *CSF analysis:* It is performed in most instances after some form of neuroimaging, especially in children with deep coma and asymmetrical neurological signs. Analyze pressure, color, cells, proteins, sugar, gram and acid-fast bacteria (AFB) staining, serology, and culture and sensitivity (C&S)
- Ammonia and lactate

SECOND LINE: NEUROIMAGING PROCEDURES

These include computed tomography (CT) scan and magnetic resonance imaging (MRI) brain.

Essential for trauma, suspected space-occupying lesions (abscess, granulomas, tumors, enclosed hemorrhages, focal seizures, papilledema, and focal neurological sign), neuroimaging has to be performed.

Other Investigations

Perform electroencephalogram (EEG), viral serology, autoimmune panel, and metabolic panel. Common EEG findings and interpretation are given in **Table 7**.

TABLE 7: Common electroencephalogram (EEG) findings and their interpretation.

EEG Findings	*Interpretation*
High voltage, slow waves	Underlying supratentorial lesion
Slowing of background activity	Metabolic coma
Triphasic waves	Hepatic coma
Periodic lateralized epileptiform discharges (PLEDS)	Herpes encephalitis and any irritating lesion lateralized to one side

MANAGEMENT

Approach to Altered Sensorium

ABCDE Approach:

- *A*—Check to see that the *Airway* is open and protected. Hypoxia is a potentially reversible cause of altered sensorium.
- *B*—Assess *Breathing*: Inadequate ventilation will lead to elevated levels of CO_2 (respiratory acidosis) and can cause altered sensorium (AS).
- *C*—Assess *Circulatory* status: Hypoperfusion starves the brain of oxygen and glucose, which leads to altered sensorium.
- *D*—Check for neurologic *Disability*: Use GCS or AVPU scale for a quick assessment of level of consciousness. Look for seizure activity. Are the pupils equal and reactive? Pay attention to spontaneous movements. Lack of movement on one side of the body might indicate stroke while lack of movement below a certain level of the body could indicate spinal cord injury. If there is any suspicion of trauma, the cervical spine should be stabilized.
- *E*—*Expose* and perform a rapid head-to-toe look for any skin rash.

Initial steps for management:

- Assessment of the ABC's
- Cardiac monitoring and pulse oximetry
- Supplement oxygen
- Bedside glucose testing
- Intravenous access
- Evaluation for signs of trauma and consider cervical spine stabilization
- Consider naloxone administration, if narcotic overdose is suspected
- *If GCS <8:* Abnormal pupil size and reaction, absent doll's eye movements, abnormal tone or posturing, hypertension with bradycardia, and abnormal respiratory pattern: *Act immediately* with following:
  - For fluid restriction, elevate the head end of bed at 30°
  - Intubate and short-term hyperventilation, 20% mannitol/furosemide/3% normal saline (NS) (if in shock)
  - Sedation, barbiturate therapy, reduced fever, high dose of corticosteroids, and decompressive craniotomy
  - *Temperature:* Treat fever and hypothermia

- *Acid-base and electrolytes imbalance:* To be corrected. *Specific antidotes:* Naloxone for opiate overdose and flumazenil for benzodiazepine overdose.
- *Stop seizures:* Specific treatment for status epilepticus and other seizure emergencies—give IV lorazepam 0.1–0.2 mg/kg, then phenytoin 20 mg/kg loading followed by maintenance with other antiseizure medications (ASM) as required.
- *Treat infections:* Appropriate antibiotic/antiviral/antimalarial therapy to be started.
- Manage agitation

Clinical Parameters to be Monitored

- Temperature
- Pulse
- Heart rate
- Blood pressure
- Coma severity by modified GCS (mGCS)
- Respiratory pattern
- Pupillary and corneal reflexes
- Extraocular movements

Signs to be monitored:

- Motor patterns
- Seizure type
- Fundus picture
    - All clinical parameters and signs must be recorded at admission and at regular intervals everyday till the child recovers from coma.
    - A low pulse pressure with elevated blood pressure may indicate raised ICP.

Principles of Treatment

The principle of treatment are as follows:

- *Regular monitoring* sensorium by GCS and maintenance of vital functions are important till the child has completely recovered. Urine output must be monitored. Vital parameters such as airway, respiration, and circulation must be maintained.
- *Maintenance of electrolytes, fluid balance, glucose homeostasis, and nutrition* is essential. In prolonged coma, intragastric feeding with a diet containing adequate calories and proteins must be instituted. Nursing care includes the care of eyes, skin, bladder, and bowel. Maintenance of normal temperature is of great importance.
- *Specific and supportive* treatment must be directed towards diagnosis.

- *Raised ICP* is controlled with judicious sedation, appropriate positioning, and osmotic agents.
- *Seizures* are treated with anticonvulsants and those that can cause respiratory depression should be avoided.
- *Infections* are to be treated with specific antimicrobials/antivirals (broad antibiotics cover along with doxycycline, azithromycin as atypical organism cover, acyclovir in children with isolated CNS involvement) (presence of systemic involvement points to diagnoses other than herpes simplex encephalitis).
- Immunotherapy in autoimmune encephalitis is done in liaison with neurologist
- Intracranial fluid, blood, or pus collections must be surgically removed whenever indicated.
- *Antidotes* with supportive measures and toxin elimination procedures will save comatose children from poisons.
- *Assisted ventilation* may be warranted whenever there is respiratory insufficiency. Respiratory support is usually required if GCS is <7; aim is to keep $PaCO_2$ levels at 35 and not produce either hypo or hypercarbia.

The management of ICP involves early recognition and a stepwise approach.

- *Step 1:* Head-end elevation (20–30 degree)
  - Avoiding neck flexion
  - Judicious sedation and analgesia
  - Maintaining normothermia
  - Prevention of hypoxia, hypercarbia, hypoglycemia, and seizures
- *Step 2:* Those who continue to show signs of raised ICP are managed with osmotic agents.
  - *Preferred osmotic agents:* IV hypertonic saline and mannitol.
- *Steps 3:* Those who have persistent signs of raised ICP are considered for more aggressive medical measures with following.
  - Barbiturate infusion
  - Surgical measures (decompressive craniectomy) as indicated
  - If the child has any features of herniation, hyperventilation (PCO_2: 25–30) for a period of 10–15 minutes along with deepening of sedation is done.
  - Additional dose of osmotic agents should be tried depending on the clinical situation.

Prognosis with altered sensorium is *good* if the treatable causes are identified early and treated appropriately and adequately.

- The *worst* prognosis is seen with the children with a GCS score of 3.
- Scores of 3–5 are *potentially fatal*, especially if accompanied by fixed pupils or absent oculovestibular responses or elevated ICP.
- Scores of 7 and above are associated with *better* chances of recovery.

The algorithmic approach to management of acute encephalopathy is given in **Flowchart 1.**

Flowchart 1: Algorithmic approach to management of acute encephalopathy.

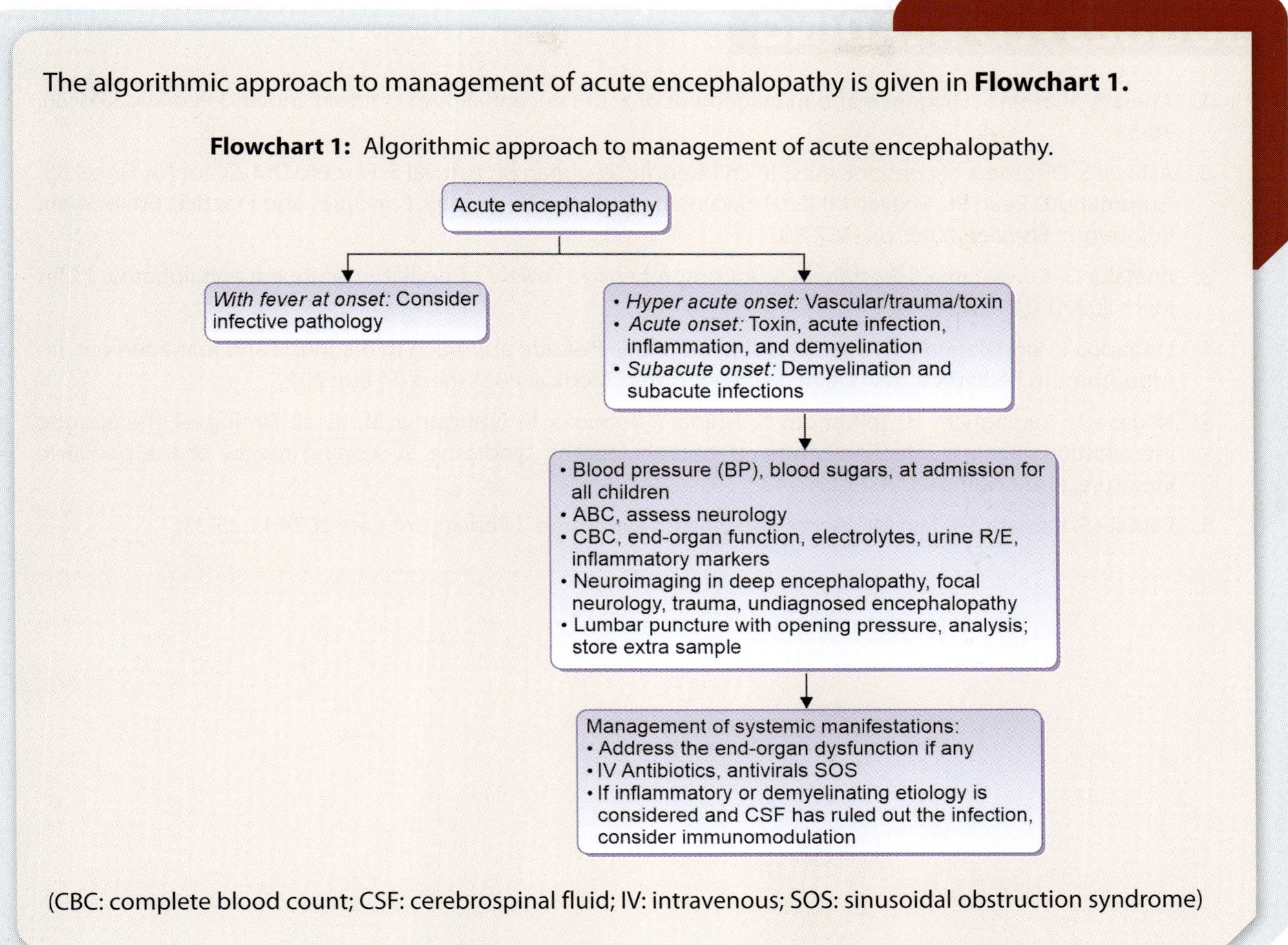

(CBC: complete blood count; CSF: cerebrospinal fluid; IV: intravenous; SOS: sinusoidal obstruction syndrome)

CONCLUSION

Acute encephalopathy is of diverse etiology, a systematic approach is essential to cover the most common causes early on to reduce the damage to brain and improve long-term outcomes.

SUGGESTED READING

1. Aneja S, Sharma S. Diagnosis and management of acute encephalitis in children. Indian J Pediatr. 2019;86: 70-5.
2. Ashwal S. Disorders of consciousness in children. In: Swaiman KF, Ashwal S, Ferriero DM, Schor NF, Finkel RS, Gropman AL, Pearl PL, Shevell MI (Eds). Swaiman's Pediatric Neurology. Principles and Practice, 6th edition. Edinburgh: Elsevier; 2018. pp. 767-80.
3. Imataka G, Kuwashima S, Yoshihara S. A Comprehensive review of pediatric acute encephalopathy. J Clin Med. 2022;11(19):5921.
4. Lingappa L, Siddaiahgari S. Afebrile encephalopathy: Bedside approach to diagnosis and management. In: Algorithms in Pediatrics. New Delhi: Jaypee Brothers Medical Publishers (P) Ltd; 2017.
5. Nagase H, Yamaguchi H, Tokumoto S, Ishida Y, Tomioka K, Nishiyama M, et al. Timing of therapeutic interventions against infection-triggered encephalopathy syndrome: A scoping review of the pediatric literature. Front Neurosci. 2023;17:1-40
6. Patnaik S, Kamath SR, Jain MK. Acute encephalitis syndrome. J Pediatr Crit Care 2024;11:25-31.

18

Pediatric Status Epilepticus

Aakash Chandran, Renu Suthar

INTRODUCTION

Pediatric status epilepticus (PSE) is the most common emergency presenting to the pediatric emergency department. The incidence of convulsive status epilepticus (CSE) ranges from 10–73 episodes/100,000 children and is most significant among children below 2 years of age.[1] The mortality in children with SE ranges between 2.7–8%, with an overall morbidity ranging from 10–20%.[2]

DEFINITION

Conventionally, CSE was defined as continuous seizure activity lasting for ≥30 minutes or ≥2 seizures during this duration without regaining consciousness between these episodes.[1] This definition was based on data from animals that irreversible neuronal damage sets in after 30 minutes of continuous seizures. However, recent data suggest that neuronal damage begins much earlier, and there is a need to redefine status epilepticus (SE).[3-5]

The International League Against Epilepsy redefined SE as "an ongoing seizure activity due to failure of mechanisms responsible for seizure termination or initiation of mechanisms provoking ongoing seizures causing prolonged seizures (after timepoint t1), and which can have long-term consequences (after timepoint t2) including neuronal death, neuronal injury, and alteration of neuronal networks, depending on the type and duration of seizures". This definition includes two operational timepoints: Timepoint t1 is the time beyond which the body's inherent mechanisms cannot control the seizure activity, and treatment should be initiated. Beyond t1, the electrical activity is regarded as "abnormally prolonged seizure". Timepoint t2 is the time duration of ongoing seizure activity beyond which there are long-term consequences; hence, treatment should be instituted aggressively to control seizures[6] **(Table 1)**.

The various terms used in PSE are defined in **Table 2**. The common etiologies of PSE are outlined in **Box 1**.

TABLE 1: Time points t1 and t2 for various seizure semiologies.		
Time points	***t1***	***t2***
Tonic-clonic status epilepticus	5 minutes	30 minutes
Focal status epilepticus with impaired consciousness	10 minutes	>60 minutes
Absence status epilepticus	10–15 minutes	Unknown

TABLE 2: Definitions of various terms used in pediatric status epilepticus.	
Terms	***Definitions***
Established status epilepticus	Status epilepticus (SE) that persists after treatment with a first-line antiseizure medication (ASM) (benzodiazepines)
Refractory status epilepticus (RSE)	SE that persists after treatment with first-line (benzodiazepines) and second-line ASM (phenytoin or levetiracetam or valproate or phenobarbitone)
New-onset refractory state epilepticus (NORSE)	Clinical condition characterized by the new onset of RSE in a child without previous/active epilepsy or other significant preexisting neurological diseases/disorders (stroke, brain tumor, drug overdoses, etc.) and without a clear acute or active structural, metabolic, or toxic cause
Febrile infection-related epilepsy syndrome (FIRES)	It is a subcategory of NORSE, applicable for all age-groups that requires a prior febrile infection/illness starting between 2 weeks and 24 hours before the onset of RSE, with or without fever at the onset of SE
Super-refractory status epilepticus (SRSE)	SE that persists for >24 hours despite treatment with anesthetic agents or recurs while weaning the anesthetic agent
Prolonged SRSE	SRSE lasting for 7 days or more, including ongoing need for anesthetic agents

BOX 1: Common etiologies of pediatric status epilepticus.

Known

Acute symptomatic
- Acute CNS infections (encephalitis, meningitis)
- Stroke
- Anoxic/hypoxic injury
- Metabolic causes (hypoglycemia, hypocalcemia, hyperglycemia, hyponatremia)
- Traumatic brain injury
- Drug-related (antiseizure medications noncompliance or withdrawal)

Remote
- Post-traumatic
- Postencephalitic
- Poststroke

Progressive
- Brain tumor
- Neurodegenerative diseases

SE in defined electroclinical syndromes (Lennox–Gestaut syndrome or Dravet syndrome)

- *Cryptogenic:* Entities like NORSE or FIRES
- *Unknown*

(CNS: central nervous system; FIRES: febrile infection-related epilepsy syndrome; NORSE: new-onset refractory state epilepticus; PSE: pediatric status epilepticus; SE: status epilepticus)

OBJECTIVES OF MANAGEMENT

- Maintain airway, breathing, and circulation.
- Seizure termination and prevention of recurrence
- Management of refractory status epilepticus (RSE) and super-refractory status epilepticus (SRSE)
- Diagnosing and initiating treatment for life-threatening causes of PSE (meningitis, encephalitis, hypoglycemia, hypocalcemia, cerebral space-occupying lesions) and ongoing search for etiology of prolonged PSE

Maintain Airway, Breathing, and Circulation

In PSE, the most common immediate cause of death is an unstable airway. Managing the airway is the first and the most crucial step in treating PSE. General measures to stabilize ABC are mentioned in **Table 3**. Seizures usually lead to catecholamine surge and increase in metabolic rate, which increases the cerebral oxygen demand; therefore, all children who are seizing should be started on oxygen. Tachycardia and elevated blood pressure are seen during the seizure episode but should return to normal once seizures are controlled. Bradycardia, poor perfusion, and hypotension are ominous signs indicating severe hypoxemia. These suggest an immediate and compelling need to establish a definitive airway and provide mechanical ventilation to the child. Indications of endotracheal intubation are mentioned in **Box 2**.

TABLE 3: General measures to stabilize ABC.

Airway	• Positioning the child on their side (recovery position) • Suctioning of easily accessible airway secretions • Securing the airway, if it is not maintainable or obstructed
Breathing	• Start oxygen • Start mechanical ventilation if respiratory depression, persistent seizures, or depressed mental status
Circulation	• Secure intravenous or intraosseous access • Obtain samples for blood glucose, calcium, culture (if indicated), levels of ASM (if already on ASM) • Maintain euvolemia and normotension • Initiate and titrate fluids and vasoactive drugs to maintain vital organ perfusion with targets to achieve normal hemodynamic parameters, peripheral perfusion, and blood pressure values for age.

(ABC: airway, breathing, circulation; ASM: antiseizure medication)

BOX 2: Indications for endotracheal intubation in status epilepticus.

All the four conditions are not mutually exclusive and are interlinked:
1. Unstable or obstructed airway
2. Respiratory depression
3. Persistent seizures
4. Depressed mental status

Seizure Termination and Prevention of Recurrence

Correctable Factors

All correctable causes for acute symptomatic seizure should be ruled out with point-of-care testing of glucose, sodium, and calcium. If any of these is abnormal, treat them appropriately.

First-line Antiseizure Medications

Benzodiazepines (BZD) are the first-line antiseizure medication (ASM) for PSE. The available options in a prehospital setting include intramuscular or buccal midazolam, buccal lorazepam, or rectal diazepam. In a hospital setting, intravenous lorazepam (0.1 mg/kg, maximum 4 mg) or intravenous/intramuscular midazolam (0.2 mg/kg, maximum 5 mg) is preferred. Diazepam can be sued in dose of 0.2–0.3 mg/kg IV stat (maximum 10 mg). If seizures do not abort within 5 minutes of a single dose of BZD, a second dose of BZD should be administered. If the seizures continue even after two doses of BZD, then second-line ASM should be initiated.

Second-line Antiseizure Medications

For seizures refractory to BZD, second-line ASM should be used. These include phenytoin/fosphenytoin, levetiracetam, valproate, or phenobarbitone. Phenytoin is administered at 20 mg/kg (maximum 1 g) in normal saline (NS) at the rate of 1 mg/kg/min. Fosphenytoin dose is 20 mg/kg (phenytoin equivalent) at the rate of 3 mg/kg/min. Levetiracetam is usually administered at 40–60 mg/kg (maximum 3 g) at 5 mg/kg/min, while valproate is given a bolus dose of 20–40 mg/kg. Phenobarbitone as a second-line ASM is considered inferior to the above three options. Nevertheless, it can be used if the above three ASMs are unavailable. The dose of phenobarbitone is 20 mg/kg in NS at the rate of 2 mg/kg/min.

Current Evidence for Second-line Antiseizure Medications

Recently, three trials evaluated efficacy of second-line ASMs in PSE. In the ConSEPT trial,[7] participants were randomized to receive either phenytoin (20 mg/kg) or levetiracetam (40 mg/kg). Authors found no statistically significant difference in the primary outcome (clinical termination of seizures 5 minutes after the completion of study drug infusion) between the two agents. The EcLIPSE trial[8] found no significant difference between phenytoin and levetiracetam regarding clinical cessation of seizures. The ESETT trial[9] compared levetiracetam, fosphenytoin, and valproate and demonstrated that all three groups had similar (52%, 49%, and 52%, respectively) efficacy for primary outcome (cessation of clinical seizures with improvement in consciousness and without additional ASM at 1 hour from the start of the ASM).

A recent meta-analysis [12 randomized controlled trials (RCTs) with 2,293 children] comparing levetiracetam and phenytoin as second-line ASM for PSE demonstrated that the cessation of seizures within 5–60 minutes was similar in both the groups (82% vs. 77.5%, respectively; $p = 0.30$). However, in the phenytoin group, there were higher seizure recurrences within 1–24 hours (16.6% vs. 9.7%, respectively; $p = 0.01$), and higher proportion of children required endotracheal intubation and mechanical ventilation (21.4% vs. 14.2%, respectively; $p = 0.04$) as compared to the levetiracetam group.[10] Another adult meta-analysis, including 9 RCTs with 1,732 patients, compared levetiracetam and phenytoin as second-line ASMs for seizure cessation and found no significant differences between the two ASMs.[11]

Management of Refractory Status Epilepticus and Super-refractory Status Epilepticus

Seizures not responding to two ASMs, one of which is BZD, are termed refractory status epilepticus. If one of the second-line ASMs does not abort the seizures, one of the other classes of second-line ASMs can be tried. Beyond the first hour of seizures' onset, second-line ASMs are less likely to work, and hence, different strategies need to be opted for seizure control. Managing RSE involve the administration of a continuous infusion of anesthetic agents like midazolam, thiopentone, high-dose phenobarbital, magnesium sulphate, ketamine, or propofol. The most used anesthetic agent is midazolam. The starting dose is 4 µg/kg/min and hiked up to 15–20 µg/kg/min. The doses of other ASMs/anesthetic agents are mentioned in **Table 4**. Tapering of anesthetic infusions is started after a seizure-free interval of 24–48 hours. RSE is usually managed in a pediatric intensive care unit (PICU) setup, with continuous EEG monitoring. Since these medications cause respiratory depression, advanced airway and mechanical ventilation should be established at this stage.[12]

Seizures that persist beyond 24 hours despite anesthetic infusion or recur during tapering of anesthetic agents are termed super-refractory status epilepticus. Management options involve a trial of other anesthetic drugs (thiopentone, pentobarbital, propofol, or ketamine). Other options include topiramate (through an orogastric/nasogastric tube) immunotherapy [steroids, intravenous immunoglobulin (IVIG), and biologicals like tocilizumab/anakinra], ketogenic diet, therapeutic hypothermia, vagal nerve stimulation, and epilepsy surgery.[13]

TABLE 4: Dosages of common antiseizure medications used in pediatric status epilepticus.

Drugs	*Dosage*
Midazolam	Stat dose: 0.15–0.2 mg/kg IV bolus (maximum 5 mg) Infusion: Start at 4 µg/kg/min, hiked up to 15–20 µg/kg/min
Lorazepam	0.1 mg/kg IV (maximum 4 mg)
Diazepam	0.2–0.3 mg/kg IV (maximum 10 mg)
Phenytoin	20 mg/kg IV (maximum 1 g) in NS at the rate of 1 mg/kg/min
Fosphenytoin	20 mg/kg IV of phenytoin equivalent at the rate of 3 mg/kg/min
Phenobarbitone	20 mg/kg IV in normal saline at the rate of 2 mg/kg/min
Levetiracetam	40–60 mg/kg IV bolus (maximum at 4500 mg) at 5 mg/kg/min followed by 20–30 mg/kg IV BD (maximum 3000 mg/day)
Valproate	20–40 mg/kg IV over 15 minutes followed by infusion of 5 mg/kg/hour
Propofol	Loading dose of 1–2 mg/kg followed by infusion dose of 1 mg/kg/hr; maximum hiked to 5 mg/kg/hr
Thiopentone	Loading dose of 5 mg/kg bolus followed by infusion dose of 1 mg/kg/hr; maximum hiked to 5 mg/kg/hr
Ketamine	Loading dose 1–2 mg/kg, followed by infusion dose of 1 mg/kg/hr; maximum hiked to 6 mg/kg/hr
Magnesium sulfate	Loading dose 50 mg/kg over 30 minutes (maximum dose 4 g/dose) followed by maintenance dose of 20 mg/kg/hr up to 40 mg/kg/hr (maximum daily dose is 40 g/day). Maintain serum magnesium levels 2–4 mmol/L
Topiramate	2–5 mg/kg/day, increased to 25 mg/kg/day at 5–10 mg/kg/day increments (enteral)

The child should be referred to a tertiary care hospital if there are one or more indications as highlighted in **Table 5**.

TABLE 5: Indications for referral to tertiary care hospital.	
Need of mechanical ventilation and children with fluid refractory and catecholamine resistant shock	Stabilize ABC before referral
Raised intracranial pressure	For monitoring and management of raised ICP
Children with RSE and SRSE	Requiring IV anesthetic medications
Need for continuous EEG monitoring	In cases with suspected NCSE
For brain imaging and other advanced tests	If not available at referring center

(ABC: airway, breathing, circulation; NCSE: nonconvulsive status epilepticus; RSE: refractory status epilepticus; SRSE: super-refractory status epilepticus)

Diagnosis and Initiating Treatment for Life-threatening Causes of Pediatric Status Epilepticus

Prolonged febrile seizures are regarded as the most common cause of PSE. This may not warrant a detailed and extensive workup. Similarly, a child with a known epileptic disorder, on anticonvulsant therapy, presenting with SE may not be worked up extensively.

However, when the etiology of PSE is not clear from history and examination, consider the laboratory investigations shown in **Table 6**.

TABLE 6: Laboratory investigations.

Investigations	*Comments*
Blood glucose, electrolytes (sodium, calcium, magnesium)	For correctable cause of acute symptomatic seizure
Complete blood count and differential	For infective etiology
Cultures	If possibility of sepsis or meningitis. It should not delay treatment
Urine and blood for toxicology screening	In case of sudden unexplained seizures
ASM levels	In children on long-term ASM therapy
Lumbar puncture	If suspicion of meningitis or encephalitis
Computed tomography (CT) head	In children with any unexplained loss of consciousness, features of raised ICP, history of trauma, or focal neurological signs. But it should not delay the treatment
Magnetic resonance imaging (MRI)	It may highlight features not identified on a CT but it is not readily available at all centers
EEG	It should be used in all cases, if feasible. Continuous EEG is preferred. It is useful to detect nonconvulsive status epileptics, guide therapy, and help in prognostication
Autoimmune panel (CSF/serum) and a CSF viral panel	In cases of prolonged PSE.
ICP monitoring	In prolonged PSE in centers where facility is available

(ASM: antiseizure medication; CSF: cerebrospinal fluid; ICP: intracranial pressure; PSE: pediatric status epilepticus)

NONCONVULSIVE STATUS EPILEPTICUS

Nonconvulsive status epilepticus (NCSE) is defined as change in behavior and/or mental status from baseline, which is associated with changes in EEG but without motor signs. Continuous EEG monitoring may be helpful in the diagnosis of NCSE. NCSE in children is often underestimated, and the frequency has been reported to be about 10–20 cases/100,000/year.[14] The incidence of NCSE in comatose patients admitted to PICU has been reported between 7–30% in different studies.[15-17] NCSE should always be suspected if there is no recovery in consciousness as expected after the seizures are stopped. The frequently observed clinical signs include changes in behavior, attention, awareness, cognition, memory, communication, and/or motor skills. The common etiologies include CNS infections, hypoxia, toxic and metabolic syndromes, and epileptic encephalopathy syndromes.

CONCLUSION

PSE is one of the most common pediatric emergencies. Time is brain; hence, prompt recognition and early initiation of therapies for seizures are paramount in limiting the morbidity and mortality associated with PSE. Assessment and stabilization of airway, breathing, and circulation is the first step followed by seizure control and prevention of seizure recurrence. First-line ASM medications include BZD and second-line medications include phenytoin/fosphenytoin, levetiracetam, and valproate. These days, levetiracetam is the preferred second-line ASM. Treatment of RSE and SRSE include time-bound use of anesthetic agents, mechanical ventilation in PICU, hemodynamic and respiratory monitoring, and continuous EEG monitoring. The time-bound management of PSE[18] is summarized in **Table 7**.

TABLE 7: Time-bound management of pediatric status epilepticus.

Time line	*Management strategies*
At arrival (0–5 minutes)	
• *Supportive care:* – Control and management of airway, breathing, and circulation – History of epilepsy/AED use • *Investigations:* – Blood for glucose, calcium, magnesium, sodium, ABG, CBC, and cultures (if febrile)	• *Management:* Intravenous first-line ASMs are preferred • *Lorazepam:* 0.1 mg/kg stat (maximum 4 mg) OR • *Midazolam:* 0.15–0.2 mg/kg stat (maximum 5 mg) OR • *Diazepam:* 0.2–0.3 mg/kg stat (maximum 10 mg) • If IV access is unavailable, intramuscular, rectal, intranasal, or buccal routes can be used
5–20 minutes	
• *Supportive care:* – Plan shifting to PICU – Raised ICP: 3% saline/mannitol	• *Management:* If seizures persist, • Intravenous second-line ASM: – *Phenytoin:* 20 mg/kg in normal saline @ 1 mg/kg/min OR – *Fosphenytoin:* 20 mg/kg of phenytoin equivalent (PE) in normal saline @ 3 mg/kg/min OR – *Valproate:* 20–40 mg/kg OR – *Levetiracetam:* 40–60 mg/kg @ 5 mg/kg/min OR – *Phenobarbitone:* 20 mg/kg in normal saline @ 2 mg/kg/min – Thiamine 100 mg IV push; Pyridoxine 100 mg IV push in children <2 years of age

Contd...

Contd...

Time line	*Management strategies*
20–60 minutes	
Supportive care: Watch for hemodynamic and respiratory parameters, cardiac arrhythmia, raised ICP, rhabdomyolysis, sepsis, and organ functions	*Management:* Consider one of the other second-line ASM that was not administered earlier
1–24 hours (RSE)	
• *Supportive care:* – Shift to PICU – Mechanical ventilation – Continuous EEG monitoring • *Investigations:* – CT head or MRI brain (as per availability and clinical stability) – Screen for neuroinfections – Metabolic testing, autoimmune panel (based on clinical suspicion)	• *Management:* Anesthetic agents • *Midazolam:* 0.2 mg/kg IV bolus followed by infusion rate of 4 µg/kg/min. If seizures persist, increase 2 µg/kg/min every 5–10 minutes till seizures stop (usual maximum is 15–20 µg/kg/min). Initiate tapering after 24 hours of seizure-free period and decrease the infusion at a rate of 1 µg/kg/min, every 3 hours OR • *Thiopentone:* 5 mg/kg bolus as loading dose followed by continuous infusion at a rate of 3–5 mg/kg/hr to achieve burst suppression. Initiate tapering after 24–48 hours of seizure-free period. OR • *High-dose phenobarbitone:* Boluses of 5–10 mg/kg every 30 minutes up to a total dose of 120 mg/kg over 24 hours with target of seizure control and EEG burst suppression, OR • *Propofol:* Loading dose of 1–2 mg/kg, followed by continuous infusion of 1–2 mg/kg/hr, maximum of 5 mg/kg/h OR • *Ketamine:* 1–2 mg/kg bolus as loading dose followed by infusion at a rate of 3–5 mg/kg/hr • *Topiramate:* 2–5 mg/kg enteral loading (orogastric/nasogastric tube) and increase by 5–10 mg/kg/day up to a maximum of 25 mg/kg/day while tapering anesthetic medications
Beyond 24 hours (SRSE)	
• Supportive care: – PICU care – Mechanical ventilation – Continuous EEG monitoring – Watch for hemodynamic and respiratory parameters, cardiac arrhythmia, raised ICP, rhabdomyolysis, sepsis, and organ functions	• *Management:* Trial of other anesthetic drugs which were not used during the previous step • *Other therapeutic options:* Ketogenic diet: Consult with dietician • *Immunotherapy:* Pulse methylprednisolone OR IVIG OR biologicals • *Other:* Vagal nerve stimulation, therapeutic hypothermia, epilepsy surgery (in selected cases)

(ABG: arterial blood gas; CBC: complete blood count; ICP: intracranial pressure PICU: pediatric intensive care unit; IVIG: intravenous immunoglobulin SRSE: super-refractory status epilepticus RSE: refractory status epilepticus AED: automated external defibrillator ASM: antiseizure medication)

REFERENCES

1. Singh RK, Gaillard WD. Status epilepticus in children. Curr Neurol Neurosci Rep. 2009;9:137-44.
2. Sofou K, Kristjánsdóttir R, Papachatzakis NE, Ahmadzadeh A, Uvebrant P. Management of prolonged seizures and status epilepticus in childhood: a systematic review. J Child Neurol. 2009;24:918-26.
3. Towne AR, Pellock JM, Ko D, DeLorenzo RJ. Determinants of mortality in status epilepticus. Epilepsia. 1994;35:27-34.
4. DeLorenzo RJ, Garnett LK, Towne AR, Waterhouse EJ, Boggs JG, Morton L, et al. Comparison of status epilepticus with prolonged seizure episodes lasting from 10 to 29 minutes. Epilepsia. 1999;40:164-9.
5. Lowenstein DH, Bleck T, Macdonald RL. It's time to revise the definition of status epilepticus. Epilepsia. 1999;40:120-2.
6. Trinka E, Cock H, Hesdorffer D, Rossetti AO, Scheffer IE, Shinnar S, et al. A definition and classification of status epilepticus—report of the ILAE Task Force on Classification of Status Epilepticus. Epilepsia. 2015;56:1515-23.
7. Dalziel SR, Borland ML, Furyk J, Bonisch M, Neutze J, Donath S et al. Levetiracetam versus phenytoin for second-line treatment of convulsive status epilepticus in children (ConSEPT): an open-label, multicentre, randomised controlled trial. Lancet. 2019;393:2135-45.
8. Lyttle MD, Rainford NEA, Gamble C, Messahel S, Humphreys A, Hickey H et al. Paediatric Emergency Research in the United Kingdom & Ireland (PERUKI) collaborative. Levetiracetam versus phenytoin for second-line treatment of paediatric convulsive status epilepticus (EcLiPSE): a multicentre, open-label, randomised trial. Lancet. 2019;393:2125-34.
9. Chamberlain JM, Kapur J, Shinnar S, Elm J, Holsti M, Babcock L, et al. Efficacy of levetiracetam, fosphenytoin, and valproate for established status epilepticus by age group (ESETT): a double-blind, responsive-adaptive, randomised controlled trial. Lancet. 2020;395:1217-24.
10. Angurana SK, Suthar R. Efficacy and Safety of Levetiracetam vs. Phenytoin as Second Line Antiseizure Medication for Pediatric Convulsive Status Epilepticus: A Systematic Review and Meta-Analysis of Randomized Controlled Trials. J Trop Pediatr. 2021;67:fmab014.
11. DeMott JM, Slocum GW, Gottlieb M, Peksa GD. Levetiracetam vs. phenytoin as 2nd-line treatment for status epilepticus: A systematic review and meta-analysis. Epilepsy Behav. 2020;111:107286.
12. Rai S, Drislane FW. Treatment of Refractory and Super-refractory Status Epilepticus. Neurotherapeutics. 2018;15:697-712.
13. Ochoa JG, Dougherty M, Papanastassiou A, Gidal B, Mohamed I, Vossler DG. Treatment of Super-Refractory Status Epilepticus: A Review. Epilepsy Curr. 2021;21:1535759721999670.
14. Hamad AP, Ferrari-Marinho T, Caboclo LO, Thomé U, Fernandes RMF. Nonconvulsive status epilepticus in epileptic encephalopathies in childhood. Seizure. 2020;80:212-20.
15. El-Rashiedy OF, Ibrahim HM, Shatla RH. Nonconvulsive status epilepticus at pediatric intensive care unit: A single center experience. J Pediatr Res Rev Rep. 2021;1-6.
16. Shahwan A, Bailey C, Shekerdemian L, Harvey AS. The prevalence of seizures in comatose children in the pediatric intensive care unit: a prospective video-EEG study. Epilepsia. 2010;51:1198-204.
17. Towne AR, Waterhouse EJ, Boggs JG, Garnett LK, Brown AJ, Smith JR Jr, DeLorenzo RJ. Prevalence of nonconvulsive status epilepticus in comatose patients. Neurology. 2000;54:340-5.
18. Srivastava K, Chakraborty B, Gupta D. Evaluation and Management of Status Epilepticus in Children. Standard Treatment Guidelines. Indian Academy of Pediatrics. 2022.

19 Central Nervous System Infections

Yankappa N, Mounika Reddy

INTRODUCTION

Central nervous system (CNS) infections in children represent medical emergencies associated with significant morbidity and mortality and are the most common cause of nontraumatic coma.

TERMINOLOGIES AND DEFINITIONS

- Central nervous system infections encompass infections of the brain, spinal cord, optic nerves, and their surrounding membranes.
- Meningitis is inflammation of the meninges.
- Encephalitis denotes inflammation of the brain parenchyma.
- Brain abscess is a localized infection within the parenchyma.
- Acute encephalitis syndrome (AES) manifests as acute fever (≤5–7 days' duration) with altered mental status or consciousness and/or new-onset seizures (excluding simple febrile seizure) or focal neurological findings resulting from CNS inflammation.

ETIOPATHOGENESIS

Etiopathogenesis of central nervous system infections is given in **Table 1**.

TABLE 1: Etiopathogenesis of central nervous system infections.

Routes of transmission	
Nasopharyngeal colonization	Bacteremia and breach of blood–brain barrier (BBB)
Invasion from contiguous focus of infection	Paranasal sinusitis, otitis media, mastoiditis, orbital cellulitis, soft-tissue infection of face or scalp, dental infection, cranial or vertebral osteomyelitis
Direct compromise of BBB	Penetrating head injuries, surgical procedures, dermal sinus tracts, myelomeningocele
Embolic spread from distant sites	Lungs (empyema, lung abscess, bronchiectasis), heart (endocarditis), skin, gastrointestinal tract infections, kidney
Predisposing conditions	
Heart disease	Congenital or acquired (e.g., rheumatic)
Medical devices	Cerebrospinal fluid (CSF) shunts, cochlear implants, prosthetic valves
CSF leak	Congenital or acquired—dural sinus, cribriform plate, middle or inner ear fistula, skull trauma, neurosurgery
Immunodeficiency	Anatomic or functional asplenia (e.g. sickle cell disease), complement deficiency, hypogammaglobulinemia, HIV infection, glucocorticoid use, diabetes mellitus, chemotherapy, immunosuppressive therapy, primary immunodeficiency
Other factors	Unvaccinated children, close contact with affected persons, travel to an endemic or epidemic area

PRIMARY ASSESSMENT

Children with CNS infections may have one or more of the following physiological derangements:

- *Airway:* Maintainable or obstructed due to pooling of secretions, loss of protective reflexes, or hypotonia of oropharyngeal muscles
- *Breathing:* Tachypnea or bradypnea, increased or reduced work of breathing (hypoventilation), conducted sounds, hypoxia (SpO_2 <94%)
- *Circulation:* Tachycardia or bradycardia, features of shock or hypertension
- *Disability:* Altered consciousness, abnormal pupillary response, focal neurological deficits, features of raised intracranial pressure (ICP), hypoglycemia or hyperglycemia
- *Exposure:* Fever or hypothermia, surface findings such as pallor, icterus, rash, bleeding manifestations

FOCUSED HISTORY AND EXAMINATION

Complete neurological examination may point to potential cause and localization of brain dysfunction. One or more of the following features may be noted:

- Nonspecific symptoms of systemic infection—fever (or hypothermia in infants), headache, myalgia, arthralgia, anorexia, poor feeding, upper respiratory symptoms, diarrhea
- Examination may reveal pallor, petechiae, purpura, rash, icterus, eschar, hepatosplenomegaly, lymphadenopathy
- Features of meningeal irritation (due to inflammation of spinal nerves and roots)—neck pain or stiffness, back pain, Kernig sign (pain and resistance to knee extension when hips are 90° flexed), Brudzinski sign (involuntary flexion of knees and hips on passive neck flexion while supine)
- Seizures (focal or generalized)—due to fever, hypoglycemia, electrolyte disturbances, cerebritis, infarction
- Focal neurological deficits (e.g., hemiparesis in brain abscess)
- Altered consciousness (irritability, lethargy, stupor, obtundation, coma)—due to hypoglycemia, electrolyte imbalance, cerebritis, raised ICP, or shock
- Features of raised ICP—headache, emesis (projectile, often worse in the morning), bulging fontanelle, sutural diastasis, vision disturbances, oculomotor (anisocoria, ptosis, dilated or poorly responsive pupils) or abducens nerve paralysis, papilledema (not seen in acute raised ICP, develops in few days), hypertension with relative bradycardia, apnea or hyperventilation, decorticate or decerebrate posturing, stupor, coma, or signs of herniation. Cushing's triad (bradycardia, irregular breathing, and hypertension) is a late and ominous sign of brain herniation. Infants may present with unexplained irritability and persistent shrill cry.
- History regarding geographic location, recent travel, trauma, animal contact, insect or dog bite, drug or toxin exposure, recent immunization, past or concurrent systemic illness, immunocompromised status, and premorbid developmental or neurological status may provide clues to etiology or alternate diagnosis.

CLINICAL FEATURES IN SPECIFIC CENTRAL NERVOUS SYSTEM INFECTIONS

Clinical features in specific central nervous system infections are given in **Table 2**.

TABLE 2: Clinical features in specific central nervous system infections.

Type of CNS infection	*Specific features*
Herpes simplex virus (HSV) infection	• Pure neurological acute encephalitis syndrome (AES) presentation with or without focal neurological findings • Behavior and personality changes, aphasia • Suggestive neuroimaging (frontotemporal changes) • Hemorrhagic cerebrospinal fluid (CSF) • Periodic lateralized epileptiform discharges (PLEDs) in EEG
Rickettsial meningoencephalitis	• Eschar, maculopapular/petechial rash, edema, effusions, lymphadenopathy, hepatosplenomegaly • Evidence of multiorgan dysfunction (hepatic dysfunction/transaminitis, acute respiratory distress syndrome, renal failure, shock, disseminated intravascular coagulation/thrombocytopenia)
Cerebral malaria	Anemia, jaundice, hypoglycemia, retinal hemorrhages, absent meningeal signs
CNS tuberculosis (TB)	• Subacute or chronic meningitis, or tuberculoma (mass lesion) • Weight loss, loss of appetite, previous or current disease elsewhere in body, or contact with TB patients
Brain abscess	Classic triad of headache, fever, and focal deficit is seen in 50% of cases

EVALUATION

- *Blood investigations:*
  - Complete blood counts (CBC) with differential count
  - Inflammatory markers such as C-reactive protein (CRP) and procalcitonin
  - Blood culture (preferably before initiating antibiotics)
  - Analysis of serum electrolytes (sodium, potassium, calcium, magnesium), blood glucose, kidney and liver function tests, coagulation profile, blood gas analysis and lactate, if needed
  - Rapid tests and serologies for malaria, scrub typhus, dengue, enteric fever, leptospirosis, and other infectious agents, as indicated

- *CSF analysis:* Lumbar puncture (LP) is recommended in a febrile patient with CNS symptoms, unless contraindicated **(Box 1)**. In that case, defer the procedure and treat empirically for infection. CSF is tested for:

BOX 1: Contraindications for lumbar puncture.

- Features of raised intracranial pressure
- Focal neurological signs
- Ongoing seizures
- Features of shock
- Infection of skin overlying the lumbar puncture site
- Thrombocytopenia (platelets < 50,000/mm^3) or coagulation abnormality (relative contraindication)

- Total and differential cell count
- Glucose and protein levels
- Gram stain and culture
- Viral and bacterial antibodies or polymerase chain reaction (PCR), where available
- Special stains [e.g., acid-fast bacilli (AFB) stain, India ink for fungi), if indicated

The CSF characteristics in various CNS infections are given in **Table 3**.

TABLE 3: CSF characteristics in various CNS infections and noninfectious conditions.

Condition	*Appearance*	*Pressure (mm H_2O)*	*Leukocytes (/mm^3)*	*Protein (mg/dL)*	*Glucose (mg/dL)*
Normal	Clear	<28	<5, ≥75% lymphocytes/ monocytes (in neonates: <20)	20–45	>50 or 75% of serum glucose
Acute bacterial meningitis	Turbid	Raised	100 to >10,000, PMN predominate	100–500	<40 or <50% of serum glucose
Partially treated bacterial meningitis	Clear/turbid	Normal/ raised	5–10,000, PMNs usual but mononuclear cells may predominate	100–500	Normal/ reduced
Viral meningitis/ meningoencephalitis	Clear	Normal/ slightly raised	<1,000, PMNs early but mononuclear cells predominate	50–200	Usually normal, <40 in some (e.g., mumps)
Tuberculosis	Clear/serous/ turbid, cobweb formation	Usually raised	10–500, PMNs early, but lymphocytes predominate	100–3000, may be higher if obstruction	Usually <50

Contd...

Contd...

Condition	*Appearance*	*Pressure (mm H_2O)*	*Leukocytes (/mm^3)*	*Protein (mg/dL)*	*Glucose (mg/dL)*
Fungal meningitis	Clear/turbid	Usually raised	5–500, PMNs early but mononuclear cells predominate	25–500	<50
Chemical meningitis	Clear	Usually raised	100 to >1000, PMNs predominate	50–100	Normal or slightly reduced
Autoimmune encephalitis	Clear	Normal	~100, lymphocytes	Normal to elevated	Normal

Notes:
- In bacterial meningitis, CSF Gram stain and culture may turn negative within 2–4 hours of antibiotic administration; however, other abnormalities usually persist for several days. PCR-based assays may detect bacterial DNA.
- Traumatic LP—CSF leukocyte count and protein concentration are significantly affected by blood in CSF; Gram stain, culture, and glucose level are unlikely to be influenced. Repeat LP at a higher interspace may produce less hemorrhagic fluid. Correction factors are unreliable.

(CSF: cerebrospinal fluid; DNA: deoxyribonucleic acid; LP: lumbar puncture; PCR: polymerase chain reaction; PMNs: polymorphonuclear cells)

- *Neuroimaging:* Computed tomography (CT) is an emergency imaging modality of choice; magnetic resonance imaging (MRI) is preferred when feasible, with greater sensitivity and specificity, and utility in prognostication. Neuroimaging preceding LP is indicated in features of raised ICP, focal neurological deficits, history of hydrocephalus, or prior neurosurgical procedures including shunt placement. Imaging should be done after adequate resuscitation and stabilization. A normal CT does not rule out raised ICP. Repeat neuroimaging may be indicated in clinical deterioration or nonresponse.
- *Additional investigations (in selected cases):* As guided by clinical suspicion
  - Urine microscopy and culture
  - Stool for ova and cysts
  - Nasopharyngeal swab PCRs
  - Chest X-ray, tuberculin test, adenosine deaminase (ADA), CSF, sputum, gastric lavage or stool for AFB staining, or cartridge-based nucleic acid amplification test (CBNAAT) for tuberculosis
  - Viral markers (HIV)
  - Electroencephalogram (EEG)
  - Meningeal or brain biopsy (or aspiration in brain abscess)
  - Metabolic, autoimmune, and genetic studies for alternative causes

DIFFERENTIAL DIAGNOSIS

Differential diagnosis is given in **Box 2**.

BOX 2: Differential diagnosis of CNS infections.

- *Infective causes:*
  - *Bacterial meningitis: Streptococcus pneumoniae, Neisseria meningitidis, Hemophilus influenzae, Staphylococcus aureus*, group B streptococcus, *Listeria monocytogenes, Escherichia coli* and other gram-negative enteric bacilli, anaerobes *(Bacteroides, Fusobacterium, Actinomyces), Rickettsia, Leptospira, Mycoplasma,* syphilis, Lyme disease, tubercular meningitis
  - *Viral meningoencephalitis:* HSV, Enterovirus, JEV, dengue, chikungunya, zika virus, WNV, varicella, EBV, CMV, measles, mumps, influenza, RSV, adenovirus, coronavirus, Nipah virus, rotavirus, astrovirus, HIV, rabies
  - *Parasitic:* Malaria, neurocysticercosis, *Toxoplasma, Acanthamoeba, Naegleria, Balamuthia*
  - *Fungal: Candida, Aspergillus, Mucor, Cryptococcus, Histoplasma, Coccidioides, Blastomyces*
  - *Septic encephalopathy:* Enteric fever, Shigella

Common pathogens depend on age, host immune status, local epidemiology

- *Noninfective causes:*
  - *Trauma:* Parenchymal injury, intracranial hemorrhage, diffuse axonal injury, abusive head trauma
  - *Immune-mediated/autoimmune:* ADEM, anti-NMDA encephalitis, NMOSD, CNS vasculitis
  - *Metabolic:* Hypoglycemia, electrolyte derangements, DKA, renal or liver failure, IEM, poisonings or envenomation, Reye's syndrome
  - Nonconvulsive status epilepticus, FIRES, NORSE
  - *Vascular:* Intracranial bleed, hemorrhagic or ischemic stroke, cerebral venous sinus thrombosis
  - CNS malformations
  - CNS malignancies, metastatic lesions
  - Neurodegeneration
  - Endocrine disorders
  - Hypertensive encephalopathy
  - Hypoxic ischemic encephalopathy
  - Pseudotumor cerebri

(ADEM: acute demyelinating encephalomyelitis; CMV: cytomegalovirus; CNS: central nervous system; DKA: diabetic ketoacidosis; EBV: Ebstein–Barr virus; FIRES: febrile infection-related epilepsy syndrome; JEV: Japanese encephalitis virus; HIV: human immunodeficiency virus; IEM: inborn errors of metabolism; HSV: herpes simplex virus; NMDA: N-methyl D-aspartate; NMOSD: neuromyelitis optica spectrum disorder; NORSE: new-onset refractory status epilepticus; RSV: respiratory syncytial virus; WNV: West Nile virus)

EMERGENCY MANAGEMENT

A high index of suspicion, prompt recognition, and timely appropriate antimicrobial therapy are paramount. Initial stabilization, evaluation, and treatment must proceed simultaneously **(Algorithm 1)**.

Algorithm 1: Emergency management of CNS infections.

Signs and symptoms of CNS infection

↓

Initial stabilization
- Stabilize airway and breathing (oxygenation, ventilation); provide respiratory support as needed
- Obtain vascular access (large bore peripheral access) and send necessary blood investigations. Treat shock and provide hemodynamic support as needed (fluids and/or vasoactive drugs)
- Initiate continuous cardiorespiratory monitoring
- Identify and treat raised intracranial pressure and seizures
- Treat fever and hypoglycemia, if present
- Start empirical antimicrobial therapy
- Supportive management for multiorgan dysfunction

↓

Contraindication to LP without neuroimaging

- Yes → Urgent noncontrast CT head
  - ↓
  - Asymmetric mass effect?
  - Evidence of herniation?
  - Features of raised ICP?
  - Alternative diagnosis to explain the clinical signs and symptoms?
    - Yes → Anti-raised ICP measures; Cause-specific investigations and management
    - No → LP and CSF evaluation
- No → LP and CSF evaluation
  - ↓
  - Broad spectrum antimicrobials
  - Specific management

(CNS: central nervous system, ICP: intracranial pressure, LP: lumbar puncture, CT: computed tomography, CSF: cerebrospinal fluid)

Prevention of secondary neurological injury is an important goal. **Box 3** gives the indications for endotracheal intubation and mechanical ventilation and **Box 4** summarizes the antiraised ICP measures.

BOX 3: Indications for endotracheal intubation in CNS infections.

- Unstable airway, impaired airway protective reflexes, or inability to manage secretions
- Impaired oxygenation and/or ventilation (hypoxic or hypercapnic respiratory failure)
- Hemodynamic instability or shock
- Glasgow Coma Scale (GCS) score ≤8
- Features of raised intracranial pressure or impending herniation

BOX 4: Management of raised intracranial pressure (ICP).

Raised ICP may be due to cell death (cytotoxic cerebral edema), cytokine-induced increased capillary vascular permeability (vasogenic cerebral edema), or increased hydrostatic pressure [interstitial edema due to cerebrospinal fluid (CSF) obstruction]

- *Tier 1 management in all cases:* Maintain euthermia, euglycemia, euvolemia, and head in midline position with elevation (15–30°); correct electrolyte and acid–base abnormalities; maintain hemoglobin around 10 g/dL; avoid and manage fever, pain, and seizures (may increase ICP); minimize handling, gentle suction, and physiotherapy; avoid bladder or bowel retention; adequate sedoanalgesia
- *Tier 2 management as indicated:* Osmotherapy (3% hypertonic saline: 0.1–1 mL/kg/hr to target serum sodium 145–155 mEq/L; 20% mannitol: 1.25–2.5 mL/kg IV bolus SOS), ventilation targeting normoxemia and $paCO_2$ 30–35 mm Hg, isotonic fluids and inotrope-vasoactives to maintain mean arterial pressure above 50th centile, mannitol bolus and short (5–10 minutes) hyperventilation in impending herniation (worsening sensorium, unequal pupils, posturing, Cushing's triad)
- *Tier 3*: Surgical intervention if applicable (CSF drainage, craniotomy)

SPECIFIC MANAGEMENT

Empirical antimicrobials: Early empirical broad-spectrum antimicrobials must be initiated using a syndromic approach, without waiting for neuroimaging or LP results (should have good activity against common organisms and achieve adequate bactericidal levels in CSF). Antimicrobials must be modified once the pathogen susceptibilities are identified or discontinued based on the clinical course and investigations **(Table 4)**.

TABLE 4: Empirical antimicrobials in central nervous system (CNS) infections.

Type of infection	*Treatment*
Bacterial meningitis	• Ceftriaxone 100 mg/kg/day IV in two divided doses (maximum 4 g/day) OR Cefotaxime 300 mg/kg/day IV in three or four divided doses (maximum 12 g/day) • Add Vancomycin 60 mg/kg/day IV in three to four divided doses (maximum 4 g/day), if suspecting beta-lactam-resistant pneumococcal infection • Add penicillin (ampicillin/amoxycillin) if suspecting *Listeria* • Duration variable, depending on isolated organism. *Neisseria meningitidis:* 5–7 days, *Hemophilus influenzae:* 7–10 days, *Streptococcus pneumoniae:* 10–14 days, gram-negative bacilli: 3 weeks or a minimum of 2 weeks beyond the first sterile cerebrospinal fluid (CSF) culture, whichever is longer. If none, give empirical antibiotics for 10–14 days • Adjunctive steroids (dexamethasone 0.15 mg/kg IV 6 hourly for 2 days, first dose given 1–2 hours before antibiotics, concurrently or soon after the first dose of antibiotics) may be added in suspected cases of pneumococcal or *Hemophilus* meningitis to reduce mortality and hearing loss. Routine steroid use for acute meningitis is not recommended
Herpes simplex virus (HSV) meningoencephalitis	• *Acyclovir:* 3 months to 12 years—500 mg/m^2 IV 8th hourly, above 12 years—10 mg/kg IV 8th hourly for 14–21 days • Stop if alternate diagnosis is confirmed or CSF HSV polymerase chain reaction (PCR) is negative on two occasions (24–48 hours apart) and MRI/EEG is not suggestive of HSV infection
Rickettsial meningoencephalitis	Doxycycline 4.4 mg/kg/day IV/oral in two divided doses (maximum 200 mg/day) or azithromycin 10 mg/kg/day IV/oral for 7 days
Cerebral malaria	Artemisinin-based combination therapy: Parenteral artesunate 3 mg/kg in child <20 kg and 2.4 mg/kg in child >20 kg IV/IM at 0, 12, 24 hours, followed by once daily parental/oral artesunate for 3–7 days (in combination with longer-acting medications like lumefantrine and mefloquine). Primaquine is added to prevent recurrence. Stop if peripheral smear and rapid diagnostic test (RDT) are negative
CNS tuberculosis	• 2 months' intensive phase (isoniazid, rifampicin, pyrazinamide, ethambutol), with 8–10 months' continuation phase (rifampicin, isoniazid, ethambutol). Steroids are recommended for at least 4 weeks; start IV dexamethasone 0.15 mg/kg 6th hourly; then switch to oral therapy with tapering • Patients with hydrocephalus and raised intracranial pressure may need a ventriculoperitoneal shunt
Brain abscess	Combination of ceftriaxone, cloxacillin or vancomycin, and metronidazole, adjusted based on culture results (usually polymicrobial infections). Parenteral antibiotics for 6 weeks
CNS shunt infections	Empiric ceftriaxone and vancomycin. Extracting the infected shunt along with external ventricular drainage or periodic ventricular taps facilitates recovery
Fungal infection	Empirical liposomal amphotericin B (3–5 mg/kg/d) IV or azoles

MONITORING

- Continuous or frequent cardiorespiratory monitoring, as indicated, based on a child's clinical condition
- Regular monitoring of Glasgow Coma Scale (GCS) and features of raised ICP
- Daily comprehensive neurological examination
- Laboratory investigations, as indicated

COMPLICATIONS (BOX 5)

Complications of CNS infections are given in **Box 5**.

BOX 5: Complications of central nervous system (CNS) infections.

- *Immediate complications:*
  - Raised intracranial pressure
  - Septic shock
  - Multiorgan dysfunction syndrome
  - Syndrome of inappropriate antidiuretic hormone (SIADH)
  - Ventriculitis
  - Hydrocephalus (due to interference with CSF flow or resorption)
  - Cerebral sinus venous thrombosis
  - Hemorrhagic/ischemic stroke
  - Extra-axial fluid collection, e.g., subdural effusions
- *Long-term complications:*
  - Visual, hearing, or focal sensorimotor deficits
  - Language delay
  - Epilepsy
  - Learning disability
  - Behavioral problems
  - Developmental delay or intellectual disability

KEY LEARNING POINTS

- CNS infections in children require immediate attention due to the high risk of morbidity and mortality.
- Combination of clinical assessment, laboratory tests, CSF examination, and neuroimaging helps in confirming the diagnosis and guiding appropriate treatment strategies.
- Stabilization of airway, breathing, and circulation while monitoring for raised ICP is key to preventing secondary brain injury.
- Prompt empirical antimicrobial therapy is crucial, followed by specific treatments based on pathogen identification and clinical monitoring.

SUGGESTED READING

1. Dorsett M, Liang SY. Diagnosis and treatment of central nervous system infections in the emergency department. Emerg Med Clin North Am. 2016;34(4):917-42.
2. Giovane RA, Lavender PD. Central nervous system infections. Prim Care. 2018;45(3):505-18.
3. Janowski AB, Hunstad DA. Central nervous system infections. In: Kleigman RM, St. Jeme III JW (Eds). Nelson Textbook of Pediatrics, 22nd edition, Vol. 2. Philadelphia: Elsevier; 2024.
4. Kneen R, Solomon T, Appleton R. The role of lumbar puncture in children with suspected central nervous system infection. BMC Pediatr. 2002;2:8.
5. Mameli C, Genoni T, Madia C, Doneda C, Penagini F, Zuccotti G. Brain abscess in pediatric age: a review. Childs Nerv Syst. 2019;35(7):1117-28.
6. Ng LFP, Solomon T. Major advances against a moving target of CNS infections. Nat Rev Neurol. 2015; 11(11):623–4.
7. Shahan B, Choi EY, Nieves G. Cerebrospinal fluid analysis. Am Fam Physician. 2021;103(7):422-8.
8. Sigfrid L, Perfect C, Rojek A, Longuere KS, Lipworth S, Harriss E, et al. A systematic review of clinical guidelines on the management of acute, community-acquired CNS infections. BMC Med. 2019;17:170.
9. Suthar R, Sankhyan N. Bacterial infections of the central nervous system. Indian J Pediatr. 2019;86(1):60-9.
10. Tunkel AR, Hartman BJ, Kaplan SL, Kaufman BA, Roos KL, Scheld WM, et al. Practice Guidelines for the Management of Bacterial Meningitis. Clin Infect Dis. 2004;39(9):1267-84.

Approach to Raised ICP and Management

Vidya Lakshmi BK, Vykunta Raju KN

INTRODUCTION

- Brain is the control center of most of the vital functions. The pressure equilibrium maintained in the brain was supposed to be in between the brain, blood, and cerebrospinal fluid (CSF), as per the Monro–Kellie doctrine. Recent studies have contradicted this assumption. The skull expands and grows in response to pathologic changes in intracranial pressure (ICP) forming the 4th factor in the form of adaptive skull.[1]
- Any fluctuation in the pressure can lead to rise in ICP in turn causing cerebral ischemia and herniation.

TERMINOLOGIES AND DEFINITIONS

- *Cerebral perfusion pressure (CPP):* It is the pressure gradient caused due to the difference between systemic mean arterial pressure (MAP) and ICP.
    - *Optimal CPP:* Children >50–60 mm Hg, infants/toddler >40–50 mm Hg[2–8]
    - CPP = MAP–ICP
    - CPP is decreased when MAP decreases or ICP increases
- Cerebral blood flow (CBF) is autoregulated and is maintained by CPP
- *Normal ICP:*[8] In older children, it is 10–15 mm Hg, in younger children, 3–7 mm Hg, and in term infants, it is 1.5–6 mm Hg
    - Sustained ICP >40 mm Hg suggests severe intracranial hypertension
    - Treatment is warranted at an ICP of >20 mm Hg for >5 minutes

ETIOPATHOGENESIS

Etiopathogenesis is given in Flowchart.

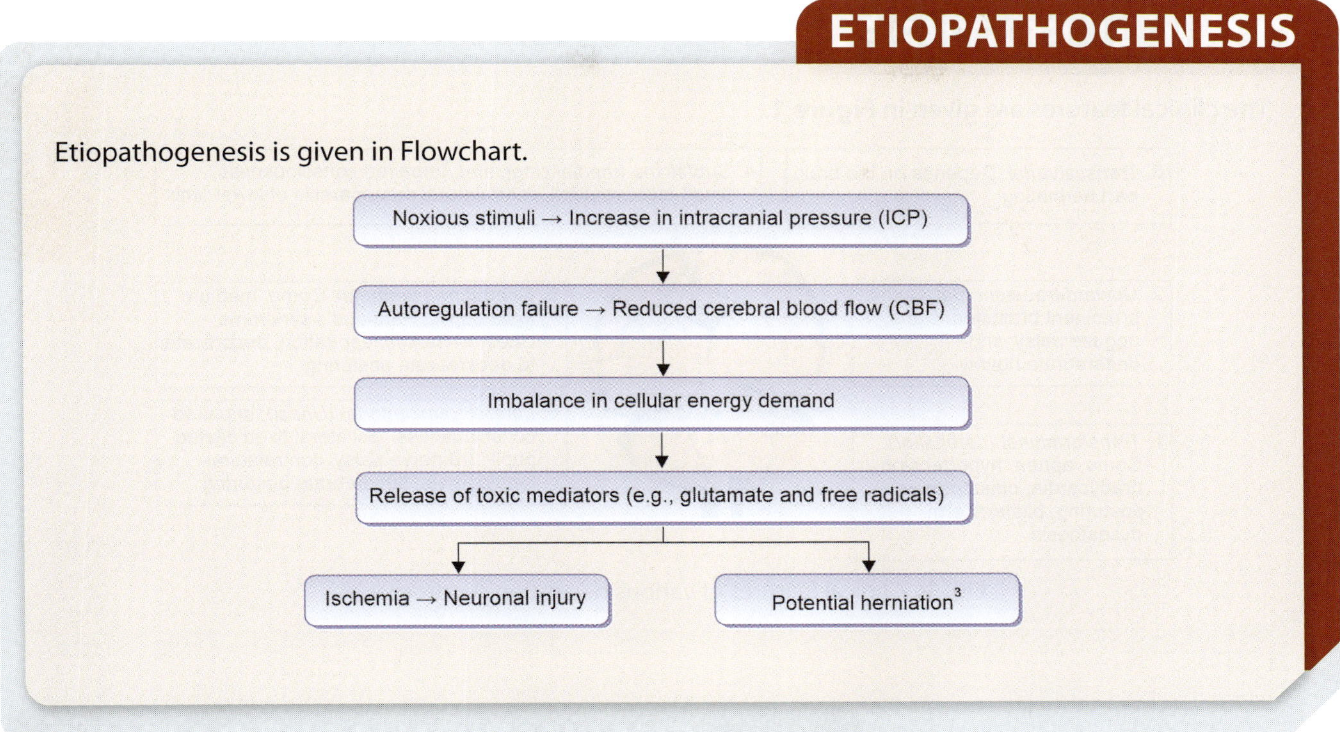

ETIOLOGY

Etiology of ICP is given in **Table 1.**

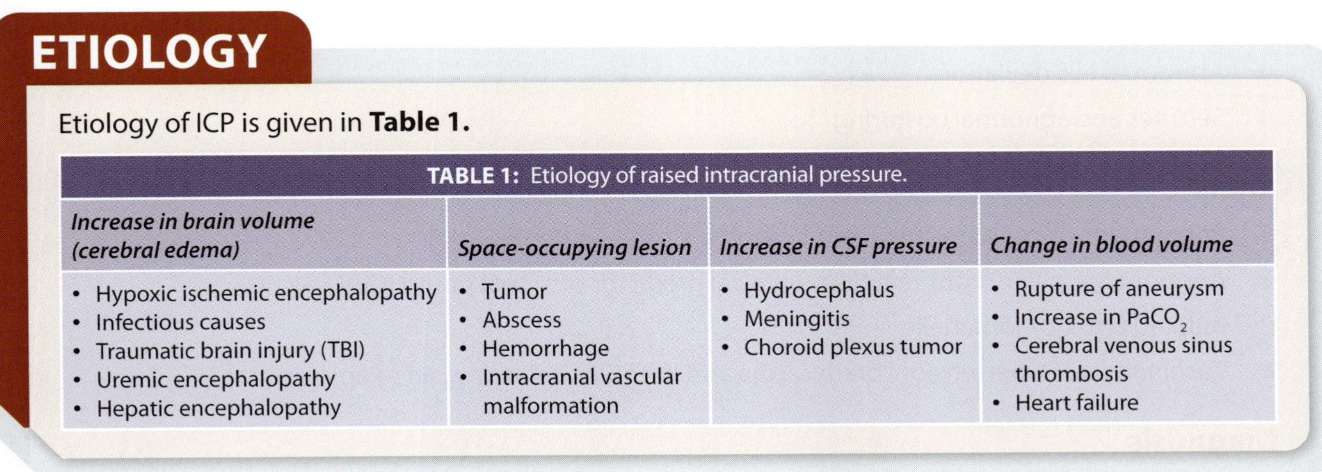

TABLE 1: Etiology of raised intracranial pressure.

Increase in brain volume (cerebral edema)	*Space-occupying lesion*	*Increase in CSF pressure*	*Change in blood volume*
• Hypoxic ischemic encephalopathy • Infectious causes • Traumatic brain injury (TBI) • Uremic encephalopathy • Hepatic encephalopathy	• Tumor • Abscess • Hemorrhage • Intracranial vascular malformation	• Hydrocephalus • Meningitis • Choroid plexus tumor	• Rupture of aneurysm • Increase in $PaCO_2$ • Cerebral venous sinus thrombosis • Heart failure

CLINICAL FEATURES

The clinical features are given in **Figure 1**.

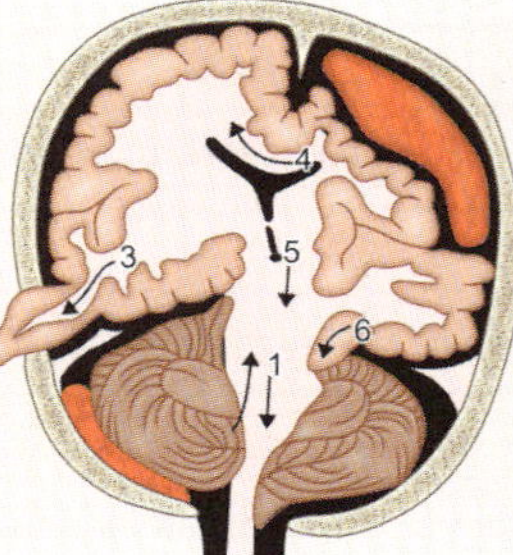

Fig. 1: Clinical features of various herniation syndromes.[4,5]

EVALUATION/APPROACH TO RAISED INTRACRANIAL PRESSURE

Symptoms

- Irritability/drowsiness
- Vomiting and headache
- Abnormal eye deviation
- Seizures and abnormal posturing.

Signs

- Impairment of consciousness and Glasgow Coma Scale (GCS) <8
- Abnormal pupillary light reactivity (clinical predictor of actual raised ICP)[7]
- Bulging anterior fontanelle
- *Cushing triad:* Hypertension, bradycardia and irregular breathing, and Papilledema

Diagnosis

- *CT scan* for
  - Ruling out the surgical cause
  - Look for midline shift/hemorrhage
- *MRI brain:* Loss of grey–white differentiation

- *Fundoscopy:* Reveals optic disc swelling
- *Lumbar puncture:*
    - CSF study for ruling out infectious cause
    - To decrease the pressure by draining CSF
- *Optic nerve sheath diameter (ONSD):* Measured by ultrasound >6 mm; suggestive of raised ICP[7]

When do you call cerebral edema and intracranial pressure?

These are defined by clinical and/or radiological measurements of ICP.

- *Clinical:* GCS <8 + 1/> of the following:
    - Unequal, dilated, or unreactive pupils
    - Loss of brain stem reflexes
    - CN palsies (III and VI)
    - Cushing's triad
- *Radiological:* –1/> of the following:
    - Effacement of the basal cisterns
    - Thin, slit-like, or completely obliterated ventricles
    - Obliterated cortical sulci
    - Shift in the midline
    - Temporal lobe or cerebellar tonsils herniation[1]
- ICP >20 mm Hg for >5 minutes

Approach Based on Etiology of Intracranial Pressure Based on Monroe–Kellie Doctrine and Management

Compartment	*Cause*	*Intervention*
Brain parenchyma	• Cerebral edema • Mass lesion	Steroids, mannitol, glycerol, frusemide, and 3% NaCl
Intravascular compartment	ICH, hematoma, decreased venous return, and increased arterial blood flow	• *PaO_2:* 90–110 mm Hg • *$PaCO_2$:* 25-30 mm Hg • *SPO_2* >90% • *Hb%:* >10 gm/dL
CSF	Hydrocephalus	Acetazolamide, frusemide, and shunt placement

(ICH: intracerebral hemorrhage, Hb: hemoglobin; PaO_2: partial pressure of oxygen; $PaCO_2$: partial pressure of carbon dioxide; SpO_2: oxygen saturation)

Goals of Management

Goals of management	*Intervention*
Decrease cerebral volume	Maintain euvolemia, hyperosmolar therapy, and evacuation of mass lesions
Decrease CSF volume	Ventriculostomy to drain CSF +/- lumbar drain
Decrease cerebral blood volume	Maintain head in the midline with the head of bed 30 degrees maintain normocarbia, hyperventilation with ventilation target: $PaCO_2$ 35–38 mm Hg/$EtCO_2$: 32–35 mm Hg.
Decrease metabolic Rate	Normothermia, sedation and analgesia, seizure management and prophylaxis, barbiturate coma, and mild-to-moderate hypothermia

(CSF: cerebrospinal fluid; $EtCO_2$: end-tidal carbon dioxide; $PaCO_2$: partial pressure of carbon dioxide)

Factors Related to Regulating Mean Arterial Pressure/Intracranial Pressure

CPP = MAP – ICP

- Optimizing CBF/CPP
- Minimizing factors that can aggravate neuronal injury or ICP elevation[3,4]
- Avoid factors that decrease MAP
  - Hypovolemia
  - Cardiogenic or septic shock
  - Hypothermia
  - Vasodilator drugs
- Avoid factors increasing ICP
  - Stimulation
  - Patient handling
  - Frequent venipuncture
  - Physiotherapy
  - Inadequate sedation
  - Head down position and neck compression
  - Alveolar hypoventilation
  - Valsalva maneuver
  - *Raised intrathoracic pressure:* Coughing and positive end-expiratory pressure (PEEP)
  - Seizure
  - Fever

TREATMENT

Maintain ABC:

- *A—airway:* Secure airway
- *B—breathing:* Oxygen or mechanical ventilation
- *C—circulation:* Ensure adequate perfusion and control hypotension or hypertension

The approach to treatment is given in Flowchart.

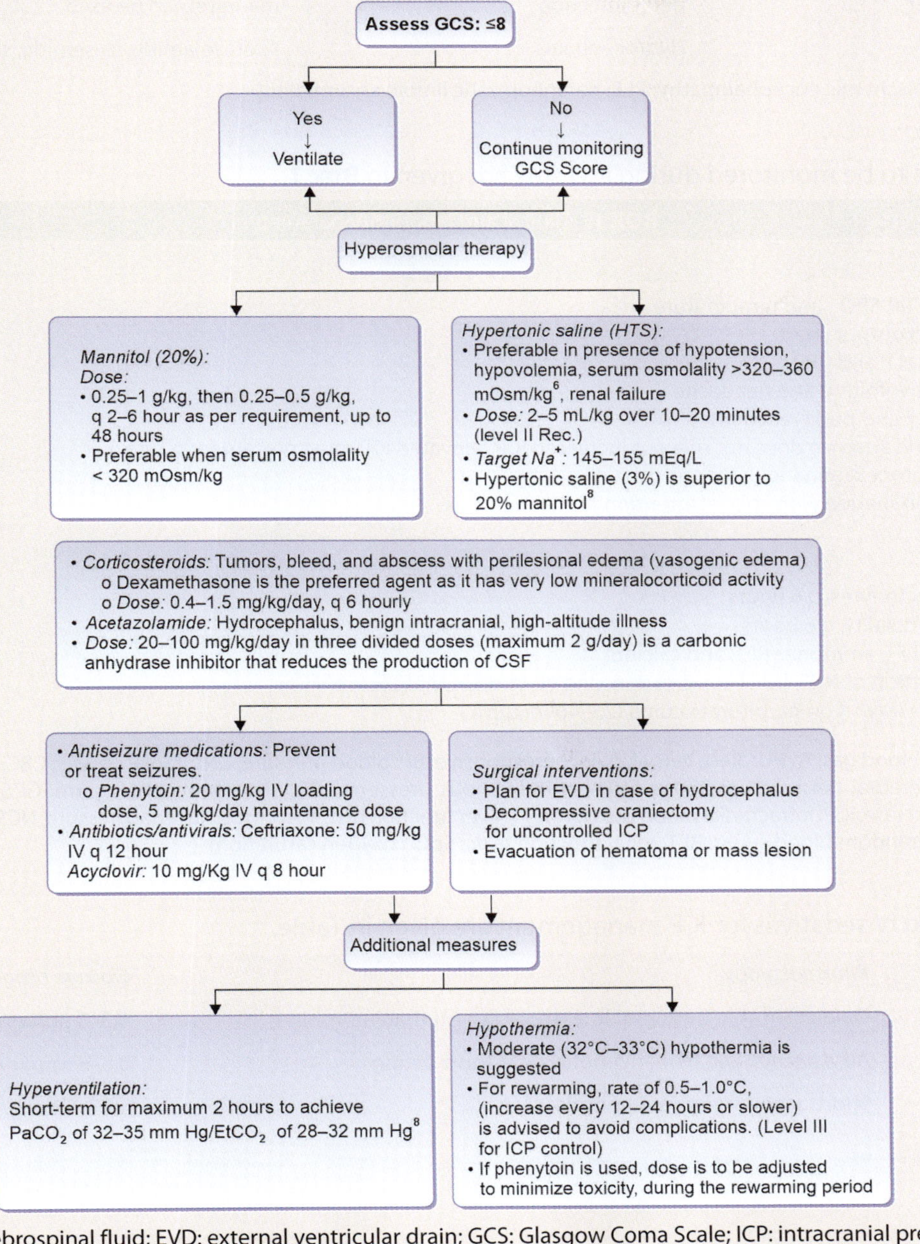

(CSF: cerebrospinal fluid; EVD: external ventricular drain; GCS: Glasgow Coma Scale; ICP: intracranial pressure)

Type of Cerebral Edema and Intervention

The types of cerebral edema and related interventions are given in Table.

Type	*Causes*	*Treatment*
Vasogenic: Affects mostly white matter	Meningitis, tumors, abscess, PLE, and hemorrhage	Responds to both steroids and osmotic agents
Cytotoxic: Affects both gray and white matter	HIE, hypoxemia, ischemia, and neuroinfection	Resistant to any medical treatment; mannitol can be used
Interstitial	Hydrocephalus	Acetazolamide, frusemide, shunt

(HIE: hypoxic-ischemic encephalopathy; PLE: paraneoplastic limbic encephalitis)

Parameters to be monitored during ICU stay are given in **Box 1**.

BOX 1: Clinical and laboratory parameters.

Clinical

- *Vitals:* HR, BP, SPO_2, and temperature
- Intake and output chart
- *CVP:* MAP, ICP and CPP
- Nausea or vomiting and headache
- GCS, AVPU, and pupil reactivity
- *Papilledema* absence does not rule out increased ICP (elevated ICP must present for >1 day)
- Ocular motor examination (3rd and 6th CN)
- Motor examination with special attention for hemiparesis

Laboratory

- ABG, q 6h
- Serum electrolytes, q 6 hours
- Serum osmolality, q 8 hours
- CBC, RBS, LFT, ammonia, RFT, and calcium
- *EEG:* Detection of NCS, burst suppression, and electrocerebral silence
- *Barbiturate level:* If on barbiturate coma (25–40 mcg/mL)

(ABG: arterial blood gas; AVPU: alert, verbal, pain, unresponsive; BP: blood pressure; CN: cranial nerves; CBC: complete blood count; CPP: cerebral perfusion pressure; CVP: central venous pressure; EEG: electroencephalogram; GCS: Glasgow coma scale; HR: heart rate; ICP: intracranial blood pressure; LFT: liver function test; MAP: mean arterial pressure; NCS: Nonconvulsive seizures; RBS: random blood sugar; RFT: renal function tests; SpO_2: oxygen saturation)

Short-acting IV sedatives for ICP management are given in Table.

Agent	*Pharmacology*	*Dosage range*
Fentanyl	*Opiate:* Short-acting, 100 times more potent than morphine	0.3–3 µg/kg/hour
Propofol	*Alkyl phenol:* Sedative–hypnotic, ultra short-acting	0.6–6 mg/kg/hour
Midazolam	Short-acting sedative–hypnotic	0.05–0.1 mg/kg/hour

The effects of drugs used for sedation are given in Table.

Drug/class	*ICP*	*CPP*	*$CMRO_2$*	*Antiepileptic action*	*Prevention of ICP increase*
Benzodiazepines	= or ↑	↓	=	+	+
Propofol	= or ↓	↓	↓	+	+
Barbiturates	= or ↓	↓	↓	+	+
Ketamine	= or ↓	=	=	0	+

(CPP: cerebral perfusion pressure; $CMRO_2$: cerebral metabolic rate of oxygen; ICP: intracranial blood pressure)

Drugs used and dosages in increased ICP are given in Table.

Drug	*Stat dose*	*Dose*	*Onset of action*	*Duration of action*	*Comments*
Mannitol	5 mL/kg	1.25–2.5 mL/kg Q6H	15 minutes	3–6 hours, Limit use <48–72 hours	*CI:* ARF, shock, active IC bleed, if serum osmolarity >320 mOsm/kg
3% NaCl	4mL/kg at 15 minutes	0.1–1 mL/kg/ hour infusion	30–60 minutes	Na level reduced over 2–3 days	• Serum Na = 160–170 mEq/L • Serum osmolarity = 360 mOsm/L
Steroids Dexamethasone	——	0.15 mg/kg/dose q 6 hour	Within hours	——	Monitor for Glucose, BP, GIT bleed
Glycerol	5 mL/kg	2 mL/kg q 6 hour	Immediately	——	Rebound
Frusemide	——	0.5–1 mg/kg	Immediately	8 hours	Volume status, serum electrolytes
Hyperventilation	——	PCO_2–mmol/L	30 minutes	2–3 hours	Cannot be used for longer time
Pentobarbital	5 mg/kg	1–2 mg/kg/hour	1–10 minutes	1–4 hours	*EEG:* Burst suppression
Thiopental	5–10 mg/kg at 30 mins	3–5 mg/kg/hour	5–10 minutes	1–1.5 hours	Do not use for sedation
Propofol	——	0.3–3 µg/kg/ hour	15–45 seconds	15 minutes	Short acting, analgesic, and sedative
Midazolam	——	0.1 mg/kg/hour	1–3 minutes	1–2 hours	For sedation
Fentanyl	0.5–10 µg/kg	1–5 µg/kg/hour		30–40 minutes	Few hemodynamic effects of all opiate
Ketamine	0.25–0.5 mg/kg	——	0.5–2 minutes	20–60 minutes	Sedation, hypnosis, and analgesia
Vecuronium	0.1 mg/kg	0.1 mg/kg /dose Q 1–2 hour	1–2 minutes	30–90 minutes	Minimal effect on HR and BP
Labetalol	0.2–1 mg/kg	0.4–1 mg/kg/ hour	1–5 minutes	Variable, about 6 hours	Interval to repeat or increase the dose 10 minutes
Nicardipine	——	0.5–5 µg/kg/min	1 minute	3 hours	Interval to repeat or increase the dose 15 minutes
Lidocaine	1–2 mg/kg	——	3 minutes	10–20 minutes	Blunts ICP spike, cough reflex during intubation

(ARF: acute renal failure; BP: blood pressure; EEG: electroencephalogram; GIT: gastrointestinal tract; IC: intracranial hemorrhage; ICP: intracranial pressure)

REFERENCES

1. Benson JC, Madhavan AA, Cutsforth-Gregory JK, Johnson DR, Carr CM. The Monro-Kellie Doctrine: A review and call for revision. AJNR Am J Neuroradiol. 2023;44(1):2-6.
2. Hawryluk GWJ, Citerio G, Hutchinson P, Kolias A, Meyfroidt G, Robba C, et al. Intracranial pressure: Current perspectives on physiology and monitoring. Intensive Care Med. 2022;48(10):1471-81.
3. Shaw E, Patel S, Davies P, Stewart C. Managing raised intracranial pressure in paediatric brain injury. PCH. 2023;33(11):350-6.
4. Sankhyan N, Vykunta Raju KN, Sharma S, Gulati S. Management of raised intracranial pressure. Indian J Pediatr. 2010;77(12):1409-16.
5. Riveros Gilardi B, Muñoz López JI, Hernández Villegas AC, Garay Mora JA, Rico Rodríguez OC, Chávez Appendini R, et al. Types of cerebral herniation and their imaging features. Radiographics. 2019;39(6):1598-610.
6. Upadhyay P, Tripathi VN, Singh RP, Sachan D. Role of hypertonic saline and mannitol in the management of raised intracranial pressure in children: A randomized comparative study. J Pediatr Neurosci. 2010;5(1):18-21.
7. Rajangam M, Bansal A, Kumar AS, Nallasamy K, Muralidharan J. SSRN. (2024). Clinical Predictors of raised intracranial pressure among children with nontraumatic coma who underwent invasive ICP monitoring. [online] Available from https://papers.ssrn.com/sol3/papers.cfm?abstract_id=4926626 [Last accessed December, 2024].
8. Rameshkumar R, Bansal A. Approach and management of children with raised intracranial pressure. J Pediatr Crit Care. 2015;2(3):13-24.

21 Acute Flaccid Paralysis

Bela Verma, Meghana Tiwary

INTRODUCTION

- Acute flaccid paralysis (AFP) is a complex clinical syndrome with a multifactorial etiology.
- Each case is an emergency, both in terms of the need for appropriate, correct treatment and AFP surveillance.
- India has been polio-free since 2014;[1] however, AFP surveillance is an important tool for the early detection and prevention of the community spread of polio.
- The number of AFP (AFP from nonpolio causes) cases in 2023 in India was 7.46/100,000 cases.[2]

TERMINOLOGIES AND DEFINITIONS

Acute flaccid paralysis is an acute onset flaccid weakness of <14 days, reaching its maximum severity in days to weeks.

An AFP case is defined as a child under 15 years presenting with sudden onset of floppy paralysis or muscle weakness due to any cause, or any person of any age with paralytic illness if a clinician suspects poliomyelitis.[3] The etiopathology of AFP is given in **Table 1**.

ETIOPATHOLOGY

TABLE 1: Etiopathology of acute flaccid paralysis.

Central causes	*Spinal*	*Anterior horn cell*	*Peripheral nerve*	*Neuromuscular junction*	*Muscle*
Brainstem encephalitis	Acute transverse myelitis	Poliomyelitis	Guillain–Barré Syndrome (radiculopathy)	Myasthenia	Viral myositis
ADEM, NMO	Acute myelopathy	Nonpolio enterovirus	Traumatic neuritis	Botulism	Hypokalemic periodic paralysis
Stroke	Cord compression syndrome	Rabies	Toxic neuropathies (diphtheria, tick bite, lead, and arsenic)	Snakebite	McArdle disease
Tumor		Varicella Zoster	Critical illness neuropathy	Organophosphorus poisoning	Polymyositis
Abscess			Drug-induced		Critical illness myopathy
Cerebral sinus Venous thrombus			acute intermittent porphyria		

(ADEM: acute disseminated encephalomyelitis; NMO: neuromyelitis optica)

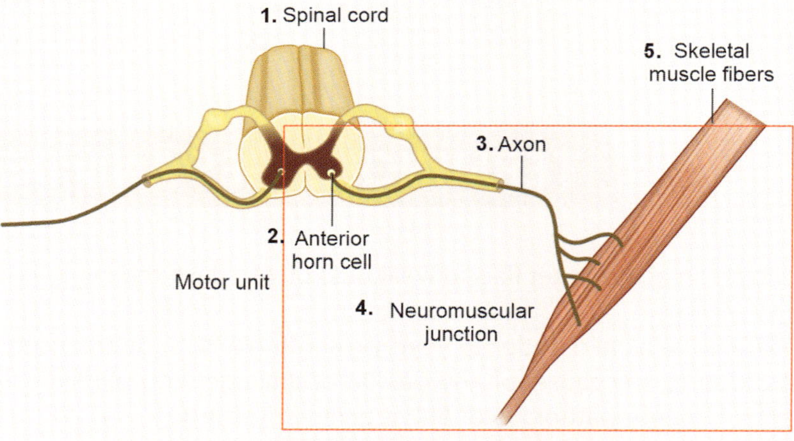

Fig. 1: Single motor unit.[4]

CLINICAL FEATURES

The clinical presentations are as follows:

- *Presenting history:*
  - Inability to walk or stand
  - Weakness of upper and lower limbs, usually associated with severe limb pain
  - Breathing difficulty
  - Difficulty in swallowing
  - Change in voice
  - Facial deviation
  - Loss of bowel/bladder control
- *Based on onset:*
  - *Hyperacute:* Few minutes—vascular pathology
  - *Acute:* Few hours—Guillain–Barré syndrome (GBS), polio, and acute transverse myelitis
  - *Insidious:* Few days—tick paralysis
- *Based on progression:*
  - *Ascending paralysis:* Lower limbs-upper limbs; can be symmetrical (GBS) or asymmetrical (polio)
  - *Descending paralysis:* Bulbar muscles-upper limbs-lower limbs-post diphtheria paralysis, and botulism
  - *Episodic paralysis:* Complete recovery between episodes-hypokalemic periodic paralysis
  - *Recurrent paralysis:* CACNA1A-related channelopathies
- *Clinical clues for diagnosis* ***(Table 2)***

TABLE 2: Clinical clues for diagnosis.

Clinical history and examination	*Diagnosis*
Preceding diarrheal illness	Guillain–Barré syndrome
History of bull neck, fever, and throat pain in preceding weeks	Postdiphtheria polyneuropathy
Recent intramuscular injection	Traumatic neuritis
Trauma to spine/neck	Traumatic myelopathy
Recent dog bite/travel to hilly areas	Rabies/tick-bite paralysis
History of consumption of canned goods/ingestion of contaminated honey	Botulism
Predominant sensory symptoms (paresthesia, numbness, tingling sensations, and abdominal pain)	*Occupational exposures:* Arsenic and lead
Similar episodes in the past, history of nonspecific abdominal pain, and photosensitivity	Acute intermittent porphyria
Sudden onset weakness in the morning after carbohydrate-rich meal in the night	Hypokalemic periodic paralysis
History of prolonged ICU stay, use of corticosteroids, and use of neuromuscular blockade drugs (e.g., vecuronium)	Critical illness polyneuropathy
Onset of weakness immediately after heavy exercise or running	Glycogen storage disorders

◈ *Diagnosis based on pattern of central nervous system involvement **(Table 3)**:* [5]

TABLE 3: Pattern of central nervous system involvement and the diagnosis.

Pattern	*Diagnosis*
Asymmetric and patchy motor weakness with complete sensory sparing	Poliomyelitis
Symmetric motor ascending weakness with or without sensory involvement	Guillain–Barré Syndrome (GBS)
Ptosis, extraocular weakness, and diplopia with diurnal variation	Myasthenia gravis (present as myasthenic crisis)
Muscle weakness with sudden ptosis, and EOM weakness	Snakebite (neurotoxic) and rabies (dumb rabies)
Bulbar onset of weakness	Postdiphtheria polyneuropathy or botulism
Cranial nerve involvement	Tick paralysis, postdiphtheria polyneuropathy, GBS, acute flaccid myelitis, and Lyme disease
Early bladder involvement (retention)	Acute transverse myelitis and GBS (15%)

The approach to diagnosing AFP is illustrated in **Flowchart 1**.

Flowchart 1: Algorithm to diagnosis.

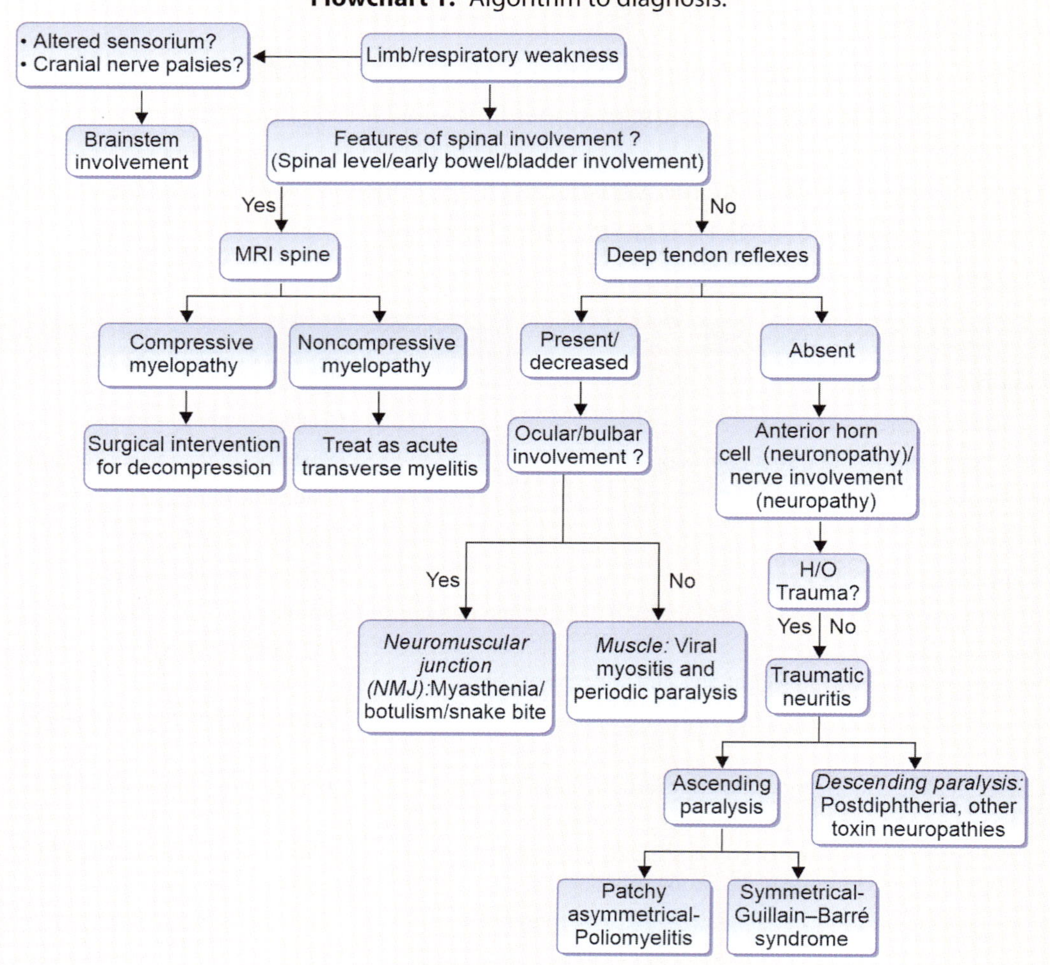

INVESTIGATIONS

- *Acute flaccid paralysis surveillance:* A country's surveillance system needs to be sensitive enough to detect at least one nonpolio AFP case each year for every 100,000 children aged under 15 years.
  - Global Polio Eradication Initiative (GPEI) aims to confirm and sequence all polioviruses *within 35 days of the onset of paralysis*. The process from onset of paralysis to the arrival of stool specimens at a World Health Organization (WHO)-accredited polio laboratory must be completed *within 14 days* **(Flowchart 2)**.

Flowchart 2: Acute flaccid paralysis surveillance.

Step 1: Finding and reporting cases with AFP

Every AFP case <15 years of age must be reported. Children diagnosed with AFP must be posted for poliovirus, even *if polio has been ruled out by a treating physician*.

↓

Step 2: Transporting stool samples for analysis
2 stool specimens are taken 24–48 hours apart, sealed in containers, and stored immediately inside a refrigerator or packed between ice packs at 4–8° C in a cold box. Specimens should arrive at the laboratory within 72 hours of collection—*reverse cold chain*.

↓

Step 3: Isolating the virus
Poliovirus is isolated from stool samples. If isolated, it must be classified as wild-type or vaccine-derived

↓

Step 4: Mapping the virus
Once the wild poliovirus has been identified, further tests are done to determine where the strain may have originated

- *Nerve conduction studies* ***(Flowchart 3):*** Test results can be normal at onset of illness; hence, it is best to repeat after 2–3 weeks.

Flowchart 3: Nerve conduction study results.

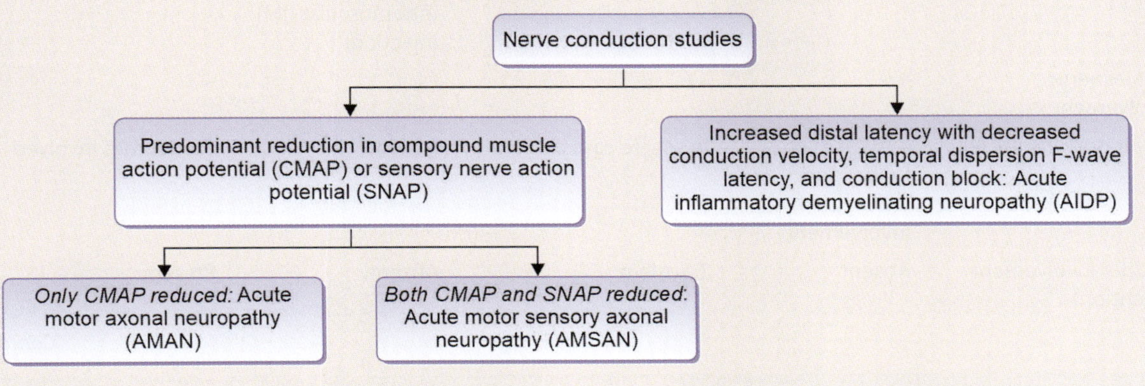

- *Cerebrospinal fluid (CSF) studies:* These help identify etiology and support the diagnosis, although does not confirm it. It is done in 2nd–3rd week of illness.
- *Magnetic resonance imaging (MRI) brain + spine:* It is a supportive investigation and can help localize various demyelinating disorders. For example, nerve root enhancement in GBS
- *Blood investigations:* Complete blood count, erythrocyte sedimentation rate (ESR), electrolytes, and creatine phosphokinase (CPK).
- *Specific investigations:* According to clinical suspicion, for example, blood-lead levels.

DIFFERENTIAL DIAGNOSIS OF ACUTE FLACCID PARALYSIS

Differential diagnoses of acute flaccid paralysis are given in **Table 4**.[6]

TABLE 4: Differential diagnosis of acute flaccid paralysis and their characteristics.

Characteristics	*Poliomyelitis*	*Guillain–Barré syndrome*	*Traumatic neuritis*	*Transverse myelitis*
Site involved	Anterior horn cell	Nerve root	Peripheral nerve	Spinal cord
Progression of paralysis	24–48 hours	Hours to days	Hours to days	Hours to days
Distribution of weakness	Asymmetric patchy	Symmetric ascending	Along distribution of involved nerve	Symmetric lower limb
Deep tendon reflexes	Absent	Absent	Decreased/absent	Absent early Hyperreflexia late
Babinski reflex	Absent	Absent	Absent	Present
Sensory involvement	Myalgia + No sensory involvement	Cramps, tingling, and hypoesthesia of palms and soles	Pain along nerve distribution (gluteal region in cases of intramuscular (IM) injection)	Anesthesia of lower limbs with sensory level
Cranial nerve involvement	+/–	+/–	–	–
Respiratory insufficiency	+ In cases of bulbar and bulbospinal involvement	In severe cases	Absent	Sometimes involved
Bladder involvement (retention)	Absent	Transient	Absent	Present

Contd...

Contd...

Characteristics	*Poliomyelitis*	*Guillain–Barré syndrome*	*Traumatic neuritis*	*Transverse myelitis*
CSF examination	Cell count raised; Protein normal/ slightly increased	<10 leukocytes, high protein, Albuminocytological dissociation	Normal	Cell count – normal/ slight increase in lymphocytes *Proteins:* normal/ slightly raised
EMG (3 weeks)	Abnormal	Normal	May be abnormal	Normal
NCV (3 weeks)	Normal	Abnormal, Demyelination/axonal	Abnormal	Normal
Sequelae	Severe asymmetrical atrophy	Symmetrical distal limb atrophy	Moderate atrophy of affected muscle	Diplegia and atrophy after many years

(CSF: cerebrospinal fluid; EMG: electromyography; NCV: nerve conduction velocity)

EMERGENCY CARE

The algorithmic approach to emergency care is given in **Flowchart 4.**

Flowchart 4: Algorithm for emergency care.[7]

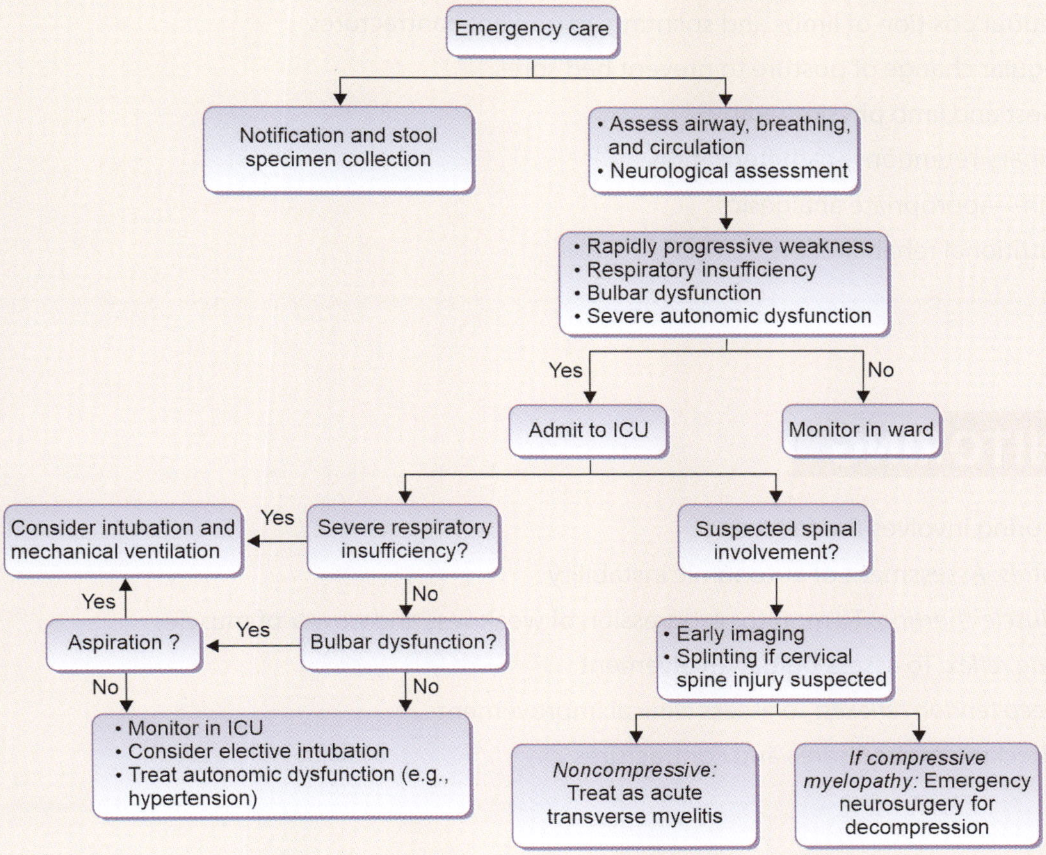

Emergency care
- → Notification and stool specimen collection
- → • Assess airway, breathing, and circulation • Neurological assessment
  - → • Rapidly progressive weakness • Respiratory insufficiency • Bulbar dysfunction • Severe autonomic dysfunction
    - No → Monitor in ward
    - Yes → Admit to ICU
      - → Severe respiratory insufficiency?
        - Yes → Consider intubation and mechanical ventilation
        - No → Bulbar dysfunction?
          - Yes → Aspiration ?
            - Yes → Consider intubation and mechanical ventilation
            - No → • Monitor in ICU • Consider elective intubation • Treat autonomic dysfunction (e.g., hypertension)
          - No → • Monitor in ICU • Consider elective intubation • Treat autonomic dysfunction (e.g., hypertension)
      - → Suspected spinal involvement?
        - → • Early imaging • Splinting if cervical spine injury suspected
          - → *Noncompressive:* Treat as acute transverse myelitis
          - → *If compressive myelopathy:* Emergency neurosurgery for decompression

SPECIFIC TREATMENT

The specific treatment for different cases of AFP is given in **Table 5.**

TABLE 5: Specific treatment.

Guillain–Barré Syndrome	Intravenous (IV) immunoglobulin 2 g/kg
Transverse myelitis	• Methylprednisolone 30 mg/kg/day for 3–5 days; • Plasma exchange or intravenous cyclophosphamide (800–1,200 mg/m^2) administered as a single pulse dose
Snakebite	Antisnake venom and trial of atropine and neostigmine
Botulism	Treatment with antitoxin
Lead poisoning	EDTA chelation therapy

(EDTA: ethylenediaminetetraacetic acid)

SUPPORTIVE MANAGEMENT

The supportive management includes:

- Neutral position of limbs and splinting to prevent contractures
- Regular change of posture to prevent bed sores
- Chest and limb physiotherapy
- Urinary retention—catheterization
- Pain—appropriate analgesics
- Nutritional rehabilitation

MONITORING

Monitoring involves the following:

- *Vitals:* Assessment of autonomic instability
- *Muscle charting:* To monitor progression of weakness and power of muscles
- *Gag reflex:* To assess bulbar involvement
- *Deep tendon reflexes:* To assess clinical improvement
- Checking for bed sores and contractures

KEY LEARNING POINTS

- AFP is a diagnostic dilemma, and it is important to carefully evaluate each case to establish a diagnosis.
- AFP surveillance is an essential part of the healthcare system and is the pillar of polio eradication in India.

REFERENCES

1. The National Department of Health, South Africa, Expanded Programme on Immunisation. (2015). EPI Diseases Surveillance Guideline, 3rd Edition (2015). [online] Available from https://www.nicd.ac.za/assets/files/EPI%20Surveillance%20Manual_15Dec2015.pdf [Last accessed November, 2024].
2. Our World in Data. (2024). Rate of acute flaccid paralysis from non-polio causes. [online] Available from https://ourworldindata.org/grapher/rate-of-acute-flaccid-paralysis-from-non-polio-causes?country=AFG~PAK~MWI~MOZ~BWA~RWA~KEN~IND [Last accessed November, 2024].
3. World Health Organization. (2023). Global guidelines for acute flaccid paralysis (AFP) surveillance in the context of poliovirus eradication. Prepublication version. [online] Available from: https://polioeradication.org/wp-content/uploads/2023/03/Global-AFP-guidelines-pre-publiucation-version-2023.pdf [Last accessed November, 2024].
4. Webster JG, Clark JW. Medical Instrumentation: Application and Design, 4th edition. Hoboken, NJ: John Wiley & Sons; 2010.
5. Clinical Approach to Paediatric Neurology [Internet]. Google Books. 2021 [cited 2024 Sep 15]. Available from: https://books.google.co.in/books/about/Clinical_Approach_to_Pediatric_Neurology.html?id=KiEuzgEACAAJ&redir_esc=y
6. Kunju M, Subir A, Eapen M. Acute flaccid paralysis beyond polio-a case-based approach. Indian Journal of Practical Paediatrics [Internet]. 2020;22(1):36. Available: https://www.ijpp.in/Files/2020/ver1/Acute%20flaccid%20paralysis%20beyond%20polio%20-%20A%20case%20based%20approach.pdf
7. Acute Flaccid Paralysis in Adults [Internet]. [cited 2024 Sep 15]. Available from: https://www.jipmer.edu.in/sites/default/files/Acute_flaccid_paralysis_Protocol-final-2.pdf

Stroke in Children

Renu Suthar, Kiran Anand

INTRODUCTION

- Stroke is defined as rapidly developing clinical signs and symptoms of focal or global disturbance of cerebral function lasting for >24 hours or leading to death with no apparent cause other than vascular origin [defined by World Health Organization (WHO)].

TERMINOLOGIES AND DEFINITIONS

Stroke in children is defined specifically by International Pediatric Stroke Study (IPSS) group.

The IPSS-defined criteria for diagnosis of arterioischemic stroke (AIS) in children include:

- Neurological deficit of acute onset or seizure alone in neonates
- Radiographic image(s)* (MRI or CT) showing cerebral parenchymal infarct(s) conforming to known arterial territory(ies) and corresponding to clinical manifestations.

  *Compared to definition of stroke in adults, radiologic evidence of infract is must for diagnosis

TYPES OF STROKES

Types of strokes depend on the blood vessels affected and are secondary to vascular occlusion or rupture. Stroke can be further classified into:

- Arterioischemic stroke (AIS)
- Cerebral sinus venous thrombosis (CSVT)
- Hemorrhagic stroke (HS)

TRANSIENT ISCHEMIC ATTACK

Transient ischemic attack (TIA) is a brief episode of neurological dysfunction resulting from focal cerebral ischemia not associated with permanent cerebral infarction.

- Typically, TIA has symptoms lasting <24 hours.
- MRI in patients with TIA may show infraction in 30–50% cases

Operation definition of TIA: TIA is a brief episode of neurological dysfunction caused by focal brain or retinal ischemia, with clinical symptoms typically lasting <1 hour and without evidence of acute infarction.

INCIDENCE

- *Incidence of acute ischemic stroke in children:* 3–25/100,000 year including neonatal stroke. The incidence of HS is 0.8/100,000 children per year and for CSVT, it is 0.6/100,000 children per year.[1]
- The incidence of stroke is less in children compared to adults, but PEDIATRIC stroke is associated with mortality in 5–10% and persistent neurological disability in one-third of children.

CLINICAL FEATURES

- *Clinical features of stroke depend on several factors:* Age of the patient, brain parenchyma supplied by the blood vessel, dominant versus nondominant hemisphere, and presence of cerebral edema and mass effect.
- Clinical features of AIS and HS are similar; however, the onset of symptoms is more catastrophic in HS; signs and symptoms of raised intracranial pressure (ICP) are more common and encephalopathy is more profound in patients with HS.

Clinical Presentation of Stroke

- Neonates with AIS present with acute onset seizure (focal clonic or generalized seizure), apnea, encephalopathy, irritability, lethargy, and hypotonia. Squint, nystagmus, and tremors are less common features.
- Children with stroke can present with acute onset hemiparesis, monoparesis, focal seizure, headache, speech impairment, focal onset movement disorder, and impaired consciousness.
- Hemiparesis, aphasia, seizure, altered consciousness, headache, and vision loss are seen in children with anterior circulation AIS. Presence of hemiparesis, vertigo, dizziness, ataxia, headache, squint, and visual field defect is suggestive of posterior circulation AIS.

- Acute onset preferential use of one hand can be an indicator of stroke in children.
    - The onset is more stuttering in thrombotic stroke and hyperacute in embolic stroke; however, the differentiation is not absolute.
- The acronym "FAST" is indicative of stroke in children and elucidated in **Box 1**.

BOX 1: The acronym "FAST" is indicative of stroke in children.

- Facial weakness
- Arm weakness
- *Speech:* Motor aphasia or incomprehension
- Time to call emergency

Clinical features of stroke depend on the vessels involved and lobar functions of the affected hemisphere. The clinical features of most common major arterial stroke in children are given in **Table 1**.

TABLE 1: Clinical features of most common major arterial stroke in children.

Blood vessel affected	*Part of cerebral parenchyma supplied by the affected blood vessel (arrow)*	*Clinical features corresponding to the cerebral parenchyma affected*
Anterior cerebral artery		• Contralateral hemiparesis affecting lower limb more than arm with sensory loss • *Dominant hemisphere:* Mutism (left in majority) • *Nondominant hemisphere:* Acute confusional state • *Bilateral infarction:* Urinary incontinence
Middle cerebral artery		• Contralateral hemiparesis, sensory loss, and hemianopia with gaze preference to affected half of the body • *Dominant hemisphere:* Aphasia and apraxia • *Nondominant hemisphere:* Hemineglect

Contd...

Contd...

Blood vessel affected	*Part of cerebral parenchyma supplied by the affected blood vessel (arrow)*	*Clinical features corresponding to the cerebral parenchyma affected*
Posterior cerebral artery		• Contralateral hemianopia (macular sparing)
Posterior circulation stroke		• Crossed hemiplegia (ipsilateral cranial nerve and opposite hemiparesis) • Vertigo, slurring of speech, diplopia, headache, nausea, vomiting, and visual field defects

DIAGNOSIS AND EVALUATION

Diagnosis and management of stroke in children should go hand in hand. In the emergency setting, the priority is immediate stabilization of the airway, breathing, circulation and preparation for an urgent neuroimaging. If the patient is within the window period for therapeutic intervention (within first 4 hours), an urgent noncontrast CT scan of the head with CT angiography should be performed. If the patient is in out-of-the-window period (>4 hours from onset or woke-up stroke), the first neuroimaging can be a noncontrast CT scan with CT angiography or MRI brain with MR angiography, depending on the availability of the imaging facility.

Neuroimaging for Diagnosis of Stroke

- *Noncontrast CT head with a CT angiography:*
    - In CT scan of the head, an established infarct appears as a hypodense area corresponding to the arterial supply of blood vessels **(Figs. 1A to C)**

- Some of the early radiological clues for diagnosis of stroke in CT scans are: Hypoattenuation of brain parenchyma, obscuration of lentiform nucleus, dense middle cerebral artery (MCA) sign, insular ribbon sign, and sulcal effacement sign.

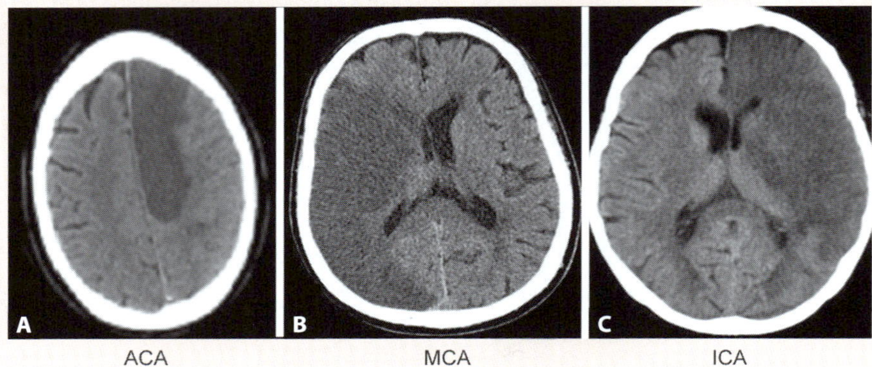

Figs. 1A to C: A noncontrast CT scan of the head showing hypodensity in the cerebral parenchyma in the distribution of (A) anterior cerebral artery (ACA), (B) middle cerebral artery (MCA), and (C) internal carotid artery (ICA).

- *MRI brain:*
  - *MRI:* T1, T2, fluid-attenuated inversion recovery (FLAIR), susceptibility-weighted imaging (SWI), diffusion-weighted imaging (DWI)/apparent diffusion coefficient (ADC), and MR angiography, if possible, within first few hours if patient is in the window period
  - If the initial CT scan is negative and suspicion of stroke is high, MRI within 24 hours (T1, T2, FLAIR, SWI, DWI/ADC, and magnetic resonance angiography (MRA) protocol)
  - MRI brain is a confirmatory neuroimaging for all children with stroke for improved diagnostic resolution, if not obtained in/at the initial imaging investigation, MRI should be obtained with MRA including arch of aorta and neck vessels.
  - Digital subtraction angiography (DSA) is required for situations where noninvasive imaging is inconclusive. In children, DSA is used for diagnosis of focal cerebral arteriopathy, dissection, moyamoya disease, venous thrombosis, aneurysms, vascular malformation, and some rare genetic syndromes. Diagnosis of Bow Hunter's syndrome requires diagnostic DSA and real-time dynamic observation of contrast injection into the vertebral artery during rotation of the patient's head.

Neurological Monitoring of Children with Stroke

Serial monitoring is required with use of age-appropriate Glasgow coma scale, Pediatric National Institute of Health Stroke Scale (PedNIHSS), or alert, voice, pain, and unresponsive (AVPU) scale to assess the child's neurological status and conscious level, respectively.

DIFFERENTIAL DIAGNOSES

Children presenting with acute onset seizures and focal neurological deficits who are suspected to have AIS ≥50% of time show etiology other than AIS. With a negative initial CT scan, further imaging with MRI brain is required for the confirmation of the diagnosis of AIS or a stroke mimic. The conditions that can mimic clinical presentation of stroke in children are also known as stroke mimics. The important stroke mimics are:

- Postictal Todd's paresis
- Viral encephalitis
- Hemiplegia–hemiconvulsion syndrome
- Infection-triggered encephalopathy syndromes
- Acute disseminated encephalomyelitis
- Sturge–Weber syndrome
- Bell's palsy
- Posterior reversible encephalopathy syndrome
- Migraine
- Alternating hemiplegia of infancy
- Hypoglycemia
- Brain tumor
- Conversion disorder

RISK FACTORS FOR STROKE IN CHILDREN

Compared to adults, the risk factors for stroke in children **(Box 2)** are heterogenous and multiple. Two or more risk factors can coexist in children. Simultaneous evaluation of stroke risk factors is important for management and prevention of stroke recurrence. The most common risk factors for stroke in children are arteriopathy and an underlying heart disease. For posterior circulation stroke, presence of anatomical abnormalities of craniovertebral junction is an important risk factor.

BOX 2: Risk factors for stroke in children.

- *Arteriopathy:*
  - *Infections:* Bacterial meningitis, tubercular meningitis, and human immunodeficiency virus (HIV)
  - Focal cerebral arteriopathy
  - Moyamoya disease
  - Cervicovertebral arterial dissection
  - Mineralizing angiopathy
  - Systemic or CNS vasculitis
- *Cardiac:*
  - Cardiac procedure and invasive angiography
  - Congenital heart disease, bacterial endocarditis, cardiomyopathy, and myocarditis
- *Prothrombotic:* Homocysteinuria, protein C and S deficiency, lupus, and anticardiolipin Anticoagulants
- *Hematological:* Iron deficiency anemia, sickle cell anemia, thalassemia, leukemia, and hemolytic uremic syndrome
- *Medication/drugs:* Chemotherapy—L-asparaginase, cocaine, and ergots
- *Other:* Inborn errors of metabolism: Fabry disease, homocystinuria, mitochondrial disorders, and organic acidemia

MANAGEMENT OF STROKE

Management of stroke in acute phase **(Box 3)** requires immediate stabilization, rapid neuroimaging, and evaluation for possibility of thrombolysis. The subacute phase management is aimed toward evaluation of risk factors and medical management and rehabilitation.

BOX 3: Management of childhood stroke in various phases.[2]

Acute phase:
- Stabilization
- Neuroimaging
- Thrombolysis
- Supportive care
- Complications

Subacute phase:
- Diagnostic workup
- Secondary prevention

Chronic phase:
- Motor disability
- Epilepsy
- Vision impairment
- Speech

Emergency Care for Stroke

- Airway protection (avoid neck manipulation if arterial dissection is suspected)
- *Breathing:* Maintain oxygen saturation (SPO_2) ≥92%.
- *Circulation:* Avoid hypotension and hypertension, target blood pressure between 50th and 95th centile for age.
- *Optimal fluid:* Avoid dehydration.
- *Normoglycemia:* Random blood sugar (RBS) should be between 140 and 180 mg/dL.
- Management of fever should be done and hyperthermia to be avoided.
- Perform serial neurological examination and monitoring with appropriate tools (GCS, APVU, and PedsNIHSS).
- Treat anemia.
- Diagnostic workup with neuroimaging should be planned simultaneously.

Medical Management of Arterioischemic Stroke in Acute Care Setting

- Start antithrombotic or anticoagulation within the first 24 hours of onset of stroke.
  - *Antithrombotic agent:* Aspirin—initial dose, 5 mg/kg/day (max 300 mg/kg/day) for 14 days, later reduce to 1–3 mg/kg/day in all cases except sickle cell disease or if anticoagulation is initiated.
  - *Anticoagulation:* Conventional heparin/low-molecular-weight heparin (LMWH) in high-risk groups such as cardioembolic stroke, arterial dissection, and hypercoagulable state
  - LMWH at 1 mg/kg/dose BD subcutaneously, monitor factor Xa levels
  - Heparin 15–20 unit/kg/hour continuous infusion and monitor international normalized ratio (INR) and activated partial thromboplastin time (APTT) levels.
- AIS in children with sickle cell disease:
  - Packed red blood cell (RBC) transfusion to keep hemoglobin (Hb) 10 gm/dL within 6 hours
  - Exchange transfusion to maintain Hb between 10 and 11 gm/dL and HbS <30%
  - Aspirin should not be routinely used in children with sickle cell disease presenting with AIS.

Thrombolysis in Children with Arterioischemic Stroke

Off-label use of tissue plasminogen activator (tPA) can be considered in children presenting with AIS within window period (evidence limited to case reports and case series).[3] Thrombolysis is safe in children >8 years of age and may be considered in selected cases between ages of 2 and 8 years. Intravenous thrombolysis in children presenting with AIS can be considered in presence of:

- An acute onset focal neurological deficit consistent with AIS
- PedNIHSS score ≥4 and ≤24
- Treatment can be administered within 4.5 hours of known onset of symptoms
- Intracranial hemorrhage has been excluded in a noncontrast CT scan
- CT demonstrates normal brain parenchyma or minimal early ischemic change, and CT angiography (CTA) demonstrates partial or complete occlusion of the intracranial artery corresponding to clinical or radiological deficit OR
- MRI and MRA showing evidence of acute ischemia on DWI plus partial or complete occlusion of the intracranial artery corresponding to clinical or radiological deficit if there are no contraindications **(Box 4)**

BOX 4: Contraindications for thrombolysis in children with arterioischemic stroke (AIS).

- Unknown time of symptoms of stroke onset
- Bleeding diathesis including platelets <100 000/μL, prothrombin time (PT) >15s, international normalized ratio (INR) >1.4 or activated partial thromboplastin time (APTT) more than upper limits of the normal range
- Systolic blood pressure >15% above the 95th percentile for age while sitting or supine
- History of prior intracranial hemorrhage
- Known cerebral arterial venous malformation, aneurysm, or neoplasm
- Prior stroke, major head trauma, surgery, GI bleed within the past 3 months
- Large infarct volume, defined as acute infarct involving one-third or more of the middle cerebral artery (MCA) territory

- Alteplase is most common thrombolytic agent used in children.
- Delay administering aspirin for 24 hours in patients where thrombolysis has been given.

Role of Mechanical Thrombectomy

Children with acute AIS with persistent neurological deficit (PedNIHSS score of ≥6) may be considered for intra-arterial clot extraction with prior IV thrombolysis, unless contraindicated, beyond an onset-to-arterial puncture time of 5 hours or in certain cases, up to 12 hours.

EARLY COMPLICATIONS OF STROKE

Early complications of stroke include:

- *Seizures and status epilepticus:* Prompt use of antiseizure medication (ASM) and electroencephalogram (EEG) monitoring should be done and managed as per the status epilepticus protocol.
- *Malignant cerebral edema:* Patients with large MCA infractions and cerebellar infracts are at risk for malignant cerebral edema and herniation. Early decompressive craniectomy can be lifesaving.
- *Extension of infraction or stroke recurrence:* It can occur in patients with arteriopathy or cardiac thrombus. Neurological monitoring and early repeat imaging are required to guide neuroprotective measures and change in treatment strategies.
- *Hemorrhagic transformation:* Large infracts of cardioembolic origin are at risk of malignant edema and hemorrhagic transformation. Serial monitoring and early repeat imaging may be warranted in case of worsening or appearance of new neurological signs and symptoms.

Decompressive hemicraniectomy should be considered a lifesaving measure in children with stroke under following circumstances:

- Clinical features suggestive of MCA infarction
- Progressive decrease in the level of consciousness (reduction in PedNIHSS score)
- An infarction of ≥50% of the MCA territory with or without additional infarction in the territory of the anterior or posterior cerebral artery on the same side

INVESTIGATIONS FOR CHILDREN WITH ARTERIOISCHEMIC STROKE

To evaluate for underlying risk factors, children with AIS should be investigated with:

- *Hematological investigations:* Complete blood counts, peripheral smear, RBC indices, iron status (iron, ferritin, and total iron binding capacity), and hemoglobinopathy screen
- *Biochemistry tests:* Fasting blood glucose, lipid profile, total plasma homocysteine, vitamin B_{12} levels, and alpha-galactosidase
- *Procoagulant state:* Lupus anticoagulant and anticardiolipin antibodies (ACLA), beta-2 glycoprotein 1 (B2gp1) testing with hematology if necessary.
- *Cardiac evaluation:* Electrocardiogram, echocardiogram, and cerebrovascular imaging from the aortic arch to vertex, with MRA or CTA
- Transcranial Doppler in patients with sickle cell disease
- Clinically evaluate all patients for history of prior infection (especially varicella-zoster virus)
- Evaluation for immunization status, dysmorphic features, neurocutaneous markers, autoimmune disease, and evidence of vascular disease in other organ systems.

MANAGEMENT OF ARTERIOISCHEMIC STROKE IN SPECIFIC SITUATIONS

The management of AIS in children includes immediate management with stabilization, neuro-imaging, and evaluation of potential thrombolysis. After the acute phase, the aim is to investigate underlying risk factors, management of risk factors, and secondary prevention of stroke. The details of management of risk factors are presented in **Table 2**.

TABLE 2: Management of specific risk factors of arterioischemic stroke (AIS) in children.

Risk factor	*Management*
Arteriopathies	
Infection-associated arteriopathy	• Diagnosis and management of central nervous system infection • *Meningitis:* IV antibiotics and antithrombotic therapy if no contraindications • *Tubercular meningitis:* Antitubercular therapy, steroids, aspirin, thalidomide, etc.
Postvaricella arteriopathy	• Intravenous acyclovir for 2 weeks • Oral steroids for 5 days and taper over 1 week followed by oral valganciclovir for 2–3 months • Aspirin • Repeat MRI and MRA imaging after 12 weeks
Moyamoya disease	• Aspirin • MRA-vessel-wall imaging/Digital subtraction angiography **(Fig. 2)** • Neurosurgery consult for revascularization surgery • Consideration of genetic testing for *RNF213* gene • *Clinical screening for genetic disorders:* ACTA-2, BRCC3/MTCPI, GUCYIA3, SAMHD1, Alagille syndrome, Down syndrome, neurofibromatosis type I, PHACE syndrome, Robinow syndrome, and Seckel syndrome
Arterial dissection	• Neck stabilization with neck collar • Dynamic CTA/DSA for suspected arterial dissection • Anticoagulation for 6–12 weeks and repeat vessel imaging after 12 weeks, aspirin may be used in cases with dissection.
Cardiac disease	• ECG, echocardiography, and Holter monitoring • Anticoagulation for 12 weeks and correction of underlying cardiac condition • LMWH/warfarin
Hypercoagulable state	• Inherited thrombophilia or acquired thrombophilia • Factor-V Leiden mutation • Prothrombin G20210A mutation • Protein C, Protein S, and antithrombin mutation • Lupus anticoagulant • Anticardiolipin antibody (IgG/IgM) • Anti-β_2 glycoprotein antibody (IgG/IgM) • Anticoagulation with LMWH or warfarin for 6–12 weeks or longer based on the risk factor

Contd...

Contd...

Risk factor	*Management*
Sickle cell anemia	• Optimal hydration, correction of hypoxemia, and systemic hypotension • Treat anemia with blood transfusion hemoglobin (Hb) >10 gm/dL • Exchange transfusion to keep HbS <30% • *Secondary prevention:* Regular blood transfusion therapy to reduce the percentage of HbS to a maximum of <30% in conjunction with measures to prevent iron overload • Screening for silent infarct with MRI brain • Neurocognitive assessment • Annual transcranial Doppler to measure MCA flow velocity

(CTA: computed tomography angiography; ECG: electrocardiogram; LMWH: low-molecular-weight heparin; MCA: middle cerebral artery; MRA: magnetic resonance angiography; MRI: magnetic resonance imaging)

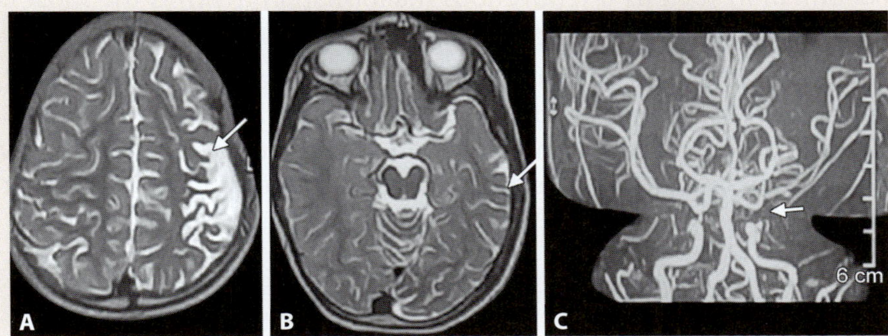

Figs. 2A to C: MRI brain T2 axial images showing acute ischemic infarct involving left middle cerebral artery (MCA) territory (A) left frontal and (B) temporal lobes with (C) MR angiography showing supraclinoid internal carotid artery narrowing on right side and nonvisualization on left side (arrowhead) with bilateral collateral formation suggestive of moyamoya disease.

Follow-up and Outcomes

- Age-appropriate rehabilitation and physiotherapy programs for children with stroke
- Detailed assessment of cognitive and language deficits for planning therapy and educational programs.
- Constraint-induced movement therapy should be considered in children with unilateral hand dysfunction after AIS.
- Long-term follow-up is required for children with stroke to assess for development of epilepsy, and cognitive, physical, and emotional concerns that may occur over time as children grow into deficits.
- Titration of ASM
- Titration of antithrombotic and anticoagulation therapy

HEMORRHAGIC STROKE IN CHILDREN

Hemorrhagic stroke in children includes intracerebral hemorrhage (ICH) and subarachnoid hemorrhages (SAH). ICH refers to bleeding into the brain parenchyma and/or ventricles, whereas SAH refers to bleeding into the subarachnoid space. About 50% strokes in childhood are HS, and among these, intraparenchymal ICH (25–75%) are common.

- The incidence of HS is 1–2/100,000 children per year
- ICH can occur following traumatic brain injury.
- Spontaneous ICH in children is secondary to a ruptured vascular malformation, brain tumor, central nervous system (CNS) infection or bleeding disorder.
- Vascular malformation accounts for 40–90% of pediatric ICH cases. In younger children, a hematological disorder or a bleeding disorder is responsible for ICH; however, in older children, vascular malformation such as arteriovenous malformation (AVM) is the most common cause of HS.
- The common presenting signs and symptoms of HS are headache, altered mental status, focal deficits like hemiparesis, seizures, and vomiting. Headache is present in 50–80% children, it is classically sudden onset and severe in nature and accompanied by nausea and vomiting. Neck pain and neck stiffness can accompany headache and suggest intraventricular or subarachnoid hemorrhage.

Diagnosis

Investigations required in acute care settings for children suspected of HS are given in **Box 5**.

Diagnosis is done as follows:

- *Neuroimaging:* An urgent noncontrast CT scan of head is required for diagnosis of HS.
- Noncontrast CT scan of head **(Fig. 3)** can diagnose almost all HS in children; however, it can miss about 5% of SAH.

BOX 5: Investigations required in acute care setting for children suspected of HS.

- Noncontrast CT head with CT angiography
- Complete blood count with platelets
- Coagulation profile
- Serum electrolytes

- MRI brain with MRA is required once patient is stabilized for detailed anatomical information of ICH and underlying vascular malformation.
- If MRA is negative, a digital subtraction angiography/ catheter angiography is required for diagnosis of vascular malformations.

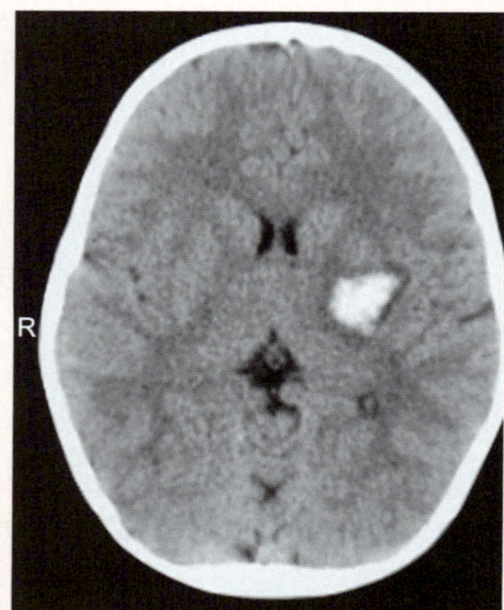

Fig. 3: Noncontrast CT scan of the head showing irregular hyperdense lesion in the left-sided putamen suggestive of acute intraparenchymal ICH.

- The common vascular malformations are AVMs, AV fistula, and cavernous malformation.
- Other hemorrhage-prone intracerebral vascular lesions include pial or dural arteriovenous fistulae, thrombosed developmental venous anomalies or sinus pericranii, sickle cell disease, moyamoya disease, and brain tumors **(Box 6)**.
- The congenital coagulation disorders associated with risk for ICH are hemophilia (factor VIII or factor IX deficiency) and rarely, factor XIII deficiency.
- Acquired hematologic disorders such as immune thrombocytopenia and leukemia in children can present with ICH.
- Vitamin K deficiency-related bleeding disorder (VKBD) is an important acquired cause of ICH in neonates and infants.

BOX 6: High-flow and low-flow vascular malformations.

- *High-flow vascular malformations:*
  - Arteriovenous malformations
  - Arteriovenous fistulas
  - Vein of Galen malformations
- *Low-flow vascular malformations:*
  - Cavernous malformations
  - Developmental venous anomalies
  - Aneurysms

Management of Hemorrhagic Stroke

The management of HS is given as follows:

- The principles of management of HS remain like AIS in children.
- Immediate stabilization should be done with focus on airway, breathing, and circulation.
- Seizure termination is done with ASM, no role of prophylactic ASM.
- Raised ICP management is done as per standard protocols.
- If hypertension, maintain blood pressure at 95th centile and cautiously use blood pressure lowering agents, as systemic hypotension can cause cerebral ischemia.
- Neurosurgery consult for all cases of ICH
- *Evacuation of the hematoma:*
  - Decompressive craniotomy may be lifesaving and functional sparing may be done in rapidly worsening raised ICP.
  - Management of underlying bleeding disorder with vitamin K, fresh frozen plasma and platelet concentrates, and factor replacement should be done.
- Vascular malformation should be managed in consultation with intervention neuroradiologist or neurosurgery team.
- ICH in children has a case fatality rate of 10–20%. Survivors have persistent neurological disability in 60% and develop epilepsy in about 20%.

CEREBRAL SINUS VENOUS THROMBOSIS

- Thrombotic occlusion of cerebral veins and/or dural venous sinuses is known as CSVT.[4]
- The incidence of CVST is 0.25–0.67 in every 100,000 children each year, neonatal age group is at higher risk.
- *Cerebral venous system has two compartments:* Cerebral veins and dural venous sinuses.
- The superficial venous system (cerebral veins) drains blood from cerebral cortex to superior sagittal sinus. The deep venous system drains blood from deep white matter and basal ganglia to the inferior sagittal sinus, which drains to straight sinus and transverse sinus. From the transverse sinus, the blood flow toward the sigmoid sinus passing through the torcular Herophili and finally into the internal jugular veins.
- Occlusion of venous channels leads to increase in the hydrostatic pressure within the veins and capillaries upstream. If the increase in venous pressure overcomes the compensatory potential of venous channels, it leads to blood–brain barrier disruption and extravasation of fluids into the cerebral parenchyma and consequent localized edema. If pressure in the venous system exceeds the arterial pressure, it can lead to cerebral ischemia and hemorrhagic infarction.
- The clinical features of CSVT are diffuse and nonspecific.
- Children with CSVT present with seizures, headaches, papilledema, altered consciousness, and focal neurologic signs. Young infants tend to present with seizures and encephalopathy.
- Diagnosis of CSVT requires a low index of suspicion.
- *CSVT should be suspected in presence of:*
  - New onset headache, papilledema, and 6th nerve palsy in children
  - CSVT must be ruled out in children with idiopathic intracranial hypertension (also commonly called pseudotumor cerebri)
  - In neonates in presence of seizures, lethargy, and encephalopathy
  - Neurological signs and symptoms in presence of fever, dehydration, hematological disorder (leukemia), acute or chronic renal or hepatic conditions, and medication use such as steroid and l-asparaginase therapy.
- *The predisposing risk factors for CSVT are:* Infections, anemia, prothrombotic disorder, and acute and chronic systemic disorders.
- "Septic" CSVT is defined as CSVT associated with head and neck infections such as otitis media, mastoiditis, sinusitis, meningitis, and intracranial abscess/empyema.
- Dehydration is the most common acute systemic illness associated with CSVT and several chronic conditions as leukemia predisposes to CSVT.

Diagnosis

Diagnosis is done as follows:

- CT scan (contrast CT scan head) (CT can miss 16–40% CSVT and can be false positive in neonates due to high hematocrit) can show empty delta sign, cord sign or IVH or parenchymal hemorrhage.
- CT venography is sensitive but increases radiation exposure.
- MRI and MR venography (sensitive and require sedation) **(Figs. 4A to C)**
- Investigations for risk factors

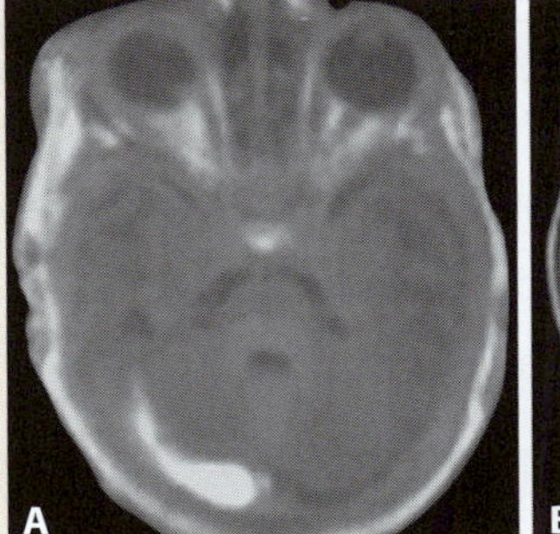

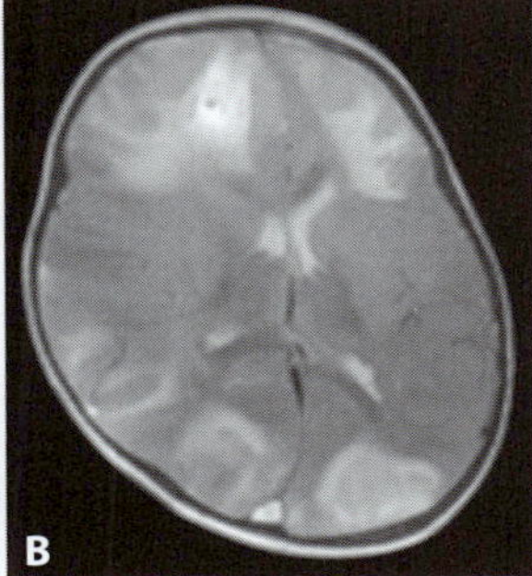

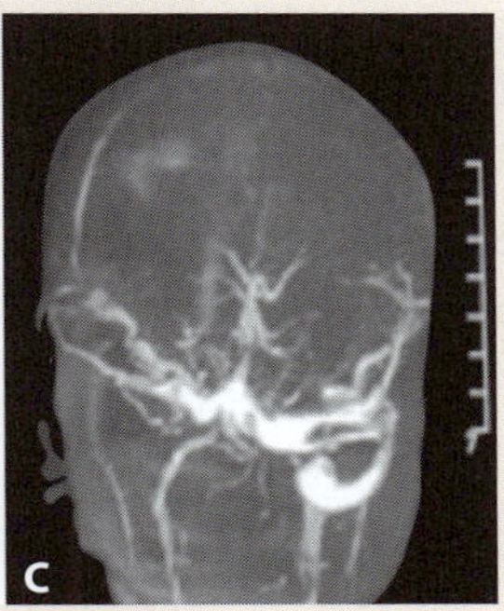

Figs. 4A to C: MRI brain. (A) T1-weighted axial section showing hyperintense right transverse sinus suggestive of thrombosis in a neonate; (B) T2-weighted MRI axial section is suggestive of multiple T2 hyperintensities over bilateral frontal, parietal, and occipital lobe with hemorrhagic changes; (C) MR venography showing nonvisualization of sagittal sinus and right transverse and sigmoid sinus suggestive of thrombosis.

Treatment

Treatment includes the following:[5]

- Management of raised ICP and seizures as per protocols
- 40–60% children with CSVT can show presence of hemorrhagic infracts with intraparenchymal and intraventricular hemorrhage.
- In term neonate IVH and asymmetric thalamic hemorrhage are frequently secondary to CSVT.
- Identification of underlying risk factors and initiation of treatment
- Anticoagulation is defined as mainstay of treatment [2018 American Heart Association (AHA) guidelines]
  - Intravenous unfractionated heparin (uFH)
  - Subcutaneous LMWH
  - Oral warfarin

- Anticoagulation remains controversial in septic CSVT.
- Presence of ICH is not a contraindication for anticoagulation therapy.
- Recently, direct oral anticoagulants (DOACs), rivaroxaban and dabigatran have been approved for use in children with venous thromboembolism.
    - Rivaroxaban is equally effective and safe for treatment of CSVT in children. In EINSTEIN-Jr CVT study, 114 children with CVT were randomized to rivaroxaban, and standard anticoagulation and weight-based doses were used. None of the 73 children randomized to rivaroxaban had recurrence of CVT compared to one in standard anticoagulation. 6.8% children had bleeding with rivaroxaban, all were nonmajor and noncerebral and one child in standard anticoagulation had major CNS bleed. In DIVESITY trial, dabigatran has been reported to have similar efficacy and safety profile for pediatric venous thromboembolism.

- Duration 6 weeks to 3 months, can be extended for 6 months in case of partial resolution.
- Repeat MRI and MRV after 3 months for resolution of thrombosis.
- Follow-up should be done for resolution and neurological monitoring.

REFERENCES

1. Ferriero DM, Fullerton HJ, Bernard TJ, Billinghurst L, Daniels SR, DeBaun MR, et al; American Heart Association Stroke Council and Council on Cardiovascular and Stroke Nursing. Management of stroke in neonates and children: A scientific statement from the American Heart Association/American Stroke Association. Stroke. 2019;50(3):e51-96.
2. Rivkin MJ, Bernard TJ, Dowling MM, Amlie-Lefond C. Guidelines for urgent management of stroke in children. Pediatr Neurol. 2016;56:8-17.
3. Royal College of Paediatrics and Child Health, NICE, Stroke Association. (2017). Stroke in childhood: Clinical guideline for diagnosis, management and rehabilitation. [online]. Available from https://www.stroke.org.uk/sites/default/files/stroke_in_childhood_clinical_guidelines.pdf [Last accessed January, 2025].
4. Mandel-Shorer N, Sabapathy CA, Krishnan P, Sharma M, Goldenberg NA, Brandão LR, et al. Cerebral sinovenous thrombosis in infants and children: A practical approach to management. Semin Pediatr Neurol. 2022;44:100993.
5. Biss TT, Chalmers EA. Addendum to British Society for Haematology guideline on the investigation, management and prevention of venous thrombosis in children. Br J Haematol. 2021;194(6):996-8.

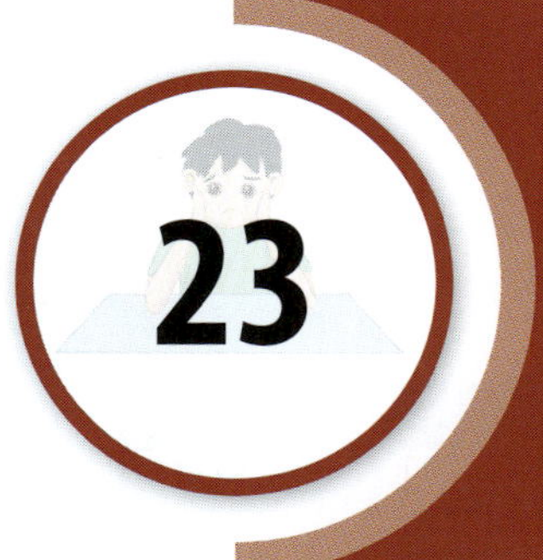

Acute Ataxia

Daisy Khera, Sneh Yadav

INTRODUCTION

- The Ataxia term has been derived from the Greek words—"a" lacking or without and "taxis" meaning order, which means lack of order.
- Ataxia refers to impaired coordination of muscle movements, affecting the ability to execute voluntary movements.
- Clinically, ataxia is characterized by a broad-based gait, inaccuracies in range and force of limb movements (dysmetria), irregularities in speed and rhythm of repetitive and alternating actions (dysdiadochokinesia), tremors that become more pronounced at the end of the movement (intention tremor), tongue incoordination leading to "scanning" speech (dysarthria), and uncoordinated eye movements (nystagmus).

DEFINITION

Acute ataxia is defined by a sudden onset of ataxia symptoms that emerge rapidly, typically within a few hours or a few (1–2) days.

ETIOPATHOLOGY

The etiopathology of acute ataxia is described in **Table 1**.

TABLE 1: Etiopathology of acute ataxia.

Types	*Cause*	*Pathology*
Acute cerebellar ataxia	Infectious/immune-mediated	• Acute postinfectious cerebellar ataxia (APCA) • Acute cerebellitis [Epstein–Barr virus (EBV), varicella, mumps, *Mycoplasma*, human herpesvirus 6 (HHV-6), and human immunodeficiency virus (HIV)] • Acute disseminated encephalomyelitis (ADEM) and multiple sclerosis (MS) • Gluten ataxia • Hashimoto encephalopathy
	Intoxications	• Antiepileptic drugs—benzodiazepines, phenytoin, and oxcarbazepine • Antihistaminic drugs • Antineoplastic/immunosuppressive agents—cyclosporine, tacrolimus alcohol, ethylene glycol, lead, mercury, thallium, and lithium
	Traumatic	• Postconcussion ataxia • Traumatic vertebral dissection
	Vascular	• Ischemic/hemorrhagic stroke
	Paraneoplastic	• Opsoclonus myoclonus syndrome (OMS) [Langerhans cell histiocytosis (LCH) neurodegeneration and neuroblastoma (NB)]
	First-event intermittent ataxia	• Maple syrup urine disease • Pyruvate dehydrogenase deficiency • Urea cycle disorders • Glucose transporter-1 (GLUT-1) deficiency
	Intracranial space occupying lesions	• Cerebellar tumor/tuberculoma/neurocysticercosis (NCC)
Acute vestibular ataxia	Acute unilateral vestibular dysfunction	• Vestibular neuritis • Labyrinthitis
Acute sensory ataxia	Inflammatory	Miller Fisher syndrome

CLINICAL FEATURES

Focal dysfunction of cerebellar vermis presents with symptoms such as truncal imbalance, nystagmus, and head waddling. Impairment of cerebellar hemisphere leads to an abnormal gait that veers toward the affected side, accompanied by asymmetry of ipsilateral extremities and a high-stepping gait. In contrast, afferent or sensory ataxia manifests as a stepping gait with sensory deficits in the extremities.

The clinical features and their possible etiology are given in **Table 2**.

TABLE 2: Clinical features and possible etiology.

Features		***Possible etiology***
Infectious (fever, rash, and recent vaccination)	10–15 days before	APCA
	2–4 weeks before	GBS
	2 days–4 weeks before	ADEM
Coexistent systemic complaints (fever/headache/vomiting)		Acute cerebellitis
Toxic exposure (suspected/observed ingestion of drugs or pesticides)		Toxic cerebellar ataxia
Feeling of dizziness, turning, and spinning		Acute vestibular ataxia
Emotional trauma (bullying, sexual/physical abuse, and death in family)		Psychogenic ataxia
Coexistent medical condition (NB, LCH, autoimmune, and cardiac)		OMS/stroke

(ADEM: acute disseminated encephalomyelitis; APCA: acute postinfectious cerebellar ataxia; GBS: Guillain–Barré syndrome; LCH: Langerhans cell histiocytosis; NB: neuroblastoma; OMS: opsoclonus myoclonus syndrome)

Acute postinfectious cerebellar ataxia: It presents with sudden onset of ataxia, typically occurring 10–15 days after a prodromal illness. APCA is characterized by purely cerebellar symptoms, including gait ataxia, dysmetria, intention tremor, hypotonia, and nystagmus.

Acute cerebellitis is a potentially life-threatening disorder characterized by more widespread neurologic symptoms than APCA. The primary symptoms include headache, vomiting, and disturbances of consciousness, ranging from somnolence to coma. These symptoms are usually the result of cerebellar swelling, which can lead to brainstem compression and hydrocephalus.

Varicella is a key pathogen known to affect the cerebellum, particularly in children. While it can occur at any age, it is most prevalent in children between 2 and 8 years. Ataxia often develops 2–6 days after the appearance of rash, but it can also manifest during the incubation period or even after the rash has resolved. Cerebellar impairment can manifest itself after mumps or infectious mononucleosis.

Inadequate intake of essential nutrients such as vitamins (thiamine, cobalamin, and vitamin E), zinc, and folate in neglected children or those suffering from intestinal disorders, can lead to symptoms of ataxia.

EVALUATION

The evaluation includes the following:

- Pediatric assessment triangle, primary assessment [airway, breathing, circulation, disability, exposure (ABCDE)]
- *Vitals:* Heart rate (HR), respiratory rate (RR), peripheral pulses, and blood pressure (BP)
- Head-to-toe examination
- Neurological examination:
  - *Mental status:* Abnormal mental status suggests toxin ingestion, ADEM, or stroke.
  - *Cranial nerve:* Ophthalmoplegia suggestive of Miller Fisher syndrome
  - *Motor:* Absent deep tendon reflexes (DTRs) suggestive of Guillain–Barré syndrome (GBS)
  - *Sensory:* Impaired proprioception in sensory ataxia
  - *Cerebellar examination:* Broad-based gait (gait ataxia), scanning speech, nystagmus, titubation, dysdiadochokinesia, hypotonia, tremors, finger-to-nose test (arm ataxia), and heel-to-shin test (leg ataxia)
  - Signs of raised intracranial pressure (ICP)
  - *Meningeal signs:* Neck rigidity, Kernig's sign, and Brudzinski sign
- Ophthalmological examination
  - Opsoclonus and saccadic movements
  - *Fundus:* Papilledema and retinopathy

INVESTIGATIONS

The investigations done for acute ataxia are as follows:

- Drug/toxin levels
- *Computed tomography (CT) head:* Cerebellar edema and hypodensity areas in cerebellar parenchyma
- *Magnetic resonance imaging (MRI) Brain:* On T-2 weighted sequences, there is hyperintense signal of the cerebellar peduncle, along with hyperintensity of the cerebellar white matter and gray matter. Additionally, there may be leptomeningeal enhancement.
- *Lumbar puncture—cerebrospinal fluid (CSF):* Pleocytosis, proteinorachia, CSF viral PCR (varicella, parainfluenza, influenza, enterovirus, and EBV)
- *Viral serology:* Measles, mumps, coxsackie virus, and HIV
- Urinary catecholamines and CT chest/abdomen
- Thyroid function test and tissue transglutaminase immunoglobulin A (IgA) test

APPROACH TO ACUTE ATAXIA

The approach to the management of acute ataxia is given in **Flowchart 1.**

Flowchart 1: Approach to the management of acute ataxia

Acute ataxia
- Post-traumatic/signs of raised ICP
  - CT/MRI
    - Anomalous
      - Hematoma
      - Hemorrhage/stroke
      - White matter lesions
      - Posterior fossa tumor/tuberculoma
    - Negative
      - Postconcussion syndrome
- Isolated
  - Toxicology screen/lumbar puncture
    - *Drug present:* Intoxication
    - No cells/no drugs
      - Consistent with post-infectious process
        - *No* Opsoclonus-myoclonus
          - Urine VMA/CT/MRI chest, abdomen
        - *Yes* Postinfectious ataxia Varicella/Mumps/Influenza A/Mycoplasma
    - Cells in CSF:
      - Viral cerebellitis/ADEM
      - Bacterial meningitis

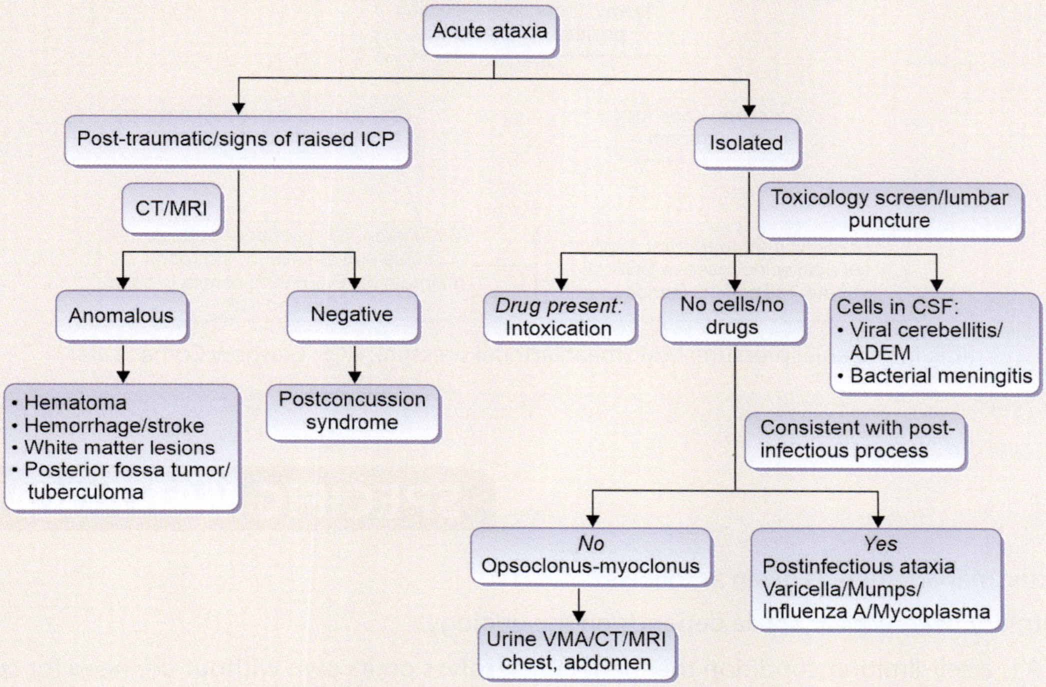

(ADEM: acute disseminated encephalomyelitis; CT: computed tomography; CSF: cerebrospinal fluid; ICP: intracranial pressure; MRI: magnetic resonance imaging; VMA: vanillylmandelic acid)

DIFFERENTIALS

The differentials include:
- Acute cerebellar ataxia
- Sensory ataxia
- Vestibular ataxia
- Acute epileptic pseudo-ataxia

EMERGENCY CARE

The emergency care for acute ataxia is given in **Flowchart 2.**

Flowchart 2: Emergency care.

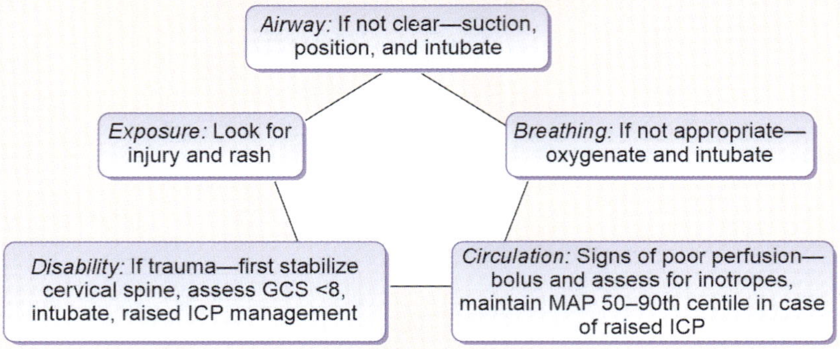

Airway: If not clear—suction, position, and intubate

Breathing: If not appropriate—oxygenate and intubate

Circulation: Signs of poor perfusion—bolus and assess for inotropes, maintain MAP 50–90th centile in case of raised ICP

Disability: If trauma—first stabilize cervical spine, assess GCS <8, intubate, raised ICP management

Exposure: Look for injury and rash

(ICP: intracranial pressure; MAP: mean arterial pressure; GCS: Glasgow Coma Scale)

SPECIFIC MANAGEMENT

The specific management is given as follows:

- Treatment of cerebellar ataxia depends on the etiology.
- APCA is a self-limiting condition that generally resolves on its own without the need for specific treatment and has an excellent prognosis.
- *Acute cerebellitis:* In case of acute cerebellitis, early diagnosis and prompt treatment are crucial. If there is suspicion of direct invasion by a specific microorganism, appropriate antimicrobial therapy should be initiated immediately. High-dose intravenous methylprednisolone (30 mg/kg/day for 3–5 days with a maximum of 1 g/day over 2 hours) can help reduce cerebellar swelling and potentially eliminate the need for surgical intervention. However, when swelling is severe causing signs of brainstem compression, surgical decompression of the posterior fossa may be life-saving procedure.
- *Vitamin supplementation:* If caused by vitamin deficiency
- *Opsoclonus myoclonus syndrome (OMS):* It currently lacks a standardized protocol for immunomodulatory therapy, and various drugs have been used in recent years. Steroids (prednisolone, adrenocorticotropic hormone (ACTH), and intravenous methylprednisolone pulses) are the most commonly used primary therapy. High-dose dexamethasone in pulses (20 mg/m^2/d over 3–5 days each month) has also shown to be beneficial. Other drugs which have shown response are intravenous immunoglobulin, cyclophosphamide, and rituximab.
- *Vascular acute cerebellar ataxia:* Early edema resulting from infarction in the posterior fossa can lead to potentially fatal complications such as brainstem compression, obstructive hydrocephalus, and herniation of the cerebellar tonsils. In cases of significant cerebellar swelling, suboccipital craniectomy should be considered to relieve pressure and prevent further deterioration.

MONITORING

Monitoring involves:

- Neurological monitoring for raised ICP/impending herniation
- Monitoring for seizures

KEY LEARNING POINTS

- Acute ataxia in childhood needs a systematic approach, detailed clinical history, and neurological examination.
- Most common cause of childhood ataxia is postinfectious cerebellar ataxia, which needs symptomatic treatment and is self-limiting.
- Acute cerebellitis is a potentially life-threatening disorder for which early diagnosis and prompt treatment are crucial.

SUGGESTED READING

1. Caffarelli M, Kimia AA, Torres AR. Acute ataxia in children: A review of the differential diagnosis and evaluation in the emergency department. Pediatr Neurol. 2016;65:14-30.
2. Kravljanac R, Golubovic A, Tadic BV, Ostojic S, Cerovic I, Savkic J. "The Red Flags" in clinical approach to acute ataxia—the experience in cohort of 76 children. Cerebellum. 2024;23(4):1321-27.
3. Lancella L, Esposito S, Galli ML, Bozzola E, Labalestra V, Boccuzzi E, et al. Acute cerebellitis in children: An eleven-year retrospective multicentric study in Italy. Ital J Pediatr. 2017;43(1):54.
4. Pavone P, Praticò AD, Pavone V, Lubrano R, Falsaperla R, Rizzo R, et al. Ataxia in children: Early recognition and clinical evaluation. Ital J Pediatr. 2017;43(1):6.
5. Thakkar K, Maricich SM, Alper G. Acute ataxia in childhood: 11-year experience at a major pediatric neurology referral center. J Child Neurol. 2016;31(9):1156-60.

24 Approach to Dizziness and Vertigo

Anita Sharma

INTRODUCTION

- Dizziness and vertigo are common problems in children with prevalence of 5.6% in school children.
- These two terms are often used interchangeably but they are two different symptoms with specific etiology and management.
- Syncope (cardiovascular cause) and vertigo (vestibular cause) are two most common groups of disorders presenting as dizziness.
- Dizziness, imbalance, and nausea are salient complaints. Symptoms are very frightening to family, and hence, important cause of emergency visits.

TERMINOLOGIES AND DEFINITIONS

- *Dizziness:* It is a general term to describe several sensations like light-headedness, impending fall, floating, or disequilibrium. There is no sensation of rotation or spinning.
- *Vertigo:* It is a sensation of rotation or spinning when no self-motion is occurring. Common symptoms are difficulty in maintaining balance, nystagmus, and nausea.
- *Presyncope (light-headedness):* Near fainting can progress to total loss of consciousness (syncope).
- *Disequilibrium:* Imbalance during standing or walking
- *Nonspecific dizziness:* Occurs in depression or anxiety

ETIOPATHOLOGY

The etiopathology is given in **Table 1**.

- Etiology of vertigo is age-dependent and helps in narrowing diagnosis.
- Serious causes of vertigo like tumors are rare and can be detected by careful clinical examination.
- Majority of vertigo and dizziness conditions in childhood are benign.
- Benign paroxysmal vertigo of childhood (BPVC), migraine, and otitis media account for 50% vertigo children.
- In children <5 years of age: BPVC (71%) is most common.
- Vestibular migraine is common in older children.
- Somatoform vertigo (functional dizziness) is common in adolescence.
- Ménière disease and head trauma are less common causes.

TABLE 1: Etiopathogenesis of different types of dizziness.

Symptom	*Causes*	*Pathogenesis*
Vertigo	Vestibular system disruption	*Two types:* 1. *Peripheral type:* Dysfunction of vestibular apparatus or vestibular nerve – *Common causes:* BPVC, labyrinthitis, vestibular neuritis (VN), otitis media, perilymph fistula, and Ménière's disease 2. *Central type:* Dysfunction of brainstem/cerebellum – *Common causes:* Vestibular migraine (VM), seizure disorder, brainstem tumor, cervical spine abnormalities, post-trauma, drugs, and demyelination disorders
Presyncope (Light-headedness)	• *Cardiogenic:* Arrhythmia • Vasovagal • Orthostatic hypotension • *Metabolic:* Hypoglycemia, dehydration, anemia	Temporary cerebral hypoperfusion
Disequilibrium	Loss of balance in legs or trunk	Peripheral neuropathy and muscle disorders
Nonspecific dizziness	Nonvertiginous dizziness	Psychiatric disorders and ocular disorders

(BPVC: benign paroxysmal vertigo of childhood)

CLINICAL FEATURES

Depend on:

- *Cause of dizziness:* True vertigo versus nonvertiginous dizziness
- *Type of vertigo:* Peripheral or central type **(Table 2)**
- Temporal pattern (acute or recurrent) and hearing status (normal or impaired) **(Table 3)**

TABLE 2: Differences between peripheral and central vertigo.

Feature	*Peripheral vertigo*	*Central vertigo*
Nystagmus	• Horizontal • Suppressed by gaze fixation	• Vertical • Not suppressed by gaze fixation
Deafness	Present (except BPVC)	No
Vertigo severity	Intense	Mild
Duration of symptoms	Episodic (very short duration)	Persistent
Other neurological signs	Absent	Present
Balance disturbance	Mild, can walk	Severe, unable to walk

(BPVC: benign paroxysmal vertigo of childhood)

TABLE 3: Characteristics of disorders causing vertigo.

Disorder	*Duration of symptoms and salient features*	*Hearing*
Acute nonrecurrent vertigo:		
• Vestibular neuritis	Imbalance for days, rare <10 years age, post-viral infection, vertigo, nausea, and nystagmus	Normal
• *Head trauma:* Labyrinth concussion	Lasts for days, common in <5 years age, vertigo/dizziness related to trauma	Often impaired SNHL
• Perilymph fistula	Attacks (seconds) provoked by coughing, sneezing, and Valsalva	Often impaired SNHL
Recurrent vertigo:		
• Vestibular migraine	Duration minutes to 72 hours, recurrent headache	Normal
• Benign paroxysmal vertigo of childhood	Common in <5 years age, episodic vertigo for seconds to minutes, no headache, family history of motion sickness or migraine present, no imaging or EEG required	Normal
• Seizure disorder	For seconds to minutes	Normal
Persistent vertigo:		
• Somatoform vertigo	Constant symptoms, school-aged, behavior problems, aggravation in certain situations, and subjective imbalance with normal examination	Normal
• Central nervous system disorders	Constant symptoms of diplopia, dysarthria, ataxia, and ocular signs	Normal
• Otitis media	Constant	Conductive deafness

(EEG: electroencephalogram; SNHL: sensorineural hearing loss)

EVALUATION

- Observe patient both during walking and running.
- Ask parents to record home videos.
- *Focused physical examination:* Examine for fever, anemia, and hydration status (for orthostatic hypotension) and abnormal head posture indicates central cause.
- *Cardiovascular examination:* Murmurs, arrhythmias, blood pressure for orthostatic hypotension.
- *Eye examination:* Pupil size, acuity, range of movement, saccades and pursuit, conjugate or disconjugate, and nystagmus.
- Ear examination:
  - Otoscopy for otitis media, tympanic membrane abnormalities
  - Hearing tests
- Neurological examination:
  - *Cranial Nerves:* Eye movement and fundus
  - *Nystagmus:* Both spontaneous and gaze evoked
  - Cerebellar signs
  - Gait and balance
  - *Signs of raised intracranial pressure:* Altered mental status and papilledema
- Psychological evaluation
- Clinical examination of vestibular functions by:
  - *Ocular motor testing:* Saccade abnormalities (hypermetric or hypometric) and pursuits; nystagmus (spontaneous/with or without fixation) and gaze-evoked
  - *Positional testing:* Both static and dynamic (by Dix-Hallpike test)
  - *Head impulse test:* For horizontal vestibuloocular reflex (VOR) function

INVESTIGATIONS

- *Blood tests:* Hemoglobin, complete blood count (CBC), glucose, electrolytes, and thyroid function test.
- *Serological test for antibodies:* Epstein–Barr virus, Herpes simplex virus, parainfluenza, and cytomegalovirus
- *Specialized tests:*
  - *Magnetic resonance imaging (MRI) brain:* If central cause suspected
  - *Magnetic resonance angiography (MRA):* In vertebrobasilar insufficiency
  - CT head if history of trauma
  - *Electrocardiograph (ECG) and echocardiogram:* To rule out cardiac cause
  - EEG in suspected seizures
  - *Audiometry:* For hearing loss
- *Vestibular function tests:* Neuronal circuits for oculomotor and vestibular function develop within the first year of life and can be tested, even in toddlers. Discontinue sedatives and vestibular suppressants 2 days before testing. Help to confirm diagnosis, differentiate between central versus peripheral vertigo and localize side of lesion.
  - *Electronystagmography (ENG):* Most widely used for recording eye movements. It is better tolerated by children over videonystagmography.
  - Videonystagmography
  - *Caloric test:* It tests each labyrinth separately with warm or cold water.
  - *Rotational chair testing:* Preferred over caloric test as it can be done with child sitting on parents' lap.
  - *Vestibular-evoked myogenic potentials (VEMP):* Evaluates vestibular function by recording electrical activity from neck muscles.
  - Computerized dynamic platform posturography

APPROACH

The approach to management of vertigo is given in **Flowchart 1**.

Flowchart 1: Management of vertigo.

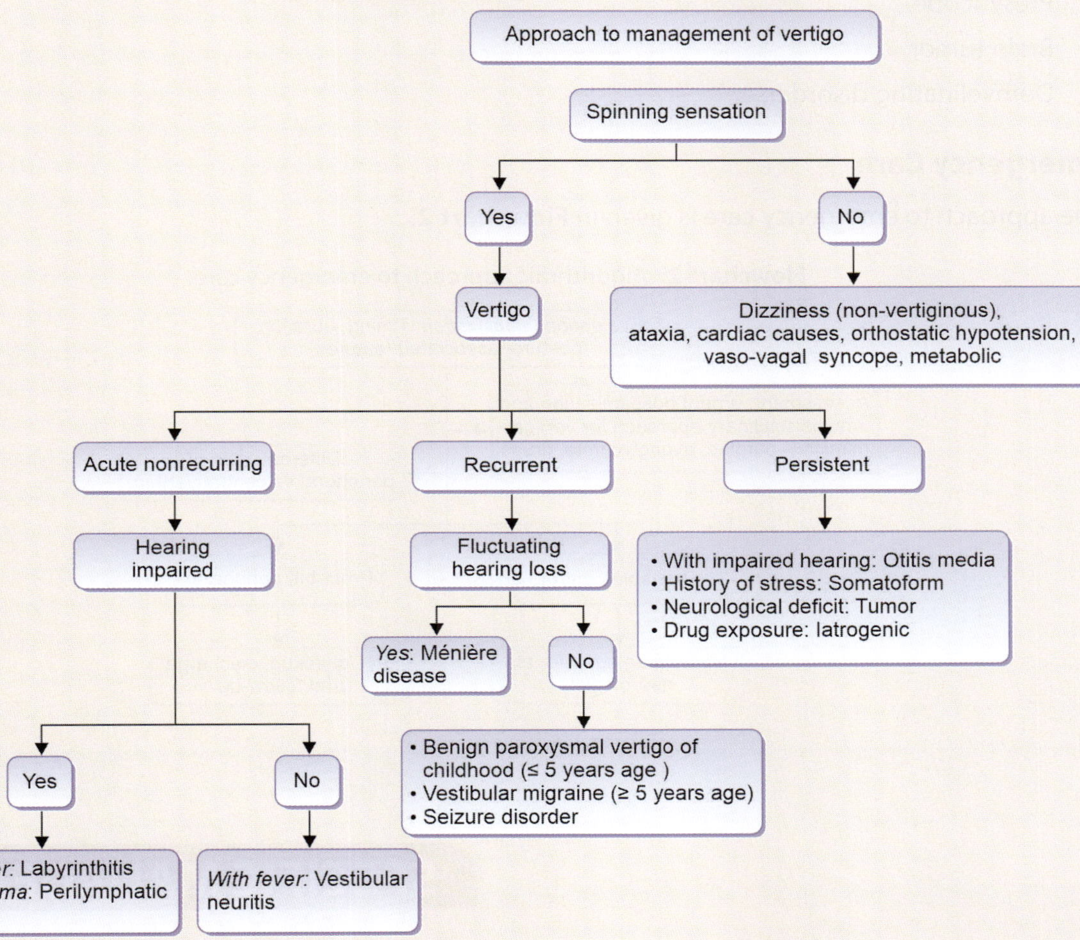

- Enquire about sensation of rotation or dizziness.
- Differentiate vertigo from other causes of dizziness.
- Classify vertigo into peripheral and central type. Rule out life-threatening central causes.
- Identify temporal pattern (Acute/recurrent/chronic) and hearing status (normal or impaired) to find etiology.
- Etiology is age-dependent.
- For evaluation, use a structured approach based on history, physical examination, and targeted investigations.

DIFFERENTIALS

- Other causes of dizziness
- Ataxia
- Presyncope
- Brain tumor
- Demyelinating disorders

Emergency Care

The approach to emergency care is given in **Flowchart 2**.

Flowchart 2: Algorithmic approach to emergency care.

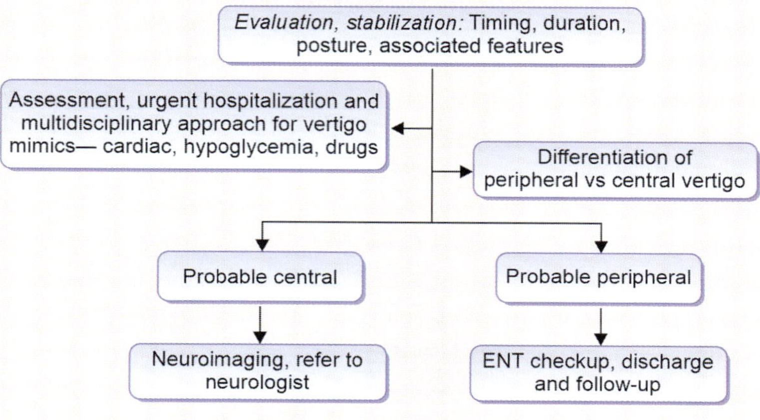

SPECIFIC MANAGEMENT

- *Acute symptom relief:*
  - *Positioning:* Keep child in safe position to avoid falls.
  - *Medications:* Vestibular suppressants (meclizine, flunarizine, and cyproheptadine) for severe vertigo.
- *Treatment of specific conditions:*
  - *BPVC:* Mostly resolves spontaneously and needs parental reassurance. Vestibular suppressants are required if frequent episodes interfere with school performance.
  - Vestibular migraine
  - *First-line therapy:* Nonpharmacological measures such as lifestyle modification, hydration, cognitive behavioral therapy, and trigger avoidance

- Vestibular rehabilitation
- Migraine prophylaxis drugs
- *Labyrinthitis:* Antibiotics if bacterial and vestibular suppressants
- *Chronic suppurative otitis media with cholesteatoma:* Mastoid exploration
- *Vestibular neuritis:* Steroids, vestibular rehabilitation, and suppressants
- *Psychogenic vertigo:* Cognitive behavioral therapy
- *Non-neurological causes:* Anemia and dehydration correction
- *Multidisciplinary care:* Cardiologist, ENT specialist, neurologist, and psychiatrist.
- *Admit:* If labyrinthitis, head trauma, brain tumor, and cardiac cause

MONITORING

Monitor for the following:

- Progression of vertigo symptoms
- Development of migraine in later life in BPVC
- Recurrence of symptoms

KEY LEARNING POINTS

- Dizziness and vertigo are two different symptoms with separate clinical implications.
- Children rarely complain of vertigo. Enquire about sensation of rotation in their vocabulary.
- Classify into peripheral and central vertigo.
- History and physical examination are helpful to rule out life-threatening central and cardiac causes.
- Majority of vertigo causes are benign. BPVC, vestibular migraine, and otitis media are common causes in children.
- Identify temporal patterns of symptoms and hearing status to find etiology.
- Suspect vestibular abnormality in any child with frequent falls, unprovoked fright, abnormal eye movement or unexplained nausea, and vomiting.

SUGGESTED READING

1. Devaraja K. Vertigo in children; a narrative review of the various causes and their management. Int J Pediatr Otorhinolaryngol. 2018;111:32-8.
2. Klaus J, Langhagena T, Heinen F. Vertigo and dizziness in children. Curr Opin Neurol. 2015;28:78-82.
3. Pellegrino N, Di Stefano V, Rotondo E, Graziosi A, Rispoli MG, Angelo Torrente A, et al. Neurological vertigo in the emergency room in pediatric and adult age: Systematic literature review and proposal for a diagnostic algorithm. Ital J Pediatr. 2022;48(1):125.
4. Vanni S, Vannucchi P, Pecci R, Pepe G, Paciaroni M, Pavellini A. Consensus paper on the management of acute isolated vertigo in the emergency department. Intern Emerg Med. 2024;19:1181-202.
5. Zwergal A, Dieterich M. Vertigo and dizziness in the emergency room. Curr Opin Neurol. 2020;33(1):117-25.

Section 5

Gastrointestinal System

Acute Liver Failure in Children

Vivin Abraham, Remya R Pai

INTRODUCTION

- Pediatric acute liver failure (PALF) is a life-threatening condition. The overall incidence of PALF is unknown.
- In the current era of advanced critical care, PALF remains a disease with high mortality.
- Developing countries face unique challenges in managing this disease owing to the lack of access to timely liver transplantation (LT).
- In addition, the outcome depends on the underlying etiology, disease severity at presentation, and—most importantly—availability of adequate supportive care.
- PALF differs significantly from acute liver failure (ALF) in adults in both clinical presentation and etiological spectrum.
- The management of PALF requires aggressive diagnostic evaluation, close monitoring, and anticipating and managing the multisystem complications to prevent organ failure, transplantation, and death.

DEFINITION

The PALF Study Group (PALFSG) Consensus entry criteria (reference) for children with ALF include (all three components required):

- Acute onset liver disease with no evidence of preexisting chronic liver disease
- Biochemical evidence of severe liver injury
- *Coagulopathy not corrected by vitamin K:*
  - Prothrombin time (PT) ≥15 or international normalized ratio (INR) ≥1.5 with encephalopathy or
  - PT ≥20 or INR ≥2 with or without encephalopathy

TERMINOLOGIES

- *Hyperacute liver failure:*
  - *Time from onset of jaundice to encephalopathy:* 0–1 week
  - Severity of coagulopathy is higher
  - *Common causes:* Hepatitis A, E, and paracetamol toxicity
- *Acute liver failure:*
  - *Time from onset of jaundice to encephalopathy:* 1–4 weeks
  - Intermediate severity of coagulopathy
- *Subacute liver failure:*
  - *Time from onset of jaundice to encephalopathy:* 4–12 weeks
  - Minimum coagulopathy
  - *Common cause:* Nonparacetamol drug-induced injury
  - Survival rate without liver transplantation is poor in this group of patients
- *Recurrent acute liver failure (ALF):*
  - Rare
  - *Neuroblastoma amplified sequence (NBAS) gene mutations:* Fever-triggered ALF

ETIOPATHOLOGY

The etiopathology of PALF is given in **Table 1**.

TABLE 1: Etiopathology of pediatric acute liver failure

<3 months	*3 months–18 years*
• Sepsis • Infections, especially herpes simplex virus and enterovirus • Hypoxic–ischemic injury (when shock/cardiac lesions are present) • Gestational alloimmune liver disease (previous term: neonatal hemochromatosis) • *Metabolic liver diseases:* Galactosemia, GSD, tyrosinemia, FXR • Hemophagocytic lymphohistiocytosis • Mitochondrial hepatopathies (DNA depletion syndromes)	• Infectious diseases (Hepatitis A, B, C, D, E, non-A, non-B viral hepatitis, dengue, malaria, leptospira, EBV, and CMV) • Drug toxicity, toxin ingestion, accidental or intentional drug overdose (paracetamol, complementary alternative medicine, tetracycline, toxic mushroom *Amanita phalloides* poisoning) • Wilson's disease and other metabolic diseases • Autoimmune hepatitis

(CMV: cytomegalovirus; EBV: Epstein–Barr virus; GSD: glycogen storage disease; FXR: Farnesoid X receptor)

Etiological Possibilities

The etiological possibilities are given in **Table 2.**

TABLE 2: Etiological possibilities.

Category	*Disease*
Infections	Hepatitis A virus, hepatitis E virus, dengue, herpes simplex, Varicella Zoster, Herpes Hominis virus type 6, cytomegalovirus, Epstein–Barr virus, enterovirus, echovirus, adenovirus, and parvovirus B19,
Drug-induced	Acetaminophen, sulfamide, sodium valproate, sulfasalazine, halothane, chemotherapy
Ischemic	Acute circulatory failure, septicemia with shock, congenital heart disease, and heat stroke
Metabolic	Galactosemia, GSD, tyrosinemia type 1, hereditary fructose intolerance, urea cycle disorders, fatty-acid oxidation disorder, primary bile acid defects, congenital disorders of glycosylation, Niemann–Pick, mitochondrial cytopathy, transaldolase deficiency, FXR deficiency, NBAS deficiency
Immune-mediated	Giant cell hepatitis, autoimmune hepatitis, gestational alloimmune liver disease (GALD) (neonates)
Hematological	Familial hemophagocytic lymphohistiocytosis, macrophage-activation syndrome, and Leukemia
Vascular	Veno-occlusive disease and Budd–Chiari syndrome

(FXR: Farnesoid X receptor; GSD: glycogen storage disease; NBAS: Neuroblastoma amplified sequence)

EVALUATION

- Initial blood tests and liver function tests (to assess liver injury)
  - Total, direct bilirubin
  - Aspartate aminotransferase (AST)/alanine aminotransferase (ALT)
  - Serum albumin
  - INR
  - Blood glucose
- *Baseline and follow-up:* Septic/renal/hematological/electrolyte/pancreatic assessment

How frequently should we monitor the patient?

- Vitals monitoring every 1–2 hours with hepatic encephalopathy (HE) or every 4 hours in cases with no HE
- *Liver function tests:* INR, ammonia, and enzymes every 8–12 hours depending on the clinical status

◈ Tests for etiological workup **(Table 3)**

TABLE 3: Etiological workup:	
Infective	
Hepatotrophic	Anti-HAV IgM, HBsAg, HBcAb IgM, and anti-HEV IgM
Nonhepatotrophic	• HSV PCR (neonates), CMV, EBV, Parvovirus (cytopenias), adenovirus, and echovirus serology/PCR • If signs present, dengue NS1/IgM, scrub typhus IgM, malaria (peripheral smear/antigen)
Metabolic	
1st line	*First-line metabolic workup:* Blood gas (pH and lactate), blood glucose (for hypoglycemia), urine for nonglucose-reducing substance, arterial ammonia, AFP, and lipid profile
Definitive	Galactose-1-phosphate uridyl transferase (Galactosemia), urinary succinylacetone (tyrosinemia), quantitative enzyme assay (hereditary fructose intolerance), mitochondrial hepatopathies (quantitative mitochondrial DNA assay, mutation analysis, lactate, lactate/pyruvate ratio, CK), fatty acid oxidation defects (plasma acylcarnitine), and urea cycle defects (ammonia and serum amino acid profile)
Wilson's disease	Serum ceruloplasmin, 24-hour urinary copper, and KF ring
Autoimmune	Immunoglobulins (IgG), autoimmune antibody profile (antinuclear antibodies, smooth muscle antibody, ANCA, liver cytosol antibodies, liver–kidney microsomal antibodies, and soluble liver antigen)
Hematological malignancy or HLH	Bone marrow examination, serum ferritin, low/absent natural killer cell activity, soluble IL-2R assay, and genetics for HLH
GALD	Serum ferritin, AFP, MRI abdomen (extrahepatic iron deposition), and lip/buccal mucosal biopsies
Budd–Chiari syndrome	Ultrasound, echocardiography, and computed tomography
Drugs and toxins	History, drug levels, and Rumack–Matthew nomogram (Paracetamol)

(AFP: alpha-fetoprotein; ANCA: antineutrophil cytoplasmic antibodies; CK: creatine kinase; CMV: cytomegalovirus; EBV: Epstein–Barr Virus; GALD: gestational alloimmune liver disease; HAV: hepatitis A vaccine; HBcAb: hepatitis B core antibody; HBsAg: hepatitis B surface antigen; HEV: hepatitis E virus; HLH: hemophagocytic lymphohistiocytosis; HSV: Herpes simplex virus; IL-2R: interleukin-2 receptor; MRI: magnetic resonance imaging; PCR: polymerase chain reaction; KF: Kayser–Fleischer)

COMPLICATIONS

Complications caused in different organ systems are given in **Table 4.**

TABLE 4: Various organ systems and related complications.

Organ system	*Complications*
Fluid and electrolyte imbalance	Hypoglycemia, hyperammonemia, hyponatremia, hypokalemia, hypocalcemia, acidosis/alkalosis, and hypophosphatemia
Sepsis	SIRS, gram-negative and gram-positive sepsis
Gastrointestinal	Bleeding and ulcers
CNS	Hepatic encephalopathy and cerebral edema leading to raised ICP
CVS	Hypotension–hypovolemic/distributive shock
RS	ARDS, pulmonary edema, pulmonary hemorrhage, pneumonia, and ventilator-associated complications
Kidney	Acute kidney injury and hepatorenal syndrome
Hematological	Cytopenias, aplastic anemia, disseminated intravascular coagulation, and hemophagocytic lymphohistiocytosis

(ARDS: acute respiratory distress syndrome; CNS: central nervous system; CVS: chorionic villus sampling; ICP: intracranial pressure; RS: Reye's syndrome; SIRS: systemic inflammatory response syndrome)

TREATMENT

Once PALF is diagnosed, supportive management should be initiated promptly, irrespective of the underlying etiology. Clinical monitoring at appropriate intervals should also be done in pediatric intensive care unit (PICU). Early transfer or contact with the liver transplant center must be considered, wherever indicated. Laboratory assessment should also be commenced immediately along with supportive treatment.

- *Initial care:*
  - Follow pediatric advanced life support (PALS) algorithm
  - Admit to PICU/refer to liver transplant center
  - Injection Vitamin K (0.3–1 mg/kg/dose), mention age-wise dosing (1 mg, 3 mg, or 5 mg, etc.)
  - Intravenous fluids (IVF)—maintain blood glucose >50 mg/dL
  - Intravenous (IV) antibiotic/antifungal (please specify stage and type of antibiotic cover) (Acyclovir, if neonate)
  - Proton pump inhibitor (PPI)/lactulose/rifaximin

◈ *Systematic care: Systematic care is given in **Table 5:***

TABLE 5: Systematic care.

Problem	*Management*
Fluid and electrolytes	• *Fluids:* Intravenous fluids (IVF) to be 90–100% of total maintenance fluids; initial fluid: One-half normal saline with 10% dextrose with 15 mEq/L potassium; avoid fluids with predetermined electrolyte. Concentration (like RL) • *Target serum glucose:* 90–120 mg/dL • *Target serum sodium:* 145–155 mEq/L, *Requirement:* 2–3 mEq/kg/day. Treat hyponatremia if symptomatic or Na <120 mEq/L or when fluid restriction is not possible • Maintain serum phosphate >3 mg/dL
Hyperammonemia and hepatic encephalopathy (HE)	• Staging of HE in children <4 years and 4 years specified separately based on mental status, reflexes, neurological signs, and EEG changes • Consider lactulose and other antibiotics like rifaximin and neomycin (insufficient data to support use in ALF) • *Ammonia-lowering agents* like LOLA and LOPA are under investigation • *Consider continuous renal replacement therapy:* Specify indications and type • *Supportive care in ICU:* Minimal stimulation; avoid unnecessary interventions, endotracheal intubation especially for stage 3 or 4 encephalopathy • Consider CT/MRI head for any acute mental status changes
Intracranial hypertension/ cerebral edema	• ICP monitoring is recommended in patients with stage III or IV encephalopathy, CT scan suggestive of edema; EEG with slowing; hyperammonia; mechanical ventilation • No recommendation on prophylactic antiseizure medication *Therapies specific for raised ICP:* Hyperosmolar therapy—mannitol: at 0.5–1.0 g/kg • Hypertonic saline to maintain serum Na 145–155 mEq/L • *Hyperventilation:* Brief (20 minutes) bursts to reduce $PaCO_2$
Coagulopathy	*IV vitamin K:* • *Platelet and/or FFP:* Only in active bleeding or invasive procedure; avoid transfusion only to improve platelet or INR • Cryoprecipitate transfusion in low fibrinogen state (<100 mg/dL) • *Recombinant factor VII:* Use before ICP monitor placement only
Gastrointestinal bleed	H2 blockers or proton pump inhibitors are recommended for prophylaxis of gastrointestinal bleed
AKI/HRS	• Continuous venovenous hemofiltration or renal replacement therapy (CRRT) is recommended in AKI • Preventive measures include maintaining fluid balance while avoiding excessive diuresis, minimizing the use of nephrotoxic medications or IV contrast, and maintaining renal perfusion pressure
Infection/SIRS	• In patients with clinical suspicion or biochemical changes, broad spectrum antibiotics should be started after obtaining blood and tracheal cultures. Discontinue when cultures turn negative. The use of intravenous (IV) antibiotics in pediatric acute liver failure (PALF) is guided by the risk of bacterial and viral infections due to immune dysfunction and systemic inflammation associated with liver failure. The specific stage of liver failure and suspected or confirmed infections influence antibiotic choices *Early Management (Empiric Coverage)* • *Bacterial sepsis:* All children with suspected PALF should receive empiric IV antibiotics at presentation if there are signs of infection. Broad-spectrum antibiotics like third-generation cephalosporins are commonly used. In neonates, IV acyclovir is added to cover herpes simplex virus

Contd...

Contd...

	• *Nosocomial infections:* In children hospitalized for PALF, pathogens such as gram-negative bacteria (e.g., *E. coli, Klebsiella*) and gram-positive organisms (Staphylococcus) are common. Empiric regimens are adjusted based on local antibiograms and infection severity *Advanced Stage or Specific Infections* • *Fungal infections: Candida* infections may require the addition of antifungal agents like fluconazole in critically ill patients • *Targeted therapy:* If a specific etiology like viral hepatitis or bacterial cholangitis is identified, treatment is tailored (e.g., antivirals for herpes or antibiotics for ascending cholangitis). *Prophylactic use:* Routine prophylactic antibiotics are not universally recommended unless there is a strong risk of secondary infections or invasive procedures. *Recommendations for Severe Disease:* In severe encephalopathy (Grade 3 or 4) or in the presence of sepsis with multi-drug-resistant organisms, escalation to carbapenems or vancomycin may be considered, guided by cultures and clinical response
Nutrition, hypoglycemia	• Enteral feeding is preferred over TPN • Restrict protein to 1gm/kg/day, if hyperammonemia is present. Lipids are to be used except if FAOD or mitochondrial disease is suspected
Problem	***Management***
Ascites	Spironolactone is the diuretic of choice for patients with ascites who have respiratory compromise or discomfort due to fluid accumulation
Plasmapheresis	Evidence in PALF is sparse. Recommended with other extracorporeal therapy as a bridge to liver transplant
Cardiorespiratory stability	• Adequate fluid resuscitation with IV normal saline • Norepinephrine is the preferred choice of vasoconstrictor agent for volume-refractory instability • Endotracheal intubation should be performed for respiratory failure or for airway protection in advanced stages of HE • Ventilator strategies include low tidal volumes (5–8 mL/kg of predicted weight) and moderately elevated PEEP levels

(ALF: acute liver failure; AKI: acute kidney injury; FAOD: fatty acid oxidation disorders; FFP: fresh frozen plasma; HRS: hepatorenal syndrome; ICP: intracranial pressure; ICU: intensive care unit; INR: international randomized ratio; LOLA: L-ornithine L-aspartate; PALF: pediatric acute liver failure; PEEP: positive end-expiratory pressure; SIRS: systemic inflammatory response syndrome; TPN: total parenteral nutrition)

- *Specific treatment:* Steroids for autoimmune hepatitis, N-acetyl cysteine (NAC) infusion for acetaminophen poisoning, and avoiding galactose-containing formula for galactosemia
- *Liver transplantation:* Liver transplantation offers a life-saving alternative to medical management in patients with PALF who have otherwise guarded prognosis. Timely liver transplantation has improved survival in patients with PALF. Currently, the indications and criteria for transplant are ill-defined. Several prognostic scoring systems like the King's College Hospital Criteria (KCHC) and Pediatric Liver Injury Unit (LIU) score have been used in children.

Liver transplantation for ALF is generally associated with poor outcomes when compared to that for chronic liver disease. The factors predicting poor outcomes following liver transplantation were age <1 year, grade IV HE, and need for dialysis prior to transplantation.

CONCLUSION

Pediatric acute liver failure remains poorly defined and incompletely studied due to its rarity and heterogeneity. It presents unique challenges, requiring prompt recognition, multidisciplinary management, and consideration of liver transplantation as a life-saving option. An equal emphasis on strategies to prevent infection and drug-related ALF is imperative. There is a critical need to develop effective prognostic scoring models and better access to liver transplant facilities in developing countries.

SUGGESTED READING

1. Abimannane A, Deepthi B, Bhowmick R, Parameswaran N. Clinical profile and outcomes of children with acute liver failure in a tertiary care center in South India: A Retrospective Study. Pediatr Gastroenterol Hepatol Nutr. 2024;27(1):43-52.
2. Anand AC, Nandi B, Acharya SK, Arora A, Babu S, Batra Y, et al. Indian National Association for the Study of the Liver Consensus Statement on Acute Liver Failure (Part 1): Epidemiology, pathogenesis, presentation and prognosis. J Clin Exp Hepatol. 2020;10(4):339-76.
3. Bhatt H, Rao GS. Management of acute liver failure: A pediatric perspective. Curr Pediatr Rep. 2018;6(3): 246-57.
4. Mishra S, Pallavi P. Diagnosis and management of pediatric acute liver failure: ESPGHAN and NASPGHAN 2022. Indian Pediatr. 2022;59(4):307-11.
5. Squires JE, Alonso EM, Ibrahim SH, Kasper V, Kehar M, Martinez M, et al. North American Society for Pediatric Gastroenterology, Hepatology, and Nutrition Position Paper on the Diagnosis and Management of Pediatric Acute Liver Failure. J Pediatr Gastroenterol Nutr. 2022;74(1):138-58.

26 Pediatric Abdominal Trauma

Chetan Ginigeri

INTRODUCTION

Trauma is the primary cause of death and disability among children older than 1 year of age, representing 60% of all childhood fatalities in both developed and developing nations. Abdominal trauma constitutes 10% of all traumatic injuries and is the third leading cause of death in children, following head and thoracic injuries. Often, abdominal injuries can lead to substantial internal bleeding without any visible external signs or changes in size. Consequently, the abdomen is the most frequent site of undetected fatal injuries in children.[1]

The mechanism of traumatic abdominal injuries is given in **Table 1**.

TABLE 1: Mechanism of traumatic abdominal injuries.[2]

Blunt abdominal trauma (85%)	• *Direct blow:* Compression injuries (consider nonaccidental injuries) • *Shearing injuries:* Seat belt injuries • *High impact/decelerating injuries:* Small bowel bucket handle injuries
Penetrating abdominal trauma (15%)	• Stab wounds • Gunshot wounds

Organs most frequently affected due to blunt abdominal trauma are given in **Box 1**.

BOX 1: Organs most frequently affected due to blunt abdominal trauma.[2]

- Spleen (40–55%)
- Liver (35–45%)
- Small intestine (5–10%)

The causes of abdominal trauma based on age are given in **Table 2**.

TABLE 2: Cause of abdominal trauma based on age.[2]

Age	*Cause*
Infants and young children	Motor vehicle collisions (MVC), drowning, suffocation, burns, falls, and abuse
School-aged children	MVC, pedestrian injuries, bicycle injuries, and firearm injuries
Adolescents	MVC, firearm injuries, falls, and intentional injuries

ANATOMICAL AND PHYSIOLOGICAL CONSIDERATIONS: HOW CHILDREN DIFFER?[2]

The implications based on anatomy and physiology are given in **Table 3.**

TABLE 3: Anatomy/physiology and its implications in children.

Anatomy/Physiology	*Implication*
Relatively large body surface area-to-body cell mass ratio	Higher susceptibility to hypothermia and insensible fluid losses, with shock often being masked
Smaller circulating blood volume	Increased risk of hemorrhagic shock
Relatively compact torso with smaller anteroposterior diameter	The force of injury is dissipated over a smaller area leading to more significant impact
Larger viscera (especially liver and spleen) extending below the costal margin	Vital organs are less protected
Less overlying fat and weaker abdominal musculature	Reduced cushion to intra-abdominal structures

INITIAL EVALUATION AND STABILIZATION (PRIMARY SURVEY)[3,4]

Any child with suspected abdominal trauma should initially be evaluated according to advanced trauma life support (ATLS) guidelines **(Table 4)**.

TABLE 4: Initial evaluation and stabilization according to advanced trauma life support (ATLS) guidelines.

Airway (C-Spine) and breathing	• *C-spine:* Manual in-line stabilization • *If spontaneously breathing:* High flow oxygen [nonrebreather mask (NRM) 100%) • Intubate and ventilate if: – Severe respiratory distress – Hemodynamic instability – Poor Glasgow Coma Scale (GCS) (<8)	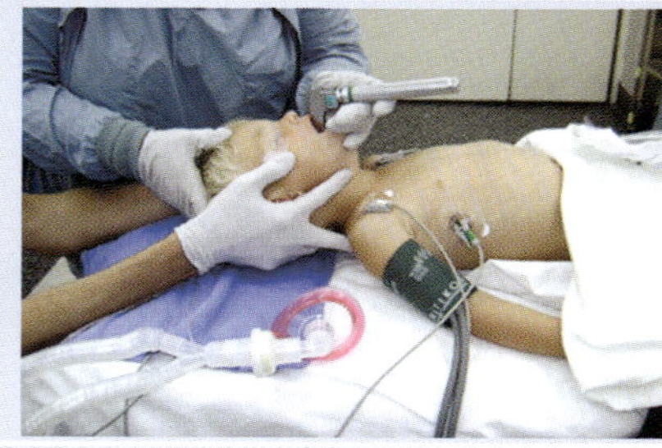
Circulation 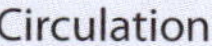	• Assess skin color, pulse, capillary refill, and blood pressure • *"Hypotension is due to hemorrhagic shock unless proved otherwise"* • *Permissive hypotension or controlled resuscitation*: Maintain blood pressure (BP) at 5th centile to maintain organ perfusion and prevent bleeding: – Warm isotonic crystalloid bolus – *If >40mL/kg crystalloid bolus is required:* Type-specific or O-negative warmed packed red blood cell (PRBC) transfusion – Activate *massive transfusion protocol (MTP):* If >20 mL/kg PRBC transfusion is required • *Extended focused assessment with sonography in trauma (E-FAST):* To identify major areas of occult hemorrhage	Permissive hypotension Minimization of crystalloids **Damage control resuscitation** 1:1:1 product ratios Early hemorrhage control

Contd...

Contd...

Disability	• Assess the level of consciousness (GCS/AVPU scale), pupillary size, and reaction • Look for lateralizing signs and spinal cord injury level • Check blood glucose	
Exposure	• Check core temperature • Cover the patient with warm blankets to prevent hypothermia	Lethal triad 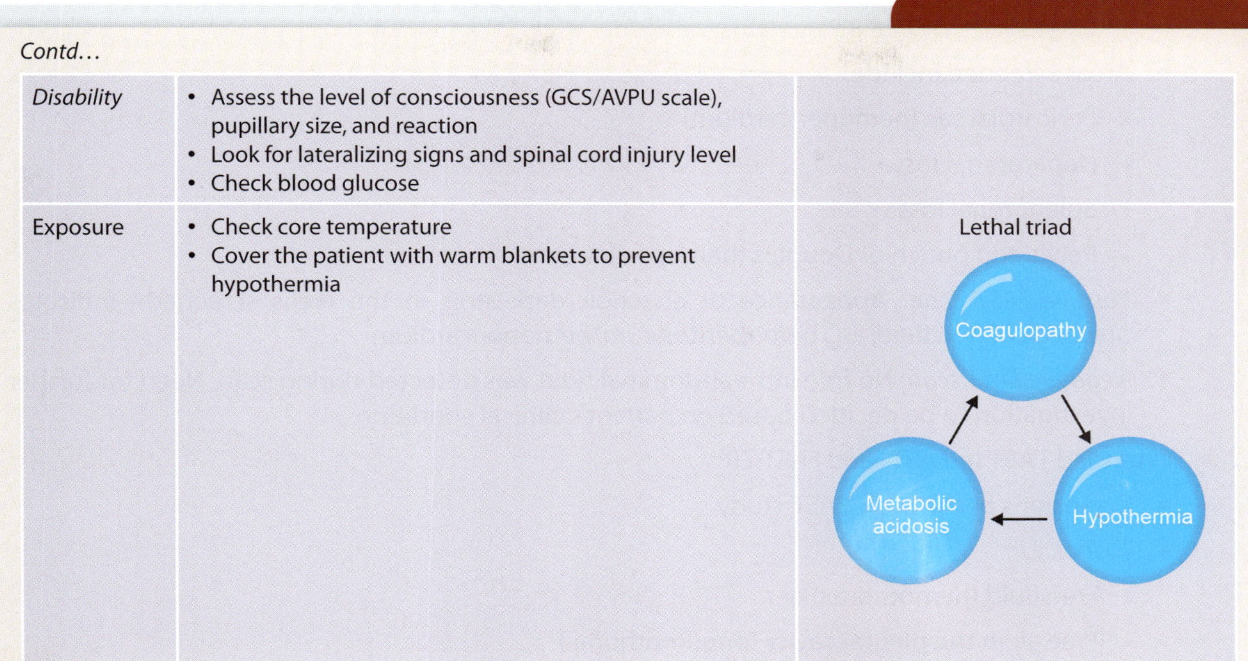

Adjuvants to Primary Survey and Resuscitation

- *Electrocardiograph (ECG) monitoring:* Monitor for dysrhythmias (secondary to blunt cardiac injury, cardiac tamponade, tension pneumothorax, and metabolic disturbances).
- *Urinary catheter:*
  - For early detection of reduced renal perfusion secondary to hypovolemia
  - *Exceptions:* Do not attempt catheterization in suspected urethral injury (blood at the urethral meatus, perineal ecchymosis, and blood in the scrotum)
- *Gastric catheters:*
  - Use to decrease gastric distension and risk of gastric aspiration
  - *Nasogastric (NG) tube:* Contraindicated in suspected case of skull fracture
- *Radiological investigations:*
  - *Triple trauma X-ray screens*: Anteroposterior (AP) chest, pelvis, and lateral cervical spine

Sonography in Abdominal Trauma

- Focused Assessment with Sonography in Trauma (FAST)[3,5]
  - Noninvasive point-of-care tests for quick detection of occult intra-abdominal hemorrhage can be done at bedside by trained emergency room (ER) physician/surgeon.

- Areas screened include:
    - Pericardial sac (hemopericardium)
    - Hepatorenal fossa
    - Splenorenal fossa
    - Pelvis and pouch of Douglas (hemoperitoneum)
- *Positive FAST scan:* Appearance of anechoic/dark strip in the areas screened—indicates presence of free fluid, i.e., hemoperitoneum/hemopericardium
- *Negative FAST scan:* No free intra-abdominal fluid was detected during scan. Need for further investigation to be decided based on patient's clinical condition.

◈ Extended-FAST (e-FAST) and FAST-ER[5]

- Extensions of the basic FAST study
- *To look for:*
    - Free fluid (hemothorax) or
    - Free air in the pleural cavity (pneumothorax)
    - Long bone fractures (hematomas)
- Less sensitive for evaluation of solid organ and hollow viscous injury

◈ *Six areas were screened:* Right upper quadrant (RUQ), left upper quadrant (LUQ), pelvic (suprapubic), cardiac (subxiphoid), and right and left anterior chest **(Figs. 1A and B)**.

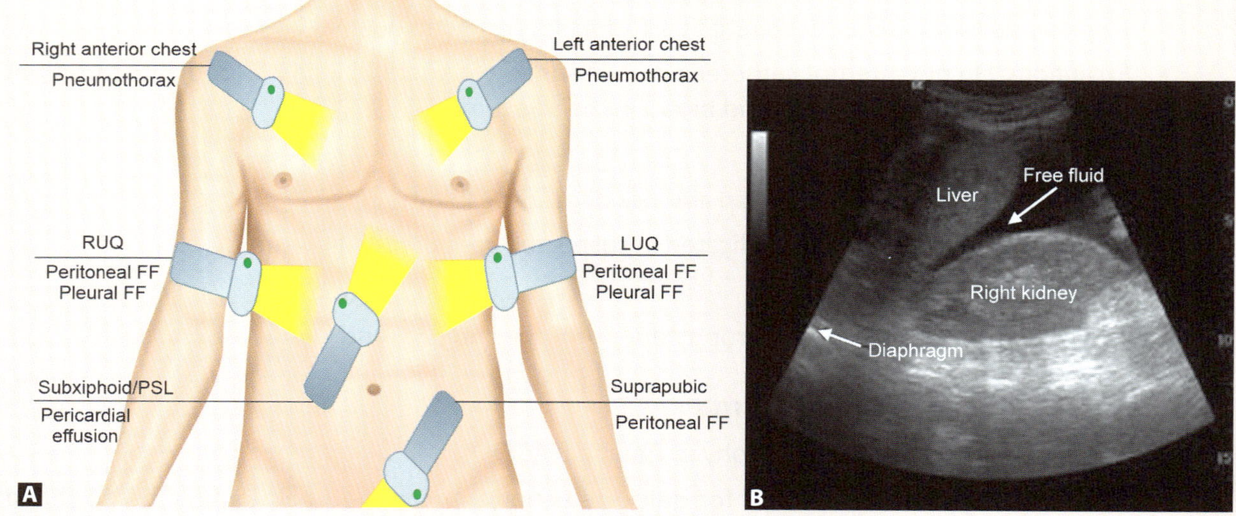

Figs. 1A and B: (A) Six areas screened; (B) Focused Assessment With Sonography in Trauma (FF: free fluid; LUQ: left upper quadrant; RUQ: right upper quadrant)

SECONDARY SURVEY

Secondary survey involves:

- Detailed head-to-toe evaluation
- SAMPLE (S: signs and symptoms; A: allergies; M: medications currently used; P: past illness; L: last meal; E: events/environment leading to the injury).

EVALUATION OF ABDOMINAL TRAUMA[2,3]

Evaluation of abdominal signs includes the physical signs given in **Box 2.**

BOX 2: Physical signs that indicate an increased risk of abdominal injury.

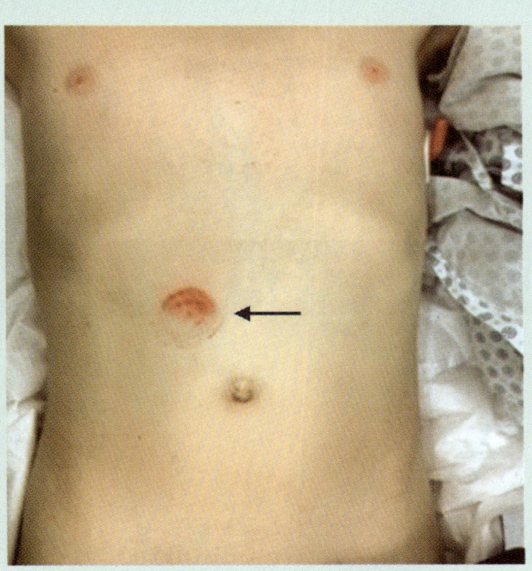

- Ecchymoses (particularly of the umbilical or flank regions), such as in handlebar injuries
- Abrasions and tire-track marks
- Seat belt sign in restrained passengers from motor vehicle collisions
- Abdominal tenderness
- Abdominal distension
- Peritoneal irritation [e.g., abdominal wall rigidity, rebound, guarding, or pain in the left shoulder induced by palpation of the left upper quadrant (Kehr's sign)]
- Absent bowel sounds indicating a prolonged ileus (greater than 4 hours)

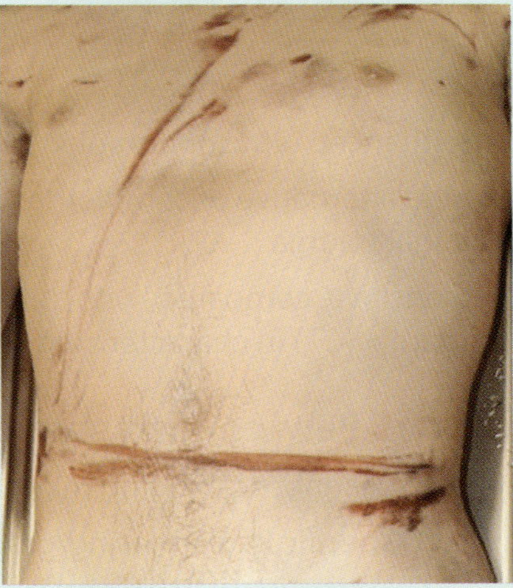

LABORATORY EVALUATION[3,4]

Laboratory investigations and associated remarks are given in **Table 5.**

TABLE 5: Laboratory evaluation.

Investigations	*Remarks*
• Complete blood count (CBC) • Blood type and crossmatch • Arterial or venous blood gas • Serum transaminases [alanine • aminotransferase (ALT) and aspartate aminotransferase (AST)] • Serum electrolytes, creatinine, and blood urea nitrogen • Blood glucose • Amylase and lipase • Prothrombin time (PT) and partial thromboplastin time (PTT) • Urinalysis	• *Serial hemoglobin and hematocrit monitoring:* Occult ongoing bleed • Elevated liver enzyme studies (AST >200 IU/L or ALT >125 IU/L) require CT of the abdomen and pelvis • *Elevated pancreatic enzymes (amylase/lipase):* CT imaging to rule out pancreatic injury • *Urine analysis (presence of gross or microscopic hematuria [>50 Red blood cells (RBCs)/high-powered field (Hpf):* Screening test for genitourinary/renal trauma

RADIOLOGICAL EVALUATION

Ultrasonography

- E-FAST
- Contrast-enhanced ultrasonography (CEUS)
  - Emerging alternative or complementary imaging modality for evaluation of low-energy blunt abdominal trauma
  - More sensitive compared with baseline ultrasound and nearly as sensitive as computed tomography (CT) in characterizing solid organ trauma

Abdominal and Pelvic Contrast-enhanced Computed Tomography

- The preferred diagnostic imaging modality to detect abdominal injuries
- Sensitive and specific in diagnosing/grading liver, spleen, and retroperitoneal injuries.

The indications for contrast-enhanced computed tomography (CECT) abdomen and pelvis are given in **Box 3**.

BOX 3: Indications for contrast-enhanced computed tomography (CECT) abdomen and pelvis.

- Abdominal wall bruising (e.g., seat belt sign, handlebar bruising, or other bruising concerning child abuse)
- Positive focused assessment with sonography in trauma (FAST) exam in a hemodynamically stable child.
- Chest radiograph findings consistent with pneumothorax or hemothorax or pulmonary contusion in patients with concerning mechanisms for abdominal injury
- Patients with distracting injuries (e.g., long bone fractures or substantial injury to the torso that warrants intervention) are at risk for abdomen injuries.
- Serum aspartate aminotransferase (AST) >200 IU/L or alanine
- aminotransferase (ALT) >125 IU/L
- Elevated serum pancreatic enzymes (amylase/lipase)
- Gross hematuria or microscopic hematuria with ≥50 RBCs per high-powered field in otherwise asymptomatic patients
- Declining hematocrit <30%
- Unclear etiology for persistent hemodynamic instability, requiring IV crystalloid fluid boluses or blood requirements

SPECIFIC INJURIES[4,6]

Specific injuries are given in **Table 6**.

TABLE 6: Specific injuries.

	Liver and spleen	*Kidney and genitourinary tract*	*Pancreas*	*Hollow viscus*	*Aorta*
General features/ comments	Most commonly injured solid organs	Contusions, hematomas, and ecchymoses of the back or flank, gross hematuria—markers	Rare	Commonly injured in penetrating trauma, blunt seat belt injury, and lumbar distraction fracture	Rare, seen in severe deceleration forces
Types of injuries	Hematoma, laceration, and vascular injury	Subcapsular, perinephric hematoma, and vascular injury	Contusion, laceration, duct injury, and transection injury	Associated with mesenteric injuries	Infra-renal aorta—Most common site
Grading name (**Fig. 2**)	AAST grade I–V	AAST grade I–V	AAST grade I–V		
Complications	Biliary fistula, bilemia, intrahepatic hematoma, vascular outflow obstruction, delayed splenic rupture, and splenic artery pseudoaneurysm	Hydronephrosis, arteriovenous (AV) fistula, pyelonephritis, and delayed hypertension	Pancreatitis, and pancreatic pseudocyst	Peritonitis	

Contd...

Contd…

	Liver and spleen	*Kidney and genitourinary tract*	*Pancreas*	*Hollow viscus*	*Aorta*
Management (according to grade)	Most often managed conservatively	Mostly conservative		Mostly surgical	Mostly surgical
Conservative	Grades I–III	Grades I–IV	Grade I–II		Endovascular stent
Surgical	• Grades IV–V/any grade with hemodynamic instability after initial resuscitation • Angioembolization—vascular injuries	• Grade V—Nephrectomy • Adjuvant (renal salvage) therapies • Angioembolization, internal drainage, and percutaneous drainage	• Grade III— distal Pancreatectomy • Grade IV—Roux-en-Y pancreatojejunostomy • Grade V—pancreatoduodenectomy	• Laparotomy, resection, and anastomosis with peritoneal drainage	Surgical repair

(AAST: American Association for the Surgery of Trauma)

*Liver injury grading: **AAST***

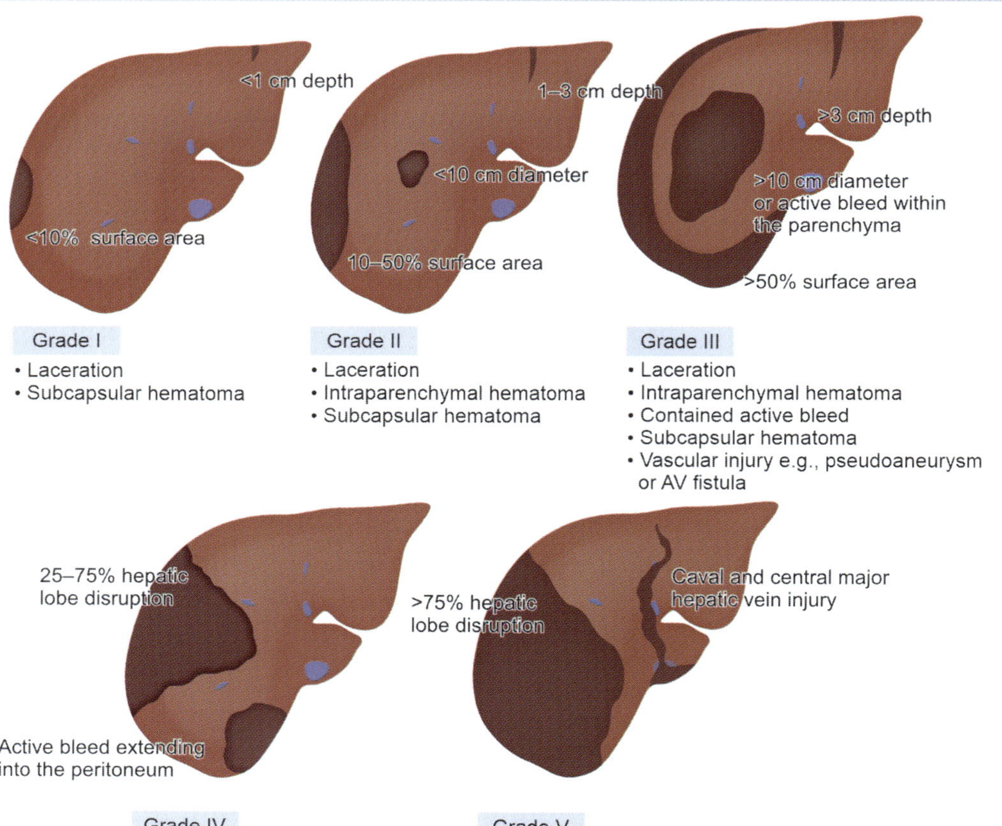

*Advance one grade for each additional injury upto grade III

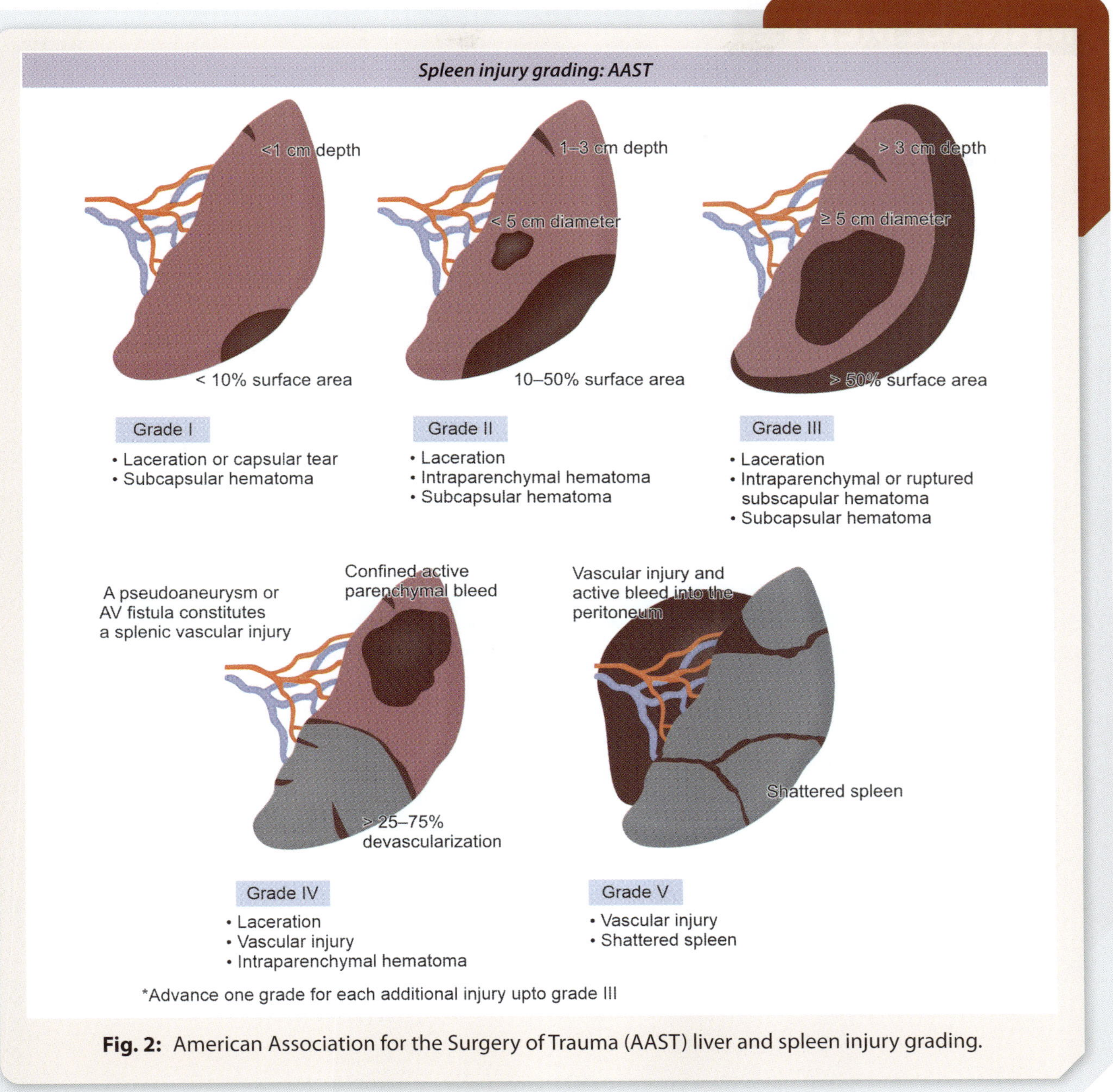

Fig. 2: American Association for the Surgery of Trauma (AAST) liver and spleen injury grading.

MANAGEMENT[3]

he algorithm for management of blunt abdomen trauma is given in **Flowchart 1.**

General Measures

- Initial stabilization
- Damage-control surgery:
  - Hemodynamically unstable children secondary to ongoing hemorrhage are at the risk of developing the lethal triad of hypothermia, acidosis, and coagulopathy.
  - Laparotomy is done with the sole aim of stopping the hemorrhage. Packing of the abdominal cavity is done to arrest the bleed from unstable injuries, and no attempt is made to correct the anatomy.
  - After 24–48 hours of supportive care in intensive care unit (ICU), once the patient is stable, child is taken up for organ-repair surgery

Definitive Management[3,4]

- Laparotomy **(Box 4)**

BOX 4: Indications.

- Blunt abdominal trauma (BAT) with hypotension with positive focused assessment with sonography in trauma (FAST)
- Hypotension with penetrating abdominal wound
- Evisceration
- Hollow viscus injury/perforation
- Free air, retroperitoneal air, or rupture of a hemidiaphragm after blunt trauma
- Peritonitis

- *Angiographic embolization: It is* an alternative to surgery in hemodynamically-*unstable* children with blunt liver or spleen injury and an arterial blush on CT imaging.

Flowchart 1: Management algorithm for blunt abdomen trauma.

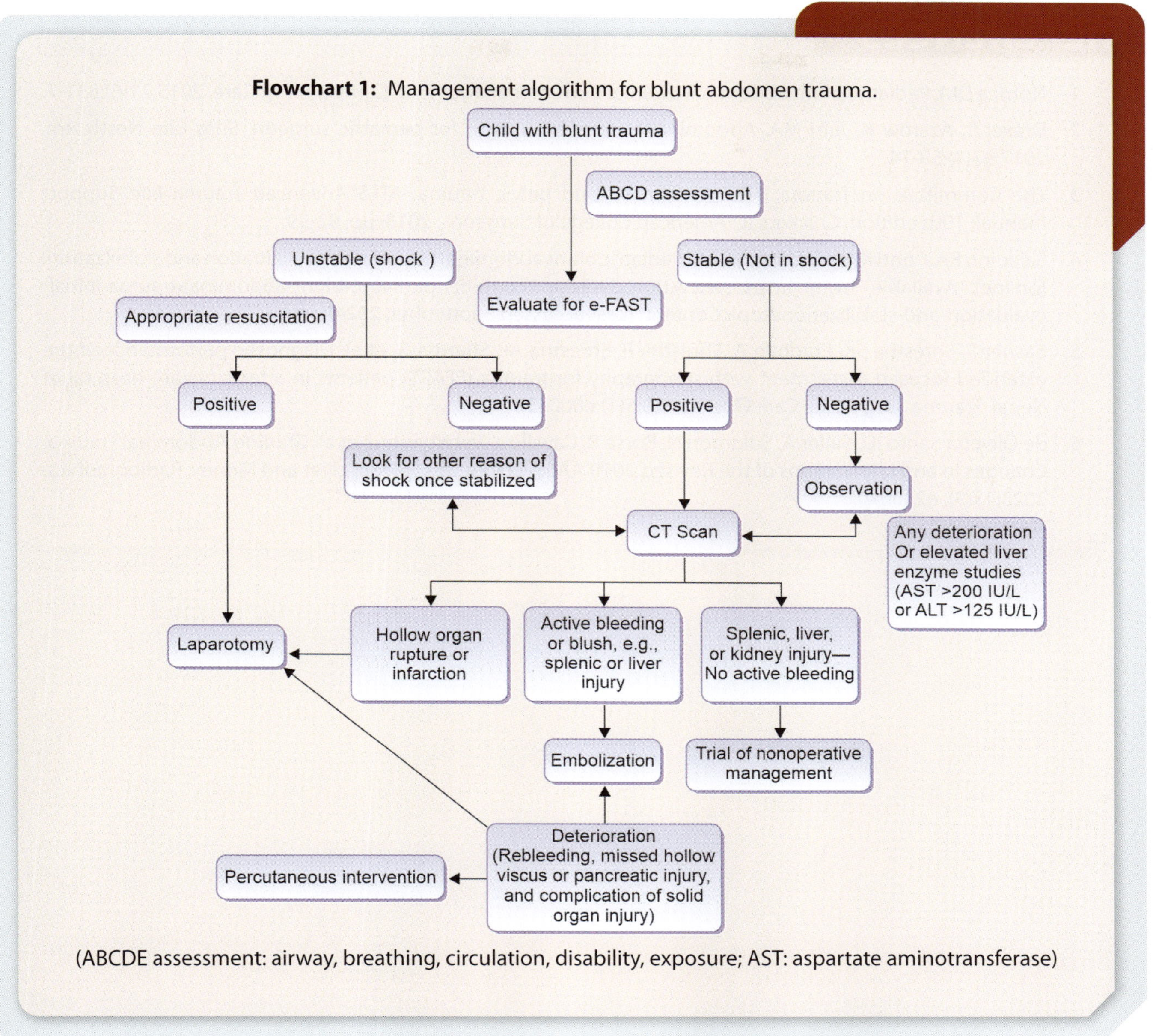

(ABCDE assessment: airway, breathing, circulation, disability, exposure; AST: aspartate aminotransferase)

REFERENCES

1. Notrica DM. Pediatric blunt abdominal trauma: Current management. Curr Opin Crit Care. 2015;21(6):531-7.
2. Drexel S, Azarow K, Jafri MA. Abdominal trauma evaluation for pediatric surgeon. Surg Clin North Am. 2017;97(1):59-74.
3. The Committee on Trauma, ACS. Abdominal and pelvic trauma. ATLS®Advanced Trauma Life Support manual; 10th edition. Chicago, IL: American College of Surgeons; 2018. pp. 82-99.
4. Saladino RA, Conti K. UpToDate. (2024). Pediatric blunt abdominal trauma: Initial evaluation and stabilization. [online] Available from https://www.uptodate.com/contents/pediatric-blunt-abdominal-trauma-initial-evaluation-and-stabilization#topicContent [Last accessed September, 2024].
5. Basnet S, Shrestha SK, Pradhan A, Shrestha R, Shrestha AP, Sharma G, et al. Diagnostic performance of the extended focused assessment with sonography for trauma (EFAST) patients in a tertiary care hospital of Nepal. Trauma Surg Acute Care Open. 2020;5(1):e000438.
6. de Oliveira Santo ID, Sailer A, Solomon N, Borse R, Cavallo J, Teitelbaum J, et al. Grading Abdominal Trauma: Changes in and Implications of the Revised 2018 AAST-OIS for the Spleen, Liver and Kidney. Radiographics. 2023;43(9): e230040.

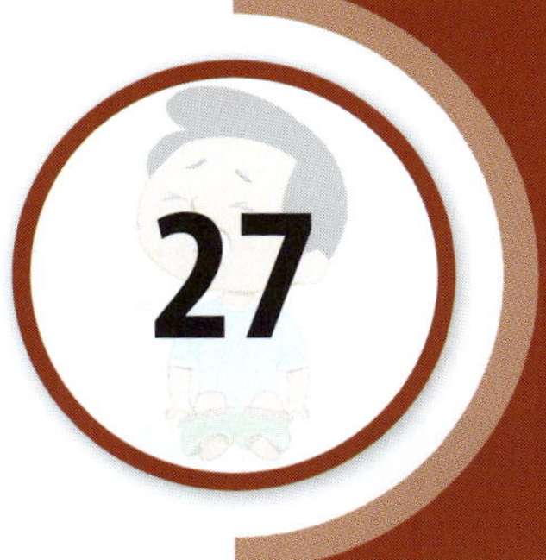

27 Constipation

Madhusudan S, Harini Chowdary Jaladi

INTRODUCTION

Childhood constipation, a common and distressing condition is responsible for 3% of visits to primary care physicians.[1,2] Indian data regarding emergency department (ED) visits is limited. Western data show about 2% of children presenting to the ED have constipation, and 14.5% of children with constipation require an ED visit.[3,4] Overall, etiology is mostly functional; only 5% of children have organic causes. Life-threatening causes of constipation are rare, and can sometimes mimic other common emergencies. Awareness is essential for prompt recognition and emergency management, and timely referral when indicated. A focused history and meticulous examination and awareness of red flag signs to recognize organic or life-threatening causes are essential in the ED. Appropriate outpatient counseling and management can prevent many ED visits, as the latter is associated with overutilization of investigations and burdening of resources.[5,6]

DEFINITION

Normal stool habits, depending on age, diet, and other factors, are variable. Therefore, a single definition for constipation may not be uniformly applicable. Constipation lasting >4 weeks is called chronic constipation and has objective criteria **(Box 1)**. Constipation <4 weeks, i.e., acute constipation, may be simply defined as any recent problem with defecation—delayed or infrequent passage, hard stools, pain, excessive straining, incomplete evacuation, involuntary soiling, or inability to pass stool at all.[7]

BOX 1: Criteria for diagnosis of chronic constipation in Indian children.[2]

More than or equal to 2 of the following occurring at least once per week for *>4 weeks*:
- Defecation frequency ≤2 times per week
- Fecal incontinence ≥1 time per week after the acquisition of toileting skills
- History of excessive stool retention
- History of painful or hard bowel movements
- Presence of a large mass in the rectum or on per abdomen examination
- History of large-diameter stools that may obstruct the toilet (this may not be elicitable for the majority of Indian children who do not use the Western type of toilet)

ETIOPATHOGENESIS

The etiology of constipation is enlisted in **Box 2**, and the pathogenesis is depicted in **Flowchart 1**.

BOX 2: Causes of constipation.

- *Surgical causes:*
  - Hirschsprung disease
  - Anorectal malformations (imperforate anus, anal stenosis, anteriorly placed rectum)
  - Intestinal obstructions
- *Neurological disorders:*
  - Spinal cord abnormalities (e.g., spina bifida, tethered cord, spinal cord injuries, tumors)
  - Autonomic neuropathy
- *Metabolic abnormalities:*
  - Hypothyroidism
  - Hypercalcemia
  - Hypokalemia
  - Diabetes mellitus
- *Gastrointestinal disorders:*
  - Cystic fibrosis
  - Inflammatory bowel disease (IBD) (e.g., Crohn's disease, ulcerative colitis)
  - Celiac disease
- *Dietary factors:* Cow's milk protein allergy
- *Toxic and medication-induced:*
  - Lead poisoning
  - Medications (e.g., opioids, anticholinergics, iron supplements)
- *Functional constipation*

Flowchart 1: Pathogenesis of constipation.

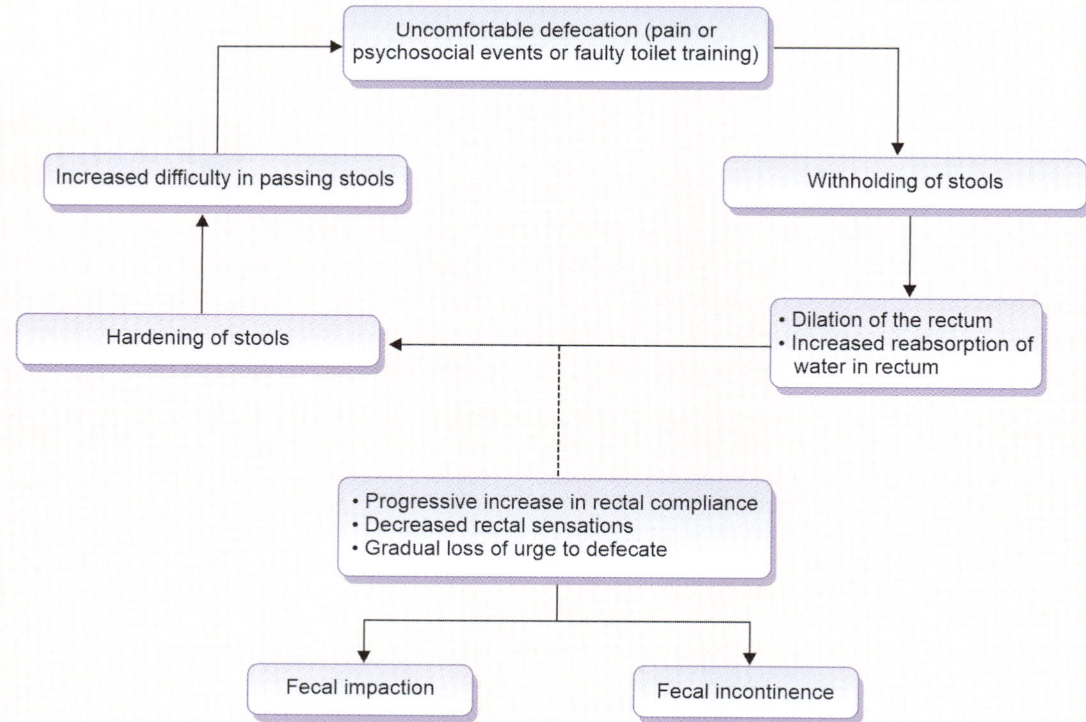

CLINICAL FEATURES

Children can present to the ED with one or more of the following:

- *Infrequent bowel movements:* Fewer than three bowel movements per week
- *Passage of hard stools:* Pictorial tools like the modified Bristol Stool Form chart can be used for assessment
- *Painful defecation:* Pain or discomfort during bowel movements
- *Straining:* Excessive effort needed to pass stools
- *Incomplete evacuation:* Feeling of incomplete bowel emptying after defecation
- Abdominal pain
- *Rectal bleeding:* Blood on the surface of stools or toilet paper, often due to anal fissures
- Fecal incontinence/encopresis in children ≥4 years or those who had previously attained bowel control

EVALUATION (FLOWCHART 2)

- Though constipation is a symptom of a disease, rather than a disease itself, evaluation, definitive diagnosis, and comprehensive management are not the purview of the ED physician. Hence, evaluation should focus on recognition of serious conditions requiring emergent management and/or relief of acute complications.
- Common conditions encountered include recent viral illnesses with dehydration, or adynamic ileus following gastroenteritis, leading to acute constipation. Anal fissures and diaper rash can lead to painful defecation and precipitate stool retention. Lead poisoning and infantile botulism are less common but serious causes.
- Recent onset of constipation associated with abdominal pain, distension, and vomiting may be suggestive of intestinal obstruction. Other than the symptoms enlisted above, use of medications or prior treatment taken for constipation, dietary habits, and family and social history regarding stressful events at home or school-related issues should be enquired.
- A thorough physical examination is essential and provides not only diagnostic clues regarding the cause, but more importantly can uncover the red flag signs, which determine further decisions in the ED. Failure to thrive suggests chronicity and underlying organic etiology. Abdominal examination should focus on identifying abdominal distension seen in surgical causes like Hirschsprung disease or intestinal obstruction, palpable fecoliths, other palpable masses or organomegaly, and features of peritonitis. Perianal area should be examined for the position of the anus, soiling with stools, presence of skin tags, and anal fissures. Digital rectal examination (DRE) is helpful in the diagnosis of anal stenosis; explosive passage of stools after withdrawing the examining finger is characteristic of Hirschsprung disease (blast sign). Routine DRE is not recommended when functional constipation is suspected.

Flowchart 2: Algorithm for approach to constipation in the emergency department (ED).

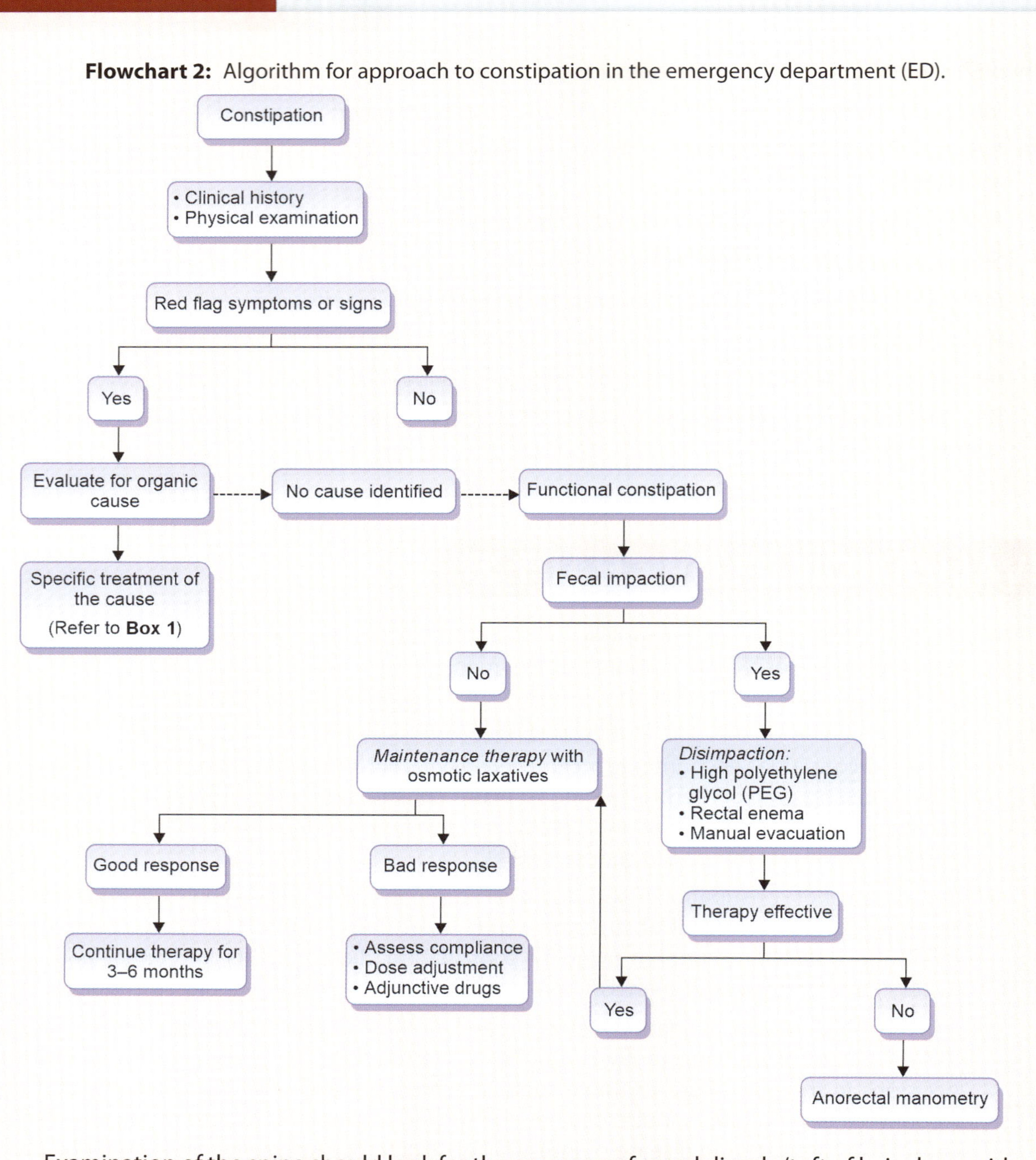

Examination of the spine should look for the presence of sacral dimple/tuft of hair along with lower-limb tone, power, and reflexes to consider spinal cord abnormalities. Identifying "red flag" symptoms and signs is important to decide management in the ED, and to differentiate between functional constipation and *constipation due and organic causes*, to provide suitable advice regarding further outpatient department (OPD) evaluation **(Box 3 and Table 1)**.

BOX 3: Red flag symptoms and signs in constipation.

- Delayed passage of meconium (beyond 48 hours of life)
- Constipation starting early during infancy
- Family history of Hirschsprung disease
- Ribbon stools
- Blood in the stools in the absence of anal fissures
- Failure to thrive
- Fever
- Bilious vomiting
- Abnormal thyroid gland
- Severe abdominal distension
- Perianal fistula
- Abnormal position of anus
- Absent anal or cremasteric reflex
- Decreased lower extremity strength/tone/reflex tuft of hair on spine
- Sacral dimple
- Gluteal cleft deviation
- Extreme fear during anal inspection anal scars

TABLE 1: Diagnostic clues and management for organic causes of constipation.

Symptoms/signs	*Possible diagnosis*	*Next step of management*
• Delayed passage of meconium • Early-onset constipation (<1 month age) • Family history of Hirschsprung disease • "Blast sign" on digital rectal examination	Hirschsprung disease	• Refer to pediatric surgery • Rectal suction biopsy for confirmation
• Passage of ribbon-like stools/decreased stool caliber • Early onset of constipation	Anal stenosis	Refer to pediatric surgery
Acute-onset constipation, abdominal pain, bilious vomiting, abdominal distension	• Intestinal obstruction • Intussusception • Volvulus	• Abdominal decompression by nasogastric tube insertion • Initial stabilization • Refer to pediatric surgery
Developmental delay, dry skin, cold intolerance, midline neck swelling	Hypothyroidism	Thyroid profile
Failure to thrive, recurrent lower respiratory tract infections, oily stools	Cystic fibrosis	Sweat chloride test
Failure to thrive, abdominal distension with or without abdominal pain, anemia with stool occult blood negative	Celiac disease	Serum TTG IgA and total IgA levels
Fever, weight loss, anemia, blood in stools	Inflammatory bowel disease	• CBC, ESR, CRP • Refer to pediatric gastroenterology
• Any lower-limb weakness • Decreased tone, strength, reflexes in lower limbs, absent cremasteric reflex • Sacral dimple/tuft of hair • Perianal fistula	Spinal cord abnormalities	MRI spine

(CBC: complete blood count; CRP: C-reactive protein; ESR: erythrocyte sedimentation rate; MRI: magnetic resonance imaging; TTG IgA: tissue transglutaminase immunoglobulin A)

INVESTIGATIONS

Though functional constipation is a clinical diagnosis, abdominal X-ray is useful for the demonstration of fecal impaction as it has therapeutic implications. Laboratory testing for organic causes like hypothyroidism, celiac disease, and hypercalcemia and allergy testing are not routinely recommended, in the absence of red flag signs or symptoms. Further evaluation on outpatient basis, including magnetic resonance imaging (MRI) spine can be done in children in whom neurological examination is suggestive of spinal abnormalities.

EMERGENCY CARE

Like any patient coming to the ED, the initial steps consist of primary assessment including vital signs, focused history and examination, identification of red flag signs, and investigations if needed. Patients with suspected peritonitis need emergent management with intravenous fluids keeping them nil by mouth, analgesics, baseline investigations in anticipation of surgery, broad-spectrum antibiotics, pediatric surgery consultation, and likely a computed tomography scan, and close hemodynamic monitoring. Patients with suspected intestinal obstruction need intravenous fluids keeping them nil by mouth, analgesics, abdominal X-ray, and pediatric surgery consultation.

SPECIFIC MANAGEMENT

Disimpaction

- It is identified by the presence of a hard mass in the lower abdomen during a physical examination, a dilated rectum filled with a large amount of stool during a rectal examination, or excessive stool in the distal colon visible on abdominal radiography.
- Disimpaction allows the rectum to restore its normal diameter and tone, enabling normal anorectal reflexes and pelvic floor coordination for stool expulsion. Oral disimpaction using high-dose polyethylene glycol (PEG) and rectal enemas are equally effective for disimpaction. Oral route is preferred as it is less invasive and has better patient tolerability **(Table 2)**.
- Phosphate enemas should not be used in children below 1 year of age. The enema may be repeated two more times, 24 hours apart, for a maximum of three doses. They should be used with caution in children with dehydration, prolonged enema retention, or renal impairment as they can rarely lead to hyperphosphatemia, hypocalcemia, and tetany.

TABLE 2: Disimpaction.		
Agent	*Dose and duration*	*Side effects*
Polyethylene glycol (powder to be reconstituted in water)	1.5–2 g/kg/day in two divided doses for 3–6 days	Loose stools, bloating/flatulence
Polyethylene glycol solution	25 mL/kg orally or by nasogastric tube over 4–6 hours	Nausea, vomiting, abdominal cramps, rarely electrolyte abnormality
Phosphate enema	• *2–18 years:* 2.5 mL/kg maximum dose: 133 mL/dose • Enema once daily for 3–6 days is recommended	• Hyperphosphatemia • Hypocalcemia

Maintenance Therapy

Following successful disimpaction maintenance laxative therapy keeps the bowel moving and empty, preventing further stool retention. The goals of maintenance therapy are to ensure stools are soft and painless, stool reimpaction, and eliminate the recurrence of stool-withholding behavior. PEG is considered as the first choice of laxative for both disimpaction and maintenance treatment.[8] Osmotic laxatives are recommended for maintenance therapy for at least 2 months' duration. The child should be symptom-free for at least 1 month before the discontinuation of maintenance therapy.

If perianal irritation or anal fissures are present, local perianal care may relieve painful defecation and decrease stool-retentive behavior.

Osmotic Laxatives

Osmotic laxatives, such as PEG, lactulose, and milk of magnesium hydroxide (MOM), contain osmotically active ions or molecules that are minimally absorbed in the small intestine, and promote water retention in the colon, thereby helping to soften stools. PEG is more effective compared to lactulose or milk of magnesia but is not approved for use in infants. Lactulose is preferred in children below 1 year of age **(Table 3)**.

TABLE 3: Osmotic laxatives for maintenance therapy.		
Agent	*Dose*	*Side effects*
Polyethylene glycol	0.5–1 g/kg/day in children >1 year of age	• Bloating • Abdominal pain/cramps • Vomiting, loose stools
Lactulose	• *Age <1 year:* 2.5 mL BD • *1–5 years:* 2.5–10 mL BD • *5–18 years:* 5–20 mL BD	• Abdominal distension • Discomfort • Flatulence
Milk of magnesia	• *2–5 years:* 0.4–1.2 g/day, once or divided doses • *6–11 years:* 1.2–2.4 g/day, once or divided doses • *12–18 years:* 2.4–4.8 g/day, once or divided doses	• Hypermagnesemia • Hypocalcemia • Hypophosphatemia

Stimulant Laxatives

Stimulant laxatives, like senna and bisacodyl, act by enhancing intestinal motility and interfering with the transport of water and electrolytes across the epithelial layer. As a result, they are commonly associated with side effects like abdominal cramps and discomfort. They are used as second-line therapy or add-on therapy in chronic constipation not responding to osmotic laxatives alone.

NONPHARMACOLOGICAL ADJUNCTIVE THERAPIES

Toilet Training

Toilet training should be started in children at 3–4 years of age. Adhere to the "Rule of 1" for toilet training: One person, follow one routine (make the child sit for 5–10 minutes in the toilet within 30 minutes of each major meal), one place, and use one word such as "pooh" or "potty". Appropriate angulation of the knees and thighs to facilitate the expulsion of stools can be achieved by squatting in an Indian toilet or using a footrest in a Western toilet seat.

Diet and Physical Activity

A high-fiber diet, decreasing consumption of animal milk, additional fluid intake, and physical activity are important long-term measures in chronic constipation. The routine use of prebiotics and biofeedback therapy is not recommended for treating childhood constipation.

KEY LEARNING POINTS

- Diagnosis of constipation is primarily clinical, based on history and physical examination.
- Use red flag signs and symptoms and diagnostic clues to identify any underlying disease responsible for constipation.
- Routine use of abdominal radiographs is not recommended for diagnosing functional constipation. However, a plain abdominal radiograph may be used if fecal impaction is suspected but a physical examination is unreliable or not possible.
- High-dose PEG at a dose of 1.0–1.5 g/kg/day for 3–6 days is recommended as the first-line treatment for children with fecal impaction. If PEG is not available, an enema once per day for 3–6 days is an alternative.
- PEG is recommended as the first-line maintenance treatment, starting at a dose of 0.5 g/kg/day, adjusted according to clinical response. Lactulose can be used if PEG is not available. The addition of enemas is not recommended for maintenance.
- Further assessment and maintenance treatment should continue on OPD basis.

REFERENCES

1. Tran DL, Sintusek P. Functional constipation in children: What physicians should know. World J Gastroenterol. 2023;29(8):1261-88.
2. Yachha SK, Srivastava A, Mohan N, Bharadia L, Sarma MS, et al.; Indian Society of Pediatric Gastroenterology, Hepatology and Nutrition Committee on Childhood Functional Constipation, and Pediatric Gastroenterology Subspecialty Chapter of Indian Academy of Pediatrics; Indian Society of Pediatric Gastroenterology, Hepatology and Nutrition Committee on Childhood Functional Constipation, and Pediatric Gastroenterology Subspecialty Chapter of Indian Academy of Pediatrics. Management of Childhood Functional Constipation: Consensus Practice Guidelines of Indian Society of Pediatric Gastroenterology, Hepatology and Nutrition and Pediatric Gastroenterology Chapter of Indian Academy of Pediatrics. Indian Pediatr. 2018;55(10):885-92.
3. Miller MK, Dowd MD, Fraker M. Emergency department management and short-term outcome of children with constipation. Pediatr Emerg Care. 2007;23(1):1-4.
4. MacGeorge CA, Simpson KN, Basco WT Jr, Bundy DG. Constipation-Related Emergency Department Use, and Associated Office Visits and Payments Among Commercially Insured Children. Acad Pediatr. 2018;18(8): 952-6.
5. Gatto A, Curatola A, Ferretti S, Capossela L, Nanni L, Rendeli C, et al. The impact of constipation on pediatric emergency department: a retrospective analysis of the diagnosis and management. Acta Biomed. 2022;92(6):e2021341.
6. Nutter A, Meckler G, Truong M, Doan Q. Constipation and paediatric emergency department utilization. Paediatr Child Health. 2017;22(3):139-42.
7. Shaw KN, Bachur RG. Fleisher and Ludwig's Textbook of Pediatric Emergency Medicine, 8th edition. Philadelphia: Wolters Kluwer; 2020.
8. de Geus A, Koppen IJN, Flint RB, Benninga MA, Tabbers MM. An Update of Pharmacological Management in Children with Functional Constipation. Paediatr Drugs. 2023;25(3):343-58.

6 Section

Infectious Disease

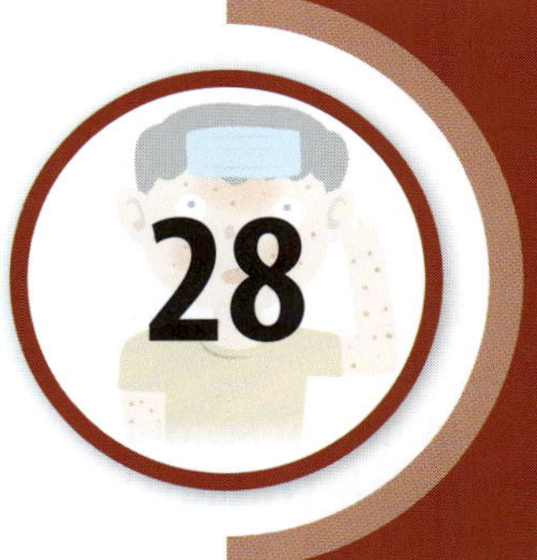

Approach to Tropical Infections

Karthi Nallasamy, Sai Charan

INTRODUCTION

- The terms "tropical fever" or "acute undifferentiated fever" collectively include acute febrile illnesses that are caused by viruses, bacteria, or protozoa, often transmitted by a vector during specific seasons of the year.
- Common etiologies include dengue, scrub typhus, malaria, leptospirosis, viral encephalitis, enteric fever, viral hepatitis, and others. The surge in these infections occurs during monsoon and post monsoon seasons (between July and December) in India.

DEFINITION

Acute undifferentiated fever that requires hospitalization and immediate management may be defined as presence of:

- Fever ≥38°C for at least 48 hours duration with onset ≤14 days
- No localizing signs (e.g., pneumonia, bronchiolitis, acute diarrheal illness, urinary tract infection, pyogenic meningitis, skin/soft tissue abscess, etc.)

AND one or more of the following:

- Clinical and/or laboratory evidence of one or more organ system involvement (hematological, respiratory, cardiac, renal, and hepatic)
- One or more systemic features such as edema, rash, organomegaly (hepatomegaly and/or splenomegaly), and encephalopathy
- A seasonal trend in incidence

This does not include children with prolonged fever, pyrexia of unknown origin, and neglected tropical diseases.

CLINICAL FEATURES

Considering the overlapping features amongst the tropical infections, a syndromic approach is better for early identification of the disease and to initiate broad-spectrum therapy.

Fever is the most consistent symptom in 90–100 % of cases. Children present in first or second week of fever with systemic signs. Examination findings include pallor, jaundice, rash **(Table 1)**, cutaneous bleeding manifestations, facial and peripheral edema due to capillary leak, hepatosplenomegaly, rapid breathing with or without recessions, and altered sensorium.

TABLE 1: Rash in common tropical infections.

Disease	*Morphology*
Dengue	• Erythrodermic or morbilliform maculopapular blanchable rash disappears in 1–5 days • Islets of white in the sea of red during recovery with pruritic
Scrub typhus	• *Eschar (5–80%):* Black necrotic area with erythematous rim—pathognomonic, seen in flexural (axilla, thighs, and perineum) • Purpuric, maculopapular rash in trunk and extremities including palms and soles
Enteric fever	Discrete faint macular rash (rose spots)
Leptospirosis	Erythematous maculopapular, but may be urticarial, petechial or purpuric

The presentation can be classified into five syndromic groups, which are not mutually exclusive and can transition from one group to another during illness (**Table 2**).

TABLE 2: Syndromic approach to tropical infections.

	Group	*Diseases*
1.	Fever without focus	• Enteric fever • Malaria • Dengue • Scrub typhus • Leptospirosis
2.	Fever with dominant respiratory features	• Scrub typhus • Influenza (H1N1) • Leptospirosis • Malaria
3.	Fever with dominant neurological features	• *Viral meningoencephalitis:* Herpes, enterovirus, Japanese encephalitis, and bacterial meningitis • Scrub typhus • Cerebral malaria • Dengue • Viral hepatitis with hepatic encephalopathy • Enteric encephalopathy—late in course of illness
4.	Fever with dominant hematological features	• *Thrombocytopenia + leukopenia + hemoconcentration:* Dengue • *Anemia + jaundice + splenomegaly:* Malaria • *Thrombocytopenia:* Dengue, scrub typhus, and malaria
5.	Involvement of hepatorenal organ systems (Jaundice, transaminitis, and coagulopathy)	• Leptospirosis • Viral hepatitis • Scrub typhus • Dengue • Malaria • Enteric fever

LABORATORY INVESTIGATIONS AND DIAGNOSTIC CLUES

Complete blood count: CBC can give clue to the diagnosis **(Table 3)**.

TABLE 3: Interpretation of complete blood count in tropical infections.

Investigations	*Remarks*
Hematocrit	• *Anemia:* Malaria • *Elevated hematocrit:* Dengue
Leukocytosis	Leptospirosis, scrub typhus, and bacterial sepsis
Leukopenia	Dengue and enteric fever
Lymphocytosis	Scrub typhus and rickettsial infections
Thrombocytopenia	Dengue, scrub typhus, and malaria
Peripheral smear	*Malaria:* Diagnosis and species identification

Urine Routine Examination

- *Hematuria and proteinuria:* Leptospirosis
- *Hemoglobinuria:* Severe malaria

Biochemistry

Biochemistry is given in **Table 4.**

TABLE 4: Biochemical findings in different tropical infections.

Biochemistry	*Findings*
LFT	• *Elevated transaminases (AST/ALT):* Viral hepatitis, dengue, scrub typhus, enteric fever, and leptospirosis • *AST/ALT >1,000:* Severe dengue and viral hepatitis • *Unconjugated bilirubin:* Elevated due to hemolysis in malaria • *Conjugated bilirubin:* Elevated in viral hepatitis and leptospirosis • Mild elevation in scrub typhus and enteric fever • Raised CPK is noted in leptospirosis
RFT	*Acute kidney injury:* Malaria, scrub typhus, and leptospirosis

(ALT: alanine aminotransferase; AST: aspartate aminotransferase; CPK: creatine phosphokinase; LFT: liver function test; RFT: renal function test)

Point-of-care investigations and rapid diagnostic tests (RDTs) are given in **Table 5**.

TABLE 5: Point-of-care investigations—rapid diagnostic tests (RDTs).

Disease	*RDT*	*Remarks*
Dengue	• RDT NS1 • RDT IgM	• *Sensitivity:* 66%, *specificity:* 97.6% • *Sensitivity:* 83%, *specificity:* 86% • IgM can persist for months. • IgM titers may be low and may not be detectable in secondary infections
Malaria	• *LDH:* Common for *Plasmodium falciparum* and *P. vivax* • Histidine rich protein (HRP-2): specific for *P. falciparum*	• 95% sensitive and specific for *P. falciparum* • *p-LDH:* Can assess response to therapy • *RDT:* Fails to identify low levels of parasitemia (<100)
Scrub typhus	RDT–IgM	• Pooled sensitivity 66% and specificity 90% • IgM can persist for months
Enteric fever	RDT–antibody in serum	• Sensitivity 69–78 % and specificity 77–90% • Turnaround time 2–4 hours
Leptospirosis	RDT–IgM	• Low specificity but sensitivity increases with disease course to 80% in second week • Can be falsely positive in coinfections with HIV, hepatitis A and B, EBV, *Salmonella, and Plasmodium*

(EBV: Epstein–Barr virus; HIV: human immunodeficiency virus; LDH: lactate dehydrogenase)

Confirmatory Test for Common Tropical Infections

- *Dengue:* NS1 enzyme-linked immunosorbent assay (ELISA)
  - IgM ELISA showing a 4-fold increase in titer is very specific.
- *Malaria:* Identification of parasites on peripheral smear remains reference standard for diagnosis (needs expertise).
- *Scrub typhus:* DNA detection by PCR in blood/eschar scrapings
  - IgM ELISA with 4-fold increase in titer/seroconversion
- *Enteric fever:* Blood culture and bone marrow culture (yield affected by antibiotic exposure). Widal titers greater than 1:160 and/or 4-fold rise in titer is highly specific, endemicity of disease decides sensitivity.
- *Leptospira:* Microscopic agglutination test (MAT) is the reference standard.
  - IgM ELISA and further confirmation with microscopic agglutination test (MAT)

TREATMENT

General principles:

- Fever control with paracetamol 15 mg/kg/dose q6 hourly
- Isotonic maintenance fluids [normal saline (NS), dextrose normal saline (DNS), and Ringer's Lactate (RL)]

Antimicrobial Therapy

- *If RDT is suggestive of malaria or peripheral smears, confirm malaria:* Inject artesunate 2.4 mg/kg (3 mg/kg if weight <20 kg) at 0, 12, and 24 hours then daily for up to 3 days.
- *If no specific diagnosis is available at the outset, empiric therapy (in children with fever and systemic features) is recommended:* Inject ceftriaxone 50 mg/kg q 12 hourly and doxycycline (Oral or IV) 2.5 mg/kg q 12 hourly.
- *In suspected acute viral meningoencephalitis without any systemic features:* Inject ceftriaxone 50 mg/kg q 12 hourly and inject acyclovir 20 mg/kg diluted in normal saline q 8 hourly.
- *Indications for pediatric intensive care unit admission:*
  - Severe plasma leakage with hypoperfusion and hypotension
  - Fluid accumulation with respiratory distress
  - Severe bleeding
  - Myocardial dysfunction
  - Acute kidney injury
  - Central nervous system (CNS) dysfunction (altered consciousness and seizures)
  - Hepatic dysfunction (ALT/AST >1,000 IU)
  - Secondary hemophagocytosis

Additional Considerations (Syndrome-based Therapy)

- *Fever with respiratory distress:*
  - Tablet oseltamivir (30–75 mg twice daily based on body weight) if there is suspicion of H1N1.
  - Ealy noninvasive respiratory support [noninvasive ventilation (NIV) and continuous positive airway pressure (CPAP)] would help in children with parenchymal involvement, fluid overload, and respiratory distress.
  - *Invasive mechanical ventilation:* Acute respiratory distress syndrome (ARDS) and lung protective ventilation strategy as per Pediatric Acute Lung Injury Consensus Conference (PALICC) recommendations.

- *Fever with thrombocytopenia:*
  - Consider platelet transfusion only if the platelet count is <20,000 or if there is clinical bleeding.
  - Avoid aspirin/anticoagulants.
- *Fever with jaundice:*
  - In addition to bilirubin and transaminase levels, perform coagulogram including prothrombin time (PT)/international normalized ratio (INR), activated partial thromboplastin time (aPTT), and serum fibrinogen.
  - Consider fresh frozen plasma (FFP)/cryoprecipitate transfusion only if there is moderate-to-severe active bleeding. Prophylactic transfusion to correct laboratory coagulation abnormalities (INR and aPTT) is not recommended.
  - If liver dysfunction is associated with encephalopathy, send serum ammonia levels.
  - *Institute liver supportive care in acute liver failure:* Measures to prevent ammonia load, continuous renal replacement therapy (CRRT), and therapeutic plasma exchange have beneficial roles.
- *Fever with encephalopathy:*
  - Early neuroimaging if Glasgow coma scale (GCS) <9
  - Intubation for airway protection if active signs of raised intracranial pressure or GCS <9
  - 3% saline bolus (5–10 mL/kg) and infusion (0.1–1 mL/kg/h) to maintain serum sodium target 145–150 mEq/L to treat raised intracranial pressure.

Etiology-specific therapy is given in **Table 6**.

TABLE 6: Etiology-specific therapy.

Disease	*Drug therapy*
Malaria	Inject artesunate 2.4 mg/kg (3 mg/kg if weight <20 kg) at 0, 12, 24 hours and then daily for up to 3 days. Convert to oral artesunate combination therapy (ACT) once oral intake is good to complete 3 days course
Scrub typhus	• *Doxycycline:* 2.5 mg/kg/dose BD (IV/oral) 5–7 days or 3 days until patient is afebrile. Or • Azithromycin (IV/oral) 10 mg/kg/day for 5 days *Dual therapy (Doxycycline + Azithromycin) may be considered in selected children with multiorgan failure.
Enteric fever	• IV ceftriaxone 50 mg/kg q 12 hourly until 48 hours after fever defervescence followed by oral cefixime (10 mg/kg q 12 hourly) for a total duration of 10–14 days *Azithromycin (IV/oral) 20 mg/kg/day for 5 days may be reserved for nonresponse after a reasonable duration (≥7 days) of ceftriaxone therapy
Leptospirosis	• *Mild disease:* Oral doxycycline 2.5 mg/kg q 12 hourly for 7 days • *Severe disease:* IV doxycycline (2.5 mg/kg q 12 hourly or IV ceftriaxone (50 mg/kg q 12 hourly) for 7 days
Herpes encephalitis	IV acyclovir 20 mg/kg q 8 hourly for 14–21 days
Dengue	• Stop empirical antimicrobial therapy • Isotonic fluids (NS, RL, or DNS)

CONCLUSION

Syndromic approach helps in narrowing down the etiology of acute undifferentiated presentation and guides initial empirical therapy. Scrub typhus and dengue are the common tropical fevers in Indian children. Active evaluation to identify the etiology coupled with organ-supportive care in intensive care facilities would improve the outcome.

SUGGESTED READING

1. Bhargava A, Raph R, Chatterjee B, Bottieau E. Assessment and initial management of acute undifferentiated fever in tropical and subtropical regions. BMJ. 2018;263:k4766.
2. Joshi S, Immanuel G, Arulrhaj S, Tiwaskar M, Vora A, Samavedam S. Roadmap for the management of acute undifferentiated febrile illness: An expert discussion and review of available guidelines. J Assoc Physicians India. 2021;69(9):11-2.
3. Singhi S, Chaudhary D, Varghese GM, Bhalla A, Karthi N, Kalantri S, et al. From: The Indian Society of Critical Care Medicine Tropical fever Group. Tropical fevers: Management guidelines. Indian J Crit Care Med. 2014;18(2):62-9.
4. Singhi S, Rungta N, Nallasamy K, Bhalla A, Peter JV, Chaudhary D, et al. for Indian Society of Critical Care Medicine Research Group. Tropical fevers in Indian intensive care units: A prospective multicenter study. Indian J Crit Care Med. 2017;21(12):811-8.

29 Tetanus

Ramesh Rajesh Pol, Rashmi Kattimani

INTRODUCTION

- Tetanus (lockjaw) is an acute spastic paralytic condition caused by *Clostridium tetani*. Tetanus cannot be eradicated easily unlike smallpox, because spores are widespread in the environment and cannot be eliminated.
- In low-income countries with unclean birth practices and immunization coverage being low, tetanus stands as a major public health problem.
- Although the World Health Organization (WHO) declared India free of maternal and neonatal tetanus in August 2015, tetanus is still a threat to children and adults. In 2021, the total number of reported cases of tetanus from India was 1,240, of which 81 were infants.

DEFINITION

Tetanus is an acute infectious disease of the nervous system characterized by muscle spasms that are caused by the toxin-producing spores of the anaerobe bacteria *C. tetani*, which usually begins in the jaw and progresses to generalized muscle spasms without any other medical cause.

MODE OF INFECTION AND PREDISPOSING FACTORS

As *C. tetani* will not grow in healthy tissues, a convergence of factors is to be present for tetanus toxin to be involved in the human host:

- Absence of antibodies (i.e., inadequate vaccination)
- A penetrating injury (inoculation of *C. tetani* spores)
- Coinfection with other bacteria
- Devitalized tissue
- A foreign body
- Localized ischemia
- Neonates (infection of the umbilical stump by retained dirt, dung, clotted blood, or serum)

ETIOPATHOGENESIS

Clostridium tetani is a gram-positive, spore-forming, obligate anaerobic bacterium, which produces a neurotoxin, i.e., tetanospasmin. The low oxidation–reduction potential of an infected injury site provides an ideal environment for the transition from spore to vegetative stage of growth, which releases toxin leading to tetanospasmin. Thus, tetanus can be considered more of a toxin-mediated process than an acute infectious process.

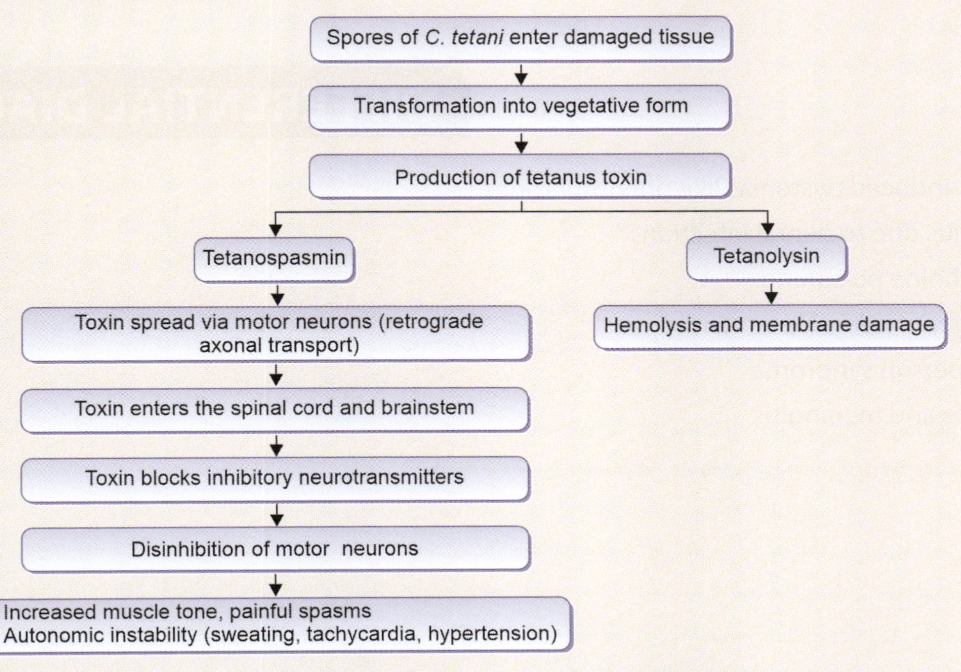

CLINICAL MANIFESTATIONS

The incubation period is approximately 8 days but may range from 3 to 21 days and is shorter in case of neonatal and cephalic tetanus. Tetanus is a descending pattern with extreme pain and there is no impairment of consciousness. The tonic and periodic spastic muscular contractions are responsible for tetanic spasms and are triggered by loud noises, touch, or light. Tetanus can present as generalized, localized, or cephalic form **(Table 1)**.

TABLE 1: Clinical manifestations of tetanus.

Generalized	*Localized*	*Cephalic*
• Most common • Trismus • Risus sardonicus (sardonic smile) • Opisthotonus • Dysuria and urinary retention • Airway obstruction and asphyxiation • Autonomic overactivity features like fever, tachycardia, labile hypertension, and diaphoresis	• Least common • Painful spasms of the muscles adjacent to the wound site • Diagnosis is difficult. Resolves spontaneously	• Seen with injuries to the head, face, or neck • Retracted eyelids • Deviated gaze • Dysphagia • Trismus • Focal cranial neuropathies (cranial nerves III, IV, VI, VII and XII)

Neonatal tetanus: This typically manifests within 3–12 days of birth. It presents as refusal to feed and difficulty in opening the mouth due to trismus and rigidity to touch, spasms with/without opisthotonus.

DIFFERENTIAL DIAGNOSIS

- Drug-induced dystonias like phenothiazines
- Trismus due to dental infection
- Strychnine poisoning
- Malignant neuroleptic syndrome
- Stiff-person syndrome
- Rabies and meningitis

DIAGNOSIS

- There is no laboratory test for the diagnosis of tetanus; an assay of antitoxin levels is not readily available and it is solely on a clinical basis.
- The *spatula test* is a simple diagnostic bedside test done by touching the oropharynx with a spatula or tongue depressor. Normally, this maneuver will elicit a gag reflex; if tetanus is present, the patient develops a reflex spasm of masseter muscle and bite spatula (positive test).

TREATMENT

Treatment of tetanus should be performed in a dark, secluded intensive care unit **(Tables 2 and 3)**.

TABLE 2: Targeted bundled intervention.

Goals	*Interventions*
Airway management	• *Intubation:* – Early intubation is often necessary. Nasal airway or nasal intubation is preferred over endotracheal intubation – Consider tracheostomy for prolonged ventilation
Halting the toxin production	• *Wound management:* – *Debridement:* Essential to remove spores and necrotic tissue • *Antimicrobial therapy:* – *Metronidazole:* 30 mg/kg/day IV every 6–8 hours for 7–10 days – *Penicillin G:* 2–4 million units IV every 4–6 hours for 7–10 days – Cephalosporins like cefazolin, cefuroxime, and ceftriaxone – *Doxycycline:* 100 mg IV every 12 hours (if *C. tetani* is suspected).
Neutralizing toxin and immunization	• *Neutralization of unbound toxin:* – *Human tetanus immune globulin (HTIG):* 500 units of IM and also infiltrated around the wound – *Alternative antitoxins*: – *Equine antitoxin (TAT):* 1,500–3,000 IU IM (after test dose for hypersensitivity). *Active immunization:* Administer a full series of tetanus and diphtheria toxoid vaccines (three doses) immediately upon diagnosis, given at a different site than HTIG
Control of muscle spasms	• *Sedation and muscle relaxation:* – *Benzodiazepines:* Diazepam—0.1–0.2 mg/kg every 3–6th hourly – *Other benzodiazepines:* Lorazepam and midazolam infusion – *Chlorpromazine:* 0.55 mg/kg/dose every 6–8 hours IM/IV along with phenobarbitone. IM is preferred and is as effective as IV • *Neuromuscular blockers:* – *Vecuronium:* Continuous infusion, monitor for neuromuscular function – *Baclofen:* Consider intrathecal (40–200 µg initial bolus followed by continuous infusion at 20 µg/hr)

Contd...

Contd…

Goals	*Interventions*
Management of autonomic dysfunction	• *Magnesium sulfate:* 40 mg/kg IV loading dose over 30 minutes followed by 1.5 g/hr (≤45 kg) or 2 g/hr (>45 kg) continuous infusion • *Beta-blockers:* Labetalol—0.25–1 mg/min IV for adrenergic blockade • Avoid propranolol alone due to the potential for sudden death.
General supportive care	• *Nutritional support:* Early enteral feeding; prophylaxis with sucralfate or acid blockers for stress ulcer prevention • *Thromboembolism prophylaxis:* Start heparin or low molecular weight heparin early • *Physical therapy:* Initiate as soon as spasms cease to prevent muscle wasting and contractures • *Monitoring:* Continuous monitoring in intensive care unit (ICU) for complications (e.g., respiratory failure, infections, thromboembolic events)

TABLE 3: Tetanus vaccination and immunoglobulin use in wound management.

Previous doses of tetanus toxoid	*Clean and minor wound*		*All other wounds*	
	Tetanus toxoid-containing vaccine	Human tetanus immune globulin	Tetanus toxoid-containing vaccine	Human tetanus immune globulin
<3 doses or unknown	Yes	No	Yes	Yes
>3 doses	Only if the last dose was given >10 years ago	No	Only if the last dose was given >5 years ago	No

COMPLICATIONS

The uncontrolled spasms may lead to rhabdomyolysis, myoglobinuria, and renal failure. Venous thrombosis, pulmonary embolism, paralytic ileus, and decubitus ulcers are considered common complications. Autonomic instability can cause unstable blood pressure, arrhythmias, and temperature instability.

PROGNOSIS

- Various severity scores can be used to predict outcomes of tetanus, such as the Ablett classification, Dakar score, and Phillips score. The frequency and severity of the illness may vary depending on the amount of toxin that reaches the central nervous system.
- The typical duration of recovery is 4–6 weeks based on regeneration of axonal nerve terminals. As tetanus toxin acts majorly on the spinal cord, there is an increased risk of neurodevelopmental disabilities. The average mortality rate is 5–35% and higher mortality is seen with neonatal tetanus and children with shorter incubation periods (<7 days).

PREVENTION

- *Clostridium tetani* spores cannot be eliminated from the environment. Immunization and treating wounds and traumatic injuries are crucial for tetanus prevention.
- According to WHO, India achieved a record high of 93% DPT booster immunization coverage in 2022, compared to 65% in 2013. Over the past 10 years, India has significantly reduced the number of new tetanus cases.
- Ensuring maternal vaccination, clean delivery, and clean umbilical cord cutting with care of the umbilical stump are crucial steps in protecting neonates from tetanus.

KEY LEARNING POINTS

- Tetanus is acquired through infection of a cut or wound with the spores of the bacterium *C. tetani* and occurs within 14 days of infection characterized by lockjaw, risus sardonicus, and opisthotonus.
- Tetanus is not transmitted from person to person and is the most dreaded yet preventable disease.
- Immunization with tetanus-toxoid-containing vaccines (TTCV) can prevent tetanus. However, children who recover from tetanus can be infected again as they do not have natural immunity.
- Treatment may involve proper wound care, ventilation, antibiotics, tetanus immunoglobulin (TIG), and supportive care.
- Diagnosis is typically made based on clinical symptoms; spatula test can be done at the bedside.

SUGGESTED READING

1. Apte NM, Karnad DR. Short report: the spatula test: a simple bedside test to diagnose tetanus. Am J Trop Med Hyg. 1995;53(4):386-7.
2. Cousins S. India is declared free of maternal and neonatal tetanus. BMJ 2015;350:h2975.
3. Geeta MG, Krishnakumar P, Mathews L. Intrathecal tetanus immunoglobulins in the management of tetanus. Indian J Pediatr. 2007;74(1):43-5.
4. Mark R. Schleiss. Tetanus. In: Kliegman RM, St Geme III JW, Blum NJ (Eds). Nelson Textbook of Pediatrics, 22nd edition. Philadelphia: Elsevier; 2024. pp. 1821-4.
5. Rodrigo C, Fernando D, Rajapakse S. Pharmacological management of tetanus: an evidence-based review. Crit Care. 2014;18(2):217.
6. Trieu HT, Anh NTK, Vuong HNT, Dao TTM, Hoa NTX, Tuong VNC, et al. Long-term outcome in survivors of neonatal tetanus following specialist intensive care in Vietnam. BMC Infect Dis. 2017;17(1):646.

30 Diphtheria

Mallanagouda M Patil, Chandrika R Doddihal

INTRODUCTION

- Diphtheria is an acute bacterial infection primarily affecting the upper respiratory tract, caused by *Corynebacterium diphtheriae* which is a gram-positive bacillus.
- It is highly contagious and can lead to severe complications such as myocarditis, neuropathy, and respiratory obstruction if untreated.
- Although largely controlled through vaccination, outbreaks still occur in areas with low immunization coverage.

TERMINOLOGIES AND DEFINITIONS

- *Diphtheria toxin:* Exotoxin inflames the epithelial mucosa, causing an exudate which can have a characteristic grayish-white "pseudomembrane" in the pharynx, nasopharynx, tonsils, or larynx (or a combination of these). The toxin disrupts protein synthesis and causes cell death leading to the breakdown of the epithelium, and subsequent spread to local lymph nodes can cause a swollen neck. Spread of the toxin in the blood can affect the myocardium, kidneys, and nervous system.
- *Pseudomembrane:* It is a hallmark feature in diphtheria, consisting of a grayish-white membrane that forms in the throat, composed of necrotic tissue, fibrin, and immune cells.
- *Carrier state:* It is a condition where individuals harbor the bacteria but do not show symptoms, potentially spreading the disease to others.

ETIOPATHOLOGY

Diphtheria is caused by toxigenic strains of *C. diphtheriae*, which produce diphtheria toxin. It has an affinity for the upper respiratory tract (nose and throat), which causes local disease and, in severe cases, airway compromise and systemic complications. Diphtheria occurs when the bacterial toxin inflames the epithelial mucosa, causing an exudate that can have a characteristic grayish-white "pseudomembrane" in the pharynx, nasopharynx, tonsils, or larynx (or a combination of these). The transmission occurs through respiratory droplets or direct contact with infected individuals.

TABLE 1: Epidemiology of Diphtheria.

Etiological Factor	*Description*
Bacterium	Toxigenic strains of *Corynebacterium diphtheria* (four biotypes—gravis, mitis, intermedius, belfanti)
Reservoir	Humans are sole reservoir*
Transmission	Respiratory droplets, contact with contaminated objects
Pathogenesis	Toxin inhibits protein synthesis, causing cell death

*In untreated patients, organisms can be present in discharges from nose, throat, eye, and skin lesions for 2–6 weeks after infection.

CLINICAL FEATURES

Patients typically present with symptoms 2–5 days following *C. diphtheria* infection, although the incubation period can range from 1 to 10 days. Clinical manifestations depend on the site of involvement.

LOCAL SYMPTOMS

- Pharyngitis with sore throat
- Formation of pseudomembrane in the throat
- Hoarseness and difficulty swallowing
- Nasal discharge (if nasopharyngeal involvement)

SYSTEMIC SYMPTOMS

- Fever and malaise
- Neck swelling (bull-neck appearance due to lymphadenopathy)
- Myocarditis leading to arrhythmias or heart failure
- Neurological complications, such as paralysis of the palate or extremities

PHYSICAL EXAMINATION

TABLE 2: Examination findings of diphtheria.

Pharyngotonsillar	• The membrane adheres to the tonsils and the pharyngeal wall extends to the uvula and down to the larynx. Attempting to remove the pseudomembrane will cause bleeding. The membrane may change colors over time—within the first few days of formation, it is bluish white. By the time, the patient • presents for treatment, it may be grayish-green or black if they have experienced bleeding • Cervical swelling caused by the edema of underlying soft tissue and enlarged lymph nodes gives the appearance of a bull neck. • Edema is brawny, pitting, warm on touch, and nonerythematous
Nasal	Nasal diphtheria, commonly seen in infants, is a mild disease. It starts with the common cold and is characterized by mild rhinorrhea and a lack of systemic symptoms. In patients with anterior nasal diphtheria, a white pseudomembrane often forms along the nasal septum
Cutaneous	Cutaneous diphtheria is typically a nonprogressive, indolent infection manifested as a superficial, ecthymic, and nonhealing ulcer with a gray-brown membrane. The extremities are more commonly affected than the trunk or head.
Rarely diphtheria can also present as vaginal, conjunctival, or otic infections.	

INVESTIGATIONS

- Need to inform the laboratory about the suspected diagnosis as special culture media like Loffler slant, tellurite plate, and blood agar plate are essential.
- Culture from throat or any mucosal or cutaneous lesion for *C. diphtheriae*
- Obtaining multiple samples from the respiratory site increases the yield of culture.
- Polymerase chain reaction (PCR) detects presence of toxin gene.
- Elek's test by immunodiffusion confirms toxin production.
- ECG to monitor for signs of myocarditis

EVALUATION

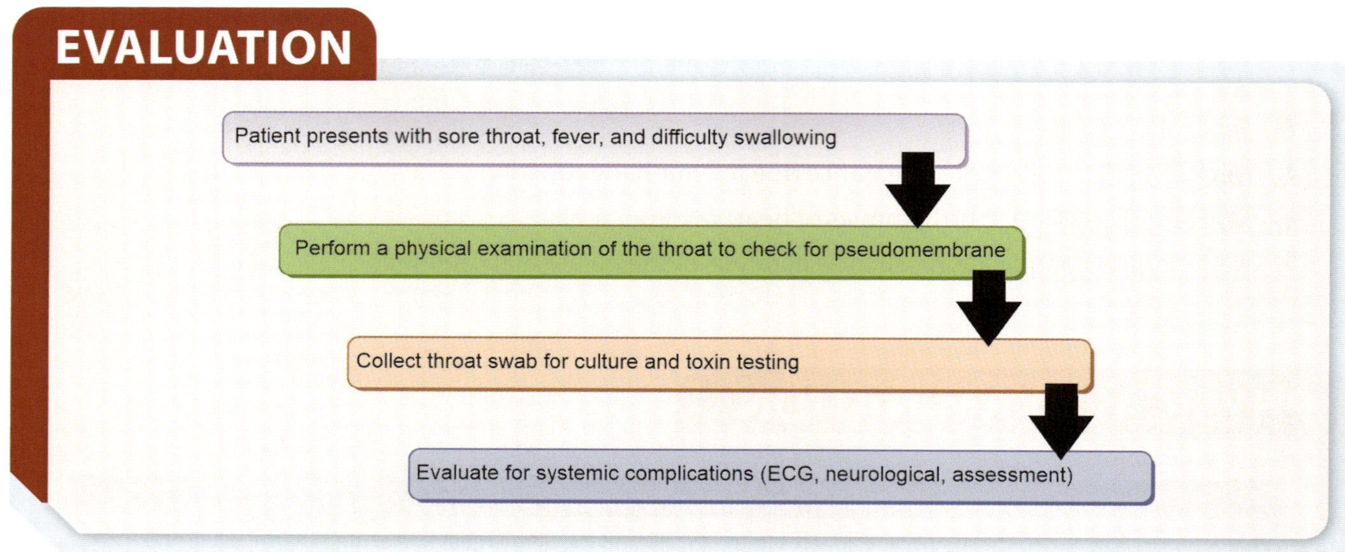

DIFFERENTIALS

- Streptococcal pharyngitis
- Infectious mononucleosis
- Epiglottitis
- Vincent's angina

MANAGEMENT

Emergency Care

- **Isolation:** Immediate isolation of suspected diphtheria case to prevent transmission
- **Antibiotic:** Initiate antibiotic therapy (erythromycin or penicillin) to eradicate the bacteria
- **Antitoxin:** Administer diphtheria antitoxin (neutralizes unbound toxin)
- **Airway:** Secure airway if signs of obstruction appear (tracheostomy may be needed)
- **Support:** Supportive care (fluids, treatment for myocarditis or neuropathy)

Specific Management

Antibiotics

Antibiotics prevent further bacterial growth and toxin production, reducing the risk of further organ damage and bacterial transmission to others. In patients with suspected or confirmed diphtheria, the World Health Organization (WHO) recommends using macrolide antibiotics (erythromycin, azithromycin) in preference to penicillin antibiotics, as recent studies have demonstrated increased resistance to penicillin over the macrolide class of antibiotics.

TABLE 3: Antibiotic therapy for diphtheria.

Antibiotics	*Doses*	*Duration*
Erythromycin (oral or IV)	40–50 mg/kg/day, maximum 2 g/day	14 days
Azithromycin (oral or IV)	10–12 mg/kg/day (maximum 500 mg/day)	
Aqueous penicillin G (IV)	100,000–150,000 units/kg/day divided into four doses	14 days
Penicillin G procaine (IM)	25,000–50,000 units/kg/day divided into two doses	14 days

Patients treated with appropriate antibiotics usually are not infectious 48 hours after treatment is initiated.

Cutaneous diphtheria: Thorough cleaning of the lesion with soap and water and antibiotic therapy for 10 days.

Antitoxin

Diphtheria antitoxin (DAT) is most effective in neutralizing extracellular toxins, and once a toxin is internalized, DAT is ineffective in preventing its intracellular consequences. The minimum effective dose of DAT has not been formally determined in humans, and doses employed in managing diphtheria assume that the duration of disease and/or severity roughly indicate the amount of circulating toxin.

In patients with suspected or confirmed diphtheria, the WHO recommends not performing routine sensitivity testing before administration of diphtheria antitoxin. However, trained staff and equipment availability must be ensured, as the risk of allergic reaction is possible.

Administration of a single dose of diphtheria antitoxin with the choice of dose based on disease severity and time since symptom onset, as suggested, is given in **Table 4**.

TABLE 4: Antitoxin dose for diphtheria.

Characteristic of diphtheria disease	*Dose of diphtheria antitoxin (IU)*
• Laryngitis *or* pharyngitis *and* • Duration <48 hours	20,000
• Nasopharyngeal disease (extensive pseudomembrane) *and* • Duration <48 hours	40,000
One or more of: • Diffuse swelling of the neck • Any disease ≥48 hours • Severe disease (respiratory distress, shock)	80,000

Note: Early treatment may reduce overall diphtheria antitoxin (DAT) usage by avoiding the higher doses required once the disease has progressed.

Treatment of Contacts

- Antimicrobial prophylaxis with oral erythromycin, 40–50 mg/kg/day for 7–10 days or single intramuscular injection of penicillin G benzathine (6 lakhs U for children weighing <30 kg and 12 lakhs U for weight >30 kg and adults)
- *Culture for C diphtheria:* If cultures are positive after chemoprophylaxis, an additional 10-day course of erythromycin must be administered.
    - Surveillance for evidence of disease for 7 days from the last exposure to an untreated patient Immunization for contacts **(Table 5)**

TABLE 5: Immunization for contacts.

Contact Status	*Immunization*
Asymptomatic, previously immunized	A booster dose of DTaP (or DT), Tdap, Td (as per age) if they have not received it within the last 5 years
Asymptomatic with less than 3 doses of vaccine, or children <7 years due for 4th dose or vaccine status unknown	A booster dose of age-appropriate vaccine
Contacts who cannot be kept under surveillance	Penicillin G benzathine and additionally a booster dose of age-appropriate vaccine if partially immunized or immunization status unknown

Immunization

Active immunization against diphtheria should be undertaken during convalescence as the disease does not confer immunity.

CASE MANAGEMENT

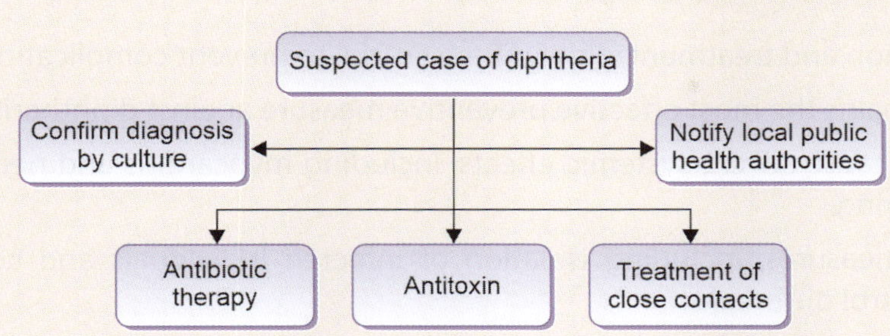

Supportive Measures

- Close monitoring for respiratory distress or airway obstruction signs
- Cardiac monitoring for myocarditis (arrhythmias or heart failure)
- Neurological monitoring for signs of paralysis or neuropathy
- Maintaining hydration

TABLE 6: Vaccination for diphtheria.

Age (completed weeks/ months/years)	*Vaccines*	*Comments*
6, 10, and 14 weeks	DTwP or DTaP	Either can be used for primary series
16–18 months	DTaP or DTwP	• Tdap is not recommended here • DTaP can be considered for boosters instead of DTwP because of its higher reactogenicity
4–6 years	DTaP or DTwP	
10–12 years	Tdap/Td	• Recommended age for Tdap is 10 years • Tdap is preferred to Td followed by Td every 10 years
Catch-up Vaccination		
Below 7 years	DTwP or DTaP	At 0, 1, and 6 months
Above 7 years	Tdap/Td	At 0, 1, and 6 months

KEY LEARNING POINTS

- Early identification and treatment with DAT are crucial to prevent complications.
- Vaccination remains the most effective preventive measure against diphtheria.
- Diphtheria can cause severe systemic effects, including myocarditis and neuropathy, requiring vigilant monitoring.
- Public health measures, including isolation of infected individuals and contact tracing, are essential to control outbreaks.

SUGGESTED READING

1. Centers for Disease Control and Prevention. Diphtheria. [online] Available from https://www.cdc.gov/diphtheria/index.html [Last accessed November, 2024].
2. Eisenberg N, Panunzi I, Wolz A, Burzio C, Cilliers A, Islam MA, et al. Diphtheria Antitoxin Administration, Outcomes, and Safety: Response to a Diphtheria Outbreak in Cox's Bazar, Bangladesh. Clin Infect Dis. 2021; 73(7):E1713-8.
3. Hennart M, Panunzi LG, Rodrigues C, Gaday Q, Baines SL, Barros-Pinkelnig M, et al. Population genomics and antimicrobial resistance in *Corynebacterium diphtheriae*. Genome Med. 2020;12(1):107.
4. MedlinePlus. Diphtheria. US National Library of Medicine. [online] Available from https://medlineplus.gov/diphtheria.html [Last accessed November, 2024].
5. Red Book. American Academy of Paediatrics. Report of Committee on Infectious Diseases, 32nd edition. New Delhi: CBS Publishers.
6. Truelove SA, Keegan LT, Moss WJ, Chaisson LH, Macher E, Azman AS, et al. Clinical and epidemiological aspects of diphtheria: a systematic review and pooled analysis. Clin Infect Dis. 2020;71(1):89-97.
7. World Health Organization. Diphtheria Vaccine: Position Paper. Weekly Epidemiological Record, 2020.
8. World Health Organization. (2023). Strengthening health emergency prevention, preparedness, response and resilience. [online] Available from https://cdn.who.int/media/docs/default-source/emergency-preparedness/who_hepr_wha2023-21051248b.pdf [Last accessed November, 2024].

31 Toxic Shock Syndrome

Swathi Rao

INTRODUCTION

- Toxic shock syndrome (TSS) is an acute, multisystem inflammatory response to an exotoxin-mediated bacterial infection. It is a rare but life-threatening condition.
- The annual incidence of TSS is estimated to be between 0.03 and 0.07/100,000 population.
- The mortality rates in streptococcal TSS and staphylococcal TSS are 4–56% and 0–22%, respectively.[1] In a recently published Indian study the mortality was 27%.[2]

ETIOLOGY

- The most common causative organisms are the toxin-producing strains of *Staphylococcus aureus* (*S. aureus*) or *Streptococcus pyogenes* [group A Streptococcus (GAS)].
- Methicillin-resistant *S. aureus* (MRSA) strains are also known to cause TSS. TSS toxin-1 (TSST-1), released by *S. aureus*, is the commonly associated toxin.

CLASSIFICATION

Toxic shock syndrome is usually classified as staphylococcal TSS and streptococcal TSS based on the causative organism. The staphylococcal TSS is further classified into menstrual TSS (m-TSS) and nonmenstrual TSS (nm-TSS)

Staphylococcal Toxic Shock Syndrome

The m-TSS usually occurs due to vaginal colonization with TSST-1-producing *S. aureus* in healthy young menstruating women who use tampons. The m-TSS cases were largely predominant in the 1980s, reduced now due to improvised tampons.

The nm-TSS can occur in patients with postoperative infection or infected nonsurgical cutaneous lesions. Postoperative TSS usually occurs 4–5 days after surgery. Blood cultures are positive for *S. aureus* in 50% of cases. The proportion of nm-TSS cases is gradually increasing over time.

Streptococcal Toxic Shock Syndrome

Toxic shock syndrome is commonly seen in 40–50% of patients with necrotizing soft-tissue infection. Blood cultures are positive in 60–86% of cases. Other sources of infection include the vagina, pharyngeal mucosa, skin, and soft tissues. Streptococcal TSS often occurs at deeper sites than staphylococcal TSS and is associated with a greater incidence of bacteremia.

PATHOPHYSIOLOGY

The bacterial exotoxins are superantigens that directly stimulate T cells by cross-linking major histocompatibility complex class II molecules causing massive T-cell activation, uncontrolled immune stimulation, and release of proinflammatory mediators. A mild infection can transform into TSS when toxins are produced in the absence of protective antibodies in the host, hence infants and children have increased susceptibility. As the age increases the risk for TSS decreases as the antitoxin antibody levels increase from 30% in children under 5 years of age to 80% by adolescence and 90–95% by adulthood.

Infants are at highest risk for developing invasive GAS infection. The skin is the most common source for developing severe infection. The risk factors for TSS are given in **Table 1**.

TABLE 1: Risk factors for toxic shock syndrome (TSS).

Staphylococcal TSS	*Streptococcal TSS*
Skin disruption: Trauma, burns, and surgery	*Viral infection:* VZV and influenza
Osteomyelitis and septic arthritis	Immunosuppression/deficiency, e.g., HIV, diabetes, drugs, and nephrotic syndrome
Respiratory infections: Influenza	Pneumonia
Septorhinoplasty and sinusitis	Malignancy and intravenous drug use

(HIV: human immunodeficiency virus; VZV: varicella-zoster virus)

CLINICAL FEATURES

The illness begins as fever, erythematous rash, and nonspecific gastrointestinal symptoms rapidly progressing to shock and multiorgan failure.[1]

The diagnostic criteria for staphylococcal TSS were proposed by the Centers for Disease Control and Prevention (CDC) in the 1980s and revised in 2011 **(Table 2)**.[3] It describes fever, hypotension, and a rash in the setting of multisystem organ failure. Desquamation often occurs 1–2 weeks after onset of illness. These criteria can help aid diagnosis in the acute clinical setting.

TABLE 2: Diagnostic criteria for staphylococcal and streptococcal TSS according to the CDC recommendations.[3]

Staphylococcal TSS	*Streptococcal TSS*
Clinical criteria	
• Fever ≥38.9°C • Rash—diffuse macular erythroderma • Desquamation—1–2 weeks after onset of the illness, particularly on palms and soles • Hypotension—systolic blood pressure <5th percentile for children • Multisystem involvement—at least 3 of the following: – Gastrointestinal: Vomiting or diarrhea – *Muscular:* Severe myalgia or elevated creatine phosphokinase twice the upper limit of normal – *Mucous membranes*: Hyperemia of any mucosal surface – *Renal:* Blood urea nitrogen or creatinine twice-upper limit of normal – *Hepatic:* Total bilirubin twice-upper limit of normal – *Hematological:* Platelets ≤ 100,000/mm^3 – Central nervous system disorientation, combativeness, or alterations in consciousness without focal neurological signs	1. Hypotension—systolic blood pressure <5th percentile by age for children 2. Two or more of the following signs: – *Renal impairment:* Creatinine greater than or equal to 2 mg/dL (>177 µmol/L) for adults or greater than or equal to twice the upper limit to normal age. If preexisting renal disease, greater than twofold elevation over the baseline level – *Coagulopathy:* Platelets ≤100,000/mm^3 or disseminated intravascular coagulation – *Hepatic involvement:* Alanine aminotransferase, aspartate aminotransferase, or total bilirubin twice the upper limit of normal. If preexisting liver disease, greater than twofold increase over the baseline level – ARDS – Generalized, erythematous, and macular rash that may desquamate – Soft-tissue necrosis, including necrotizing fasciitis or myositis or gangrene
Laboratory criteria	
Negative results on the following tests: • Blood, throat or CSF (blood culture may be positive for *S. aureus*) • Rise in titer to Rocky Mountain spotted fever, leptospirosis, or measles.	*Isolation of group A β-hemolytic streptococci:* • From a normally sterile site (blood, CSF, joint, pericardial, pleural, peritoneal fluid, and tissue biopsy) • From a nonsterile site (throat, vagina, and sputum)
Case classification: • *Probable TSS:* A case that meets 4 of the 5 clinical and the laboratory criteria. • *Confirmed TSS:* A case that meets all 5 clinical criteria (including desquamation) and laboratory criteria.	*Case classification:* • *Probable TSS:* A case that fulfills clinical case definition and isolation of group A β-hemolytic streptococci from a normally nonsterile site in the absence of other etiology for the illness. • *Definite TSS:* a case that fulfills clinical case definition and isolation of group A β-hemolytic streptococci from a normally sterile site.

(ARDS: adult respiratory distress syndrome; CSF: cerebrospinal fluid; TSS: toxic shock syndrome)

LABORATORY EVALUATION

The diagnosis of TSS is mainly clinical as there is no gold standard test to diagnose. As a part of diagnostic criteria,[3] there are a few recommended investigations and salient laboratory findings that are described in **Table 3**.

TABLE 3: Laboratory findings in TSS.

Parameter	*Remarks*
Complete blood count	Leukocytosis/leukopenia and thrombocytopenia
Lactate	High lactate >2 mmol/L indicates the need for fluid resuscitation Lactate >2 mmol/L despite fluid resuscitation indicates the need for vasopressors
Creatinine	2 × upper limit of normal indicates AKI
Liver function tests	Raised bilirubin/ALT/AST >2 × upper limit of normal indicates liver dysfunction Albumin is low
Coagulation profile	Prolonged
Electrolytes	Life-threatening hypocalcemia is prominent throughout the disease Hyponatremia is common
Blood grouping and cross-matching	At admission May require fresh frozen plasma transfusion
Creatine phosphokinase (CPK)	Greater than two times the upper limit of normal is classical
Blood culture, wound swab culture and sensitivity	To isolate the causative organism

(AKI: acute kidney injury; ALT: Alanine aminotransferase; AST: aspartate aminotransferase; TSS: toxic shock syndrome)

MANAGEMENT

Early recognition of the clinical syndrome is essential to improve the outcome. The initial resuscitation must start immediately in the emergency department **(Flowchart 1)**.

The principles of management of TSS are:

- Resuscitation in the emergency department
- Targeted antibiotics
- Source control and eradication of toxin production
- Adjunctive treatment

Resuscitation in Emergency Department

The initial assessment and stabilization of a child with TSS must be done in the emergency department before shifting the child to the pediatric intensive care unit (PICU). If there is shock, high-flow oxygen is started and IV/IO access is established immediately. Blood should be drawn for culture and sensitivity, blood gas analysis (baseline lactate levels), and fluid resuscitation must be started.

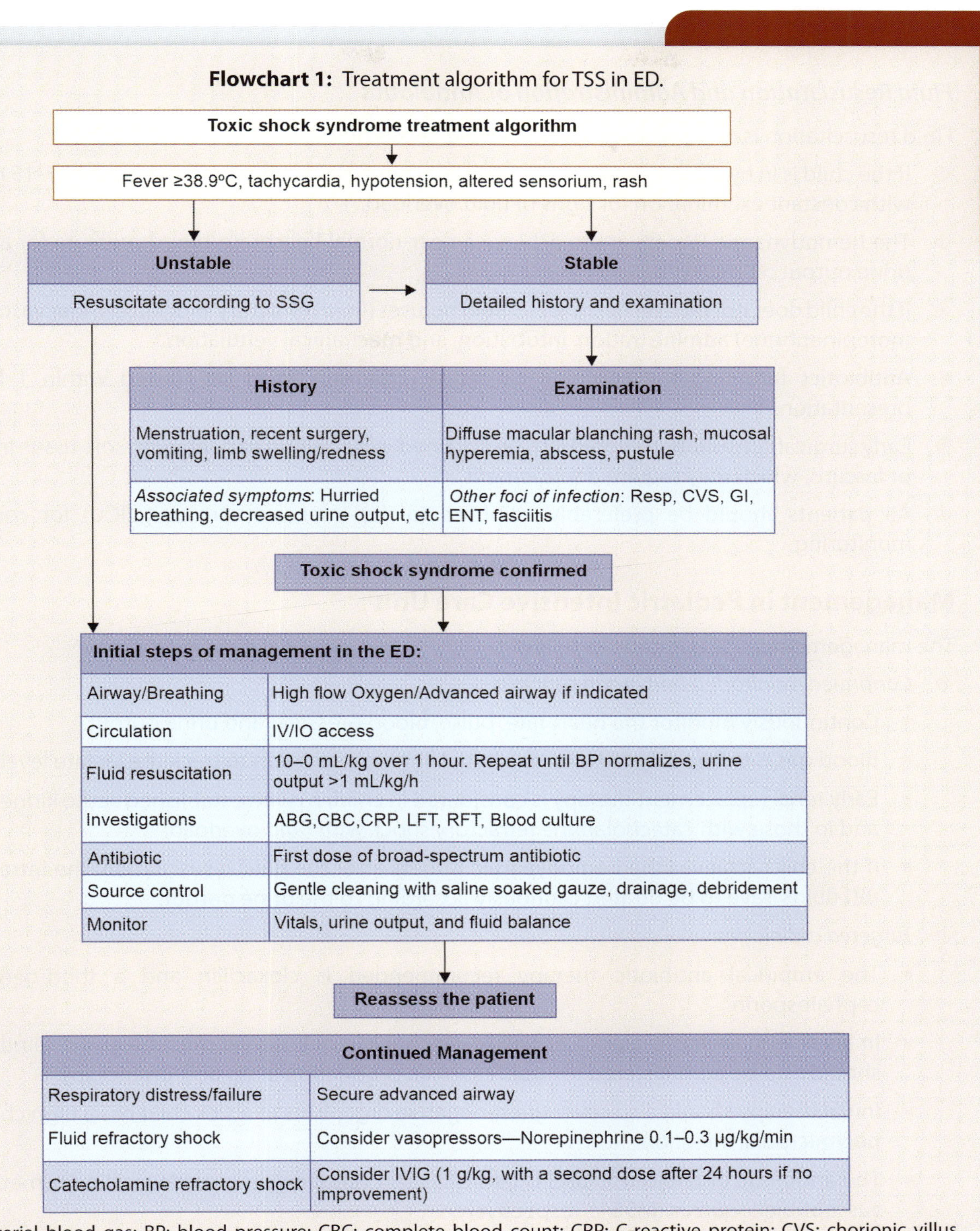

Flowchart 1: Treatment algorithm for TSS in ED.

(ABG: arterial blood gas; BP: blood pressure; CBC: complete blood count; CRP: C-reactive protein; CVS: chorionic villus sampling; ED: emergency department; GI: gastrointestinal; IVIG: intravenous immunoglobulin; LFT: liver function test; RFT: renal function test; SSG: Surviving Sepsis guidelines; TSS: toxic shock syndrome)

Fluid Resuscitation and Administration of Antibiotics

Fluid resuscitation is done according to Surviving Sepsis guidelines:[4,5]

- If the child is in hypotensive shock, 10–20 mL/kg normal saline bolus is given over 10–15 minutes with constant examination for signs of fluid overload.
- The hemodynamic targets are to achieve a near-normal heart rate/blood pressure for age, and urine output >1 mL/kg/h.
- If the child does not recover despite 2–3 fluid boluses (fluid refractory shock), consider vasopressor (norepinephrine) administration, intubation, and mechanical ventilation.[4]
- Antibiotics targeting the common causative organisms must be started within 1 hour of presentation.
- Early surgical consultation should also be obtained, especially in patients with soft-tissue infection or fasciitis, which may require debridement.
- All patients should be preferably admitted to the intensive care unit (ICU) for continued monitoring.

Management in Pediatric Intensive Care Unit

The management in PICU is done as follows:

- *Continued monitoring and organ support:*
  - Continuously monitor the heart rate, pulse, blood pressure, and urine output.
  - Blood gas is to be repeated after the initial fluid resuscitation to track the lactate levels.
  - Early renal replacement therapy is considered in children with established acute kidney injury and in those with catecholamine refractory shock with fluid overload.
  - If the child achieves the hemodynamic targets after the fluid resuscitation, the intravenous (IV) fluids have to be titrated cautiously according to the urine output.
- *Targeted antibiotics:*
  - The empirical antibiotic therapy recommended is cloxacillin and a third-generation cephalosporin.
  - In areas with high prevalence of MRSA, vancomycin or linezolid must be given. Clindamycin should also be administered to suppress toxin production as an add-on therapy.
  - Initial therapy should also cover gram-negative organisms as a sick child has a high chance of polymicrobial infection.
  - The antibiotic of choice for GAS is penicillin and clindamycin plus cloxacillin for methicillin-susceptible *S. aureus* (MSSA), respectively.
  - Once the organism is identified and sensitivity reports are available, antibiotics should be optimized and narrowed in the spectrum.
  - The recommended duration of treatment is 7–14 days.

- *Source control and eradication of toxin production:* Emergent surgical consultation should be obtained for wound debridement and drainage of the abscesses in nm-TSS and streptococcal TSS. Appropriate cultures must be collected from the suspected source. In the case of m-TSS, the foreign bodies (tampon, intrauterine device, menstrual cup, etc.) must be removed immediately. A vaginal or cervical sample must be collected to detect *S. aureus*.
- *Adjunctive treatment:* IV immunoglobulin (IVIG) is recommended in TSS with shock refractory to fluids and vasopressors. A dose of 2 g/kg is accepted in most studies. Corticosteroids are currently not recommended as adjunctive therapy for TSS.

KEY LEARNING POINTS

- TSS is a rare but life-threatening condition.
- Early recognition and timely resuscitation are the keys to improve the otherwise poor outcome.
- A high index of suspicion is required in children with skin and subcutaneous infection, necrotizing fasciitis, and young menstruating girls.
- Emergent surgical consultation for wound debridement and source control is crucial.
- Administration of targeted antibiotics must be done immediately after diagnosis.
- Fluid resuscitation is done according to Surviving Sepsis guidelines.
- IV immunoglobulin is beneficial in most of the patients.

REFERENCES

1. Atchade E, De Tymowski C, Grall N, Tanaka S, Montravers P. Toxic shock syndrome: A Literature Review. Antibiotics. 2024;13(1):96.
2. Angurana SK, Awasthi P, KCS, Nallasamy K, Bansal A, Jayashree M. Clinical profile, intensive care needs, and short-term outcome of toxic shock syndrome among children: A 10-year single-centre experience from North India. Indian J Pediatr. 2023;90(4):334-40.
3. Wilkins AL, Steer AC, Smeesters PR, Curtis N. Toxic shock syndrome: The seven Rs of management and treatment. J Infect. 2017;74:S147-52.
4. Weiss SL, Peters MJ, Alhazzani W, Agus MSD, Flori HR, Inwald DP, et al. Surviving sepsis campaign international guidelines for the management of septic shock and sepsis-associated organ dysfunction in children. Pediatr Crit Care Med. 2020;21(2):e52.
5. Miranda M, Nadel S. Pediatric sepsis: A summary of current definitions and management recommendations. Curr Pediatr Rep. 2023;11(2):29-39.

32 Management of Septic Shock

Rajeshwari Nataraj, Suchitra Ranjit

INTRODUCTION

Sepsis presents as a life-threatening clinical syndrome due to a dysregulated host response to infection and is characterized by systemic inflammation, immune dysregulation, and microcirculatory derangements. The specific clinical features depend on where the patient falls on the continuum that ranges from sepsis to septic shock and multiple organ dysfunction syndrome (MODS).

DEFINITION

Criteria to Identify Children with Sepsis (Table 1)

- Sepsis in children is identified using the Phoenix sepsis criteria, which has two or more points in the Phoenix Sepsis Score, indicating potentially life-threatening organ dysfunction of the respiratory, cardiovascular, coagulation, and/or neurological systems in children with suspected or confirmed infection.
- The new Phoenix Sepsis Score is a composite four-organ system model including criteria for cardiovascular, respiratory, neurological, and coagulation dysfunction.[1]
- Septic shock occurs in a subset of sepsis patients with cardiovascular dysfunction, operationalized by a cardiovascular score of at least 1 point of the Phoenix sepsis score among children with sepsis **(Table 1)**.

TABLE 1: Phoenix sepsis score.[a]

Variables	*0 points*	*1 points*	*2 points*	*3 points*
Respiratory (0–3 points)	$PaO_2:FiO_2 \geq 400$ or $SpO_2:FiO_2 \geq 292$[b]	$PaO_2:FiO_2 < 400$ on any respiratory support or $SpO_2:FiO_2 < 292$ on any respiratory support[b,c]	$PaO_2:FiO_2 = 100–200$ and IMV or $SpO_2:FiO_2 = 148–220$ and IMV[b]	$PaO_2:FiO_2 < 100$ and IMV or $SpO_2:FiO_2 < 148$ and IMV[b]

Contd...

Contd...

Cardiovascular (0–6 points)	• No vasoactive medications[d] • Lactate < 5 mmol/L	• 1 point each (up to 3) • One Vasoactiv medication • Lactate 5–10.9 mmol/L[e]	• Points each (up to 6) ≥2 • Vasoactive medications[d] • Lactate ≥11 mmol/L[e]	
Age based[f] **<1 mo**nths **1–11 mo**nths **1–<2 y**ears **2–<5 y**ears **5–<12 y**ears **12–17 y**ears	MAP (mm Hg) • >30 • >38 • >43 • >44 • >48 • >51	MAP (mm Hg) • 17–30 • 25–38 • 31–43 • 32–34 • 36–48 • 38–51	MAP (mm Hg) • <17 • <25 • <31 • <32 • <36 • <38	
Coagulation (0–2 points)[h]	• Platelets ≥100 × 10^3/μL • International normalized ratio ≤1.3 • D-dimer ≤2 mg/L FEU fibrinogen ≥100 mg/dL	• 1 point each (maximum 2 points) • Platelets <100 × 10^3/μL • International normalized ratio >1.3 • D-dimer >2 mg/L FEU Fibrinogen <100 mg/d		
Neurological (0–2 points)[i]	Glasgow Coma Scale score >10; pupils reactive[j]	Glasgow Coma Scale score ≤10[j]	Fixed pupils bilaterally	
• **Phoenix sepsis criteria** • **Sepsis** • **Septic shock**	• Suspected infection and Phoenix Sepsis Score ≥2 points • Sepsis with ≥1 cardiovascular point(s)			

[FEU: fibrinogen equivalent units; IMV: invasive mechanical ventilation; INR: international normalized ratio of prothrombin time; MAP: mean arterial pressure; $PaO_2:FiO_2$: arterial partial pressure of oxygen to fraction of inspired oxygen ratio; SpO_2: oxygen saturation measured by pulse oximetry (only SpO_2 of 97%)]

[a]The score may be calculated in the absence of some variables (e.g., even if lactate level is not measured and vasoactive medications are not used, a cardiovascular score can still be ascertained using blood pressure). It is expected that laboratory tests and other measurements will be obtained at the discretion of the medical team based on clinical judgment. Unmeasured variables contribute no points to the score. Ages are not adjusted for prematurity, and the criteria do not apply to birth hospitalizations, neonates whose postconceptional age is younger than 37 weeks, or those 18 years of age or older.

[b]$SpO_2:FiO_2$ ratio is only calculated if SpO_2 is 97% or less.

[c]The respiratory dysfunction of 1 point can be assessed in any patient receiving oxygen, high-flow, noninvasive positive pressure, or IMV respiratory support, and includes a $PaO_2:FiO_2$ ratio of <200 and an $SpO_2:FiO_2$ ratio of <220 in children who are not receiving IMV. For children receiving IMV with a $PaO_2:FiO_2$ <200 and $SpO_2:FiO_2$ <220, see criteria for 2 and 3 points.

[d]Vasoactive medications include any dose of epinephrine, norepinephrine, dopamine, dobutamine, milrinone, and/or vasopressin (for shock).

[e]Lactate reference range is 0.5–2.2 mmol/L. Lactate can be arterial or venous.

[f]Age is not adjusted for prematurity, and the criteria do not apply to birth hospitalizations, children whose postconceptional age is younger than 37 weeks, or those 18 years or older.

[g]Use measured MAP preferentially (invasive arterial if available or noninvasive oscillometric), and if measured MAP is not available, a calculated MAP (1/3 × systolic + 2/3 × diastolic) may be used as an alternative.

[h]*Coagulation variable reference ranges*: Platelets 150–450 × 10^3/μL; D-dimer <0.5 mg/L FEU; fibrinogen, 180–410 mg/dL. The INR reference range is based on the local reference prothrombin time.

[i]The neurological dysfunction subscore was pragmatically validated in both sedated and non-sedated patients and those receiving or not receiving IMV support.

[j]The Glasgow Coma Scale score measures levels of consciousness based on verbal, eye, and motor response (range 3–15, with a higher score indicating better neurological function).

EARLY RECOGNITION OF SEPTIC SHOCK (FLOWCHART 1)

Recognition of sepsis in children is challenging, since the presentation may be subtle in early stages, and the implementation of a recognition bundle is important for early recognition. A simple checklist to screen with an emphasis on the clinician-defined spectrum of disease allows early recognition of and intervention for sepsis.

Flowchart 1: Early recognition of septic shock.

Severe sepsis/septic shock: Clinical emergency
Signs and symptoms can be subtle and can deteriorate rapidly

Early recognition

Check age-appropriate values	Trends with treatment and over time are important
Temperature <36°C or >38.5°C	Temperature may be high, normal, or low
Tachycardia* disproportionate to fever	Each degree rise in temperature >100°C will raise HR by 10% from baseline
Tachypnea* (usually effortless, unless underlying lung pathology is present)	• Determine if tachypnea is "effortless/silent" or associated with ↑ work of breathing • Trends in respiratory status ± liver span may be useful
Blood pressure* SBP <5th centile*	• SBP, MAP, and DBP may be normal or low • Pulse pressure may be normal, narrow, or wide • Hypotension can be a late manifestation
Capillary refill time >3 seconds or <1 second	Delayed or brisk
Peripheral pulses	Weak or absent or bounding
Central pulses	Normal or bounding
Decreased urine output	History may be useful
Decreased conscious level	Agitation, restlessness, or drowsiness

Immediate treatment

- Provide oxygen if saturations <92%
- Obtain IV or IO access
- Obtain blood cultures and blood gas (include glucose and lactate)
- Correct hypoglycemia and hypocalcemia
- Give first dose antibiotics based on the focus and etiology of infection
- Fluid resuscitation: 10 + 10 mL/kg Ringer's or saline

Look for red flag signs

- Age <3 months, immunocompromised, and recent hospitalization (last 3 months)
- Hypothermia, mottled skin, CFT >5 seconds, cyanosis
- Macular erythema
- Hypotension and low urine output
- Tachypnea with grunting
- Unarousable/poor response to pain/inappropriate cry

→

- Immediate referral to higher center
- Telephonic consultation with the PICU team
- Consider the need of intubation, if expertise available

**Reference value*	*Age <1 year*	*1–5 years*	*5–10 years*	*10–16 years*	*16–18 years*
Heart rate (>beats/min)	180	140	120	100	90
Systolic blood pressure <5th centile (mm Hg)	<70	70 + (age × 2)	70 + (age × 2)	90	90
Respiratory rate (>breaths/min)	50	40	30	30	16

(CFT: clot formation time; DBP: diastolic blood pressure; HR: heart rate; IO: intraosseous; IV: intravenous; MAP: mean arterial pressure; PICU: pediatric intensive care unit; SBP: systolic blood pressure)

MANAGEMENT OF SEPTIC SHOCK (FLOWCHART 2)

Flowchart 2: Algorithmic approach to the management of septic shock.

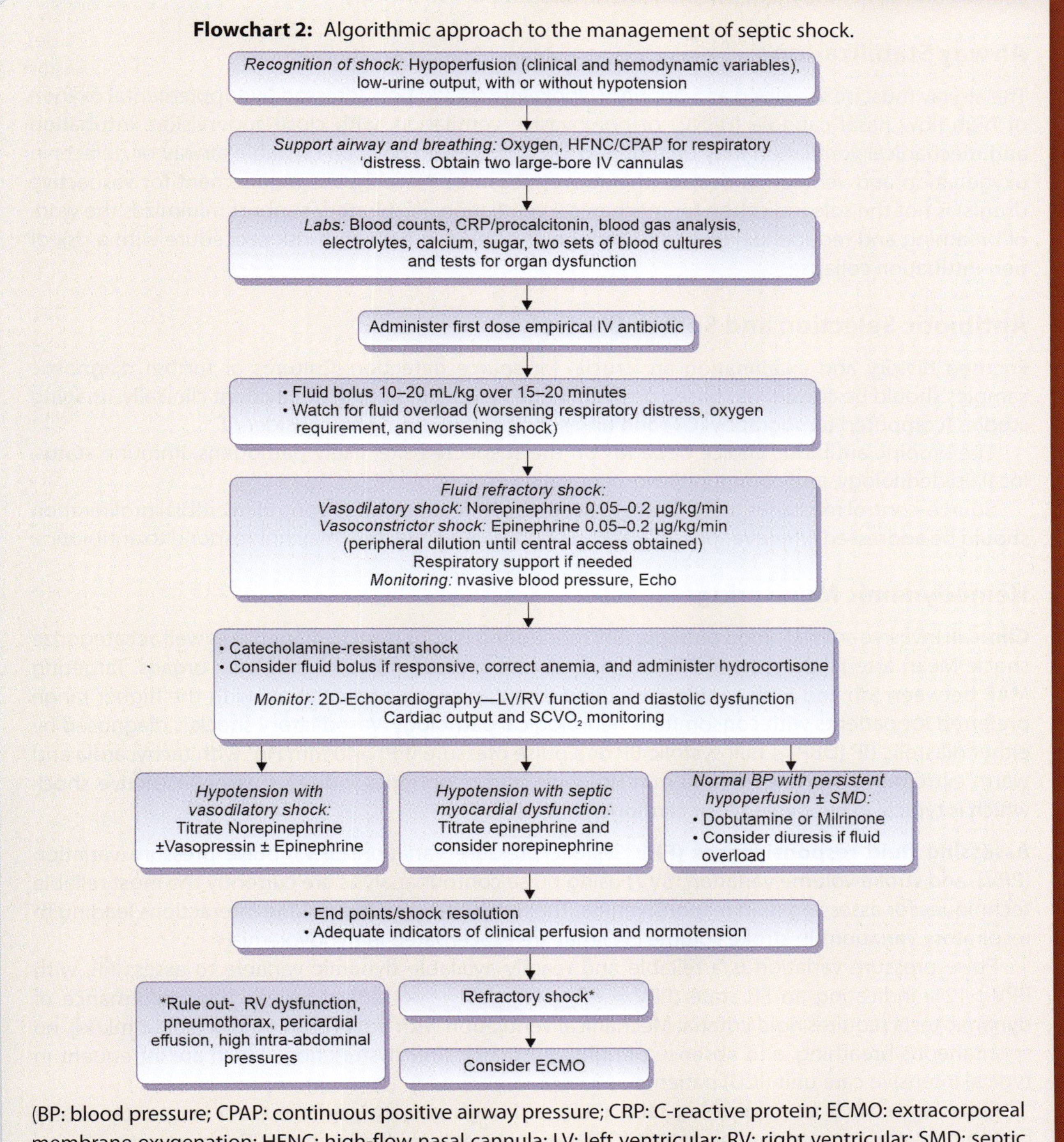

(BP: blood pressure; CPAP: continuous positive airway pressure; CRP: C-reactive protein; ECMO: extracorporeal membrane oxygenation; HFNC: high-flow nasal cannula; LV: left ventricular; RV: right ventricular; SMD: septic myocardial dysfunction)

Key strategies of septic shock management include early recognition, timely appropriate antibiotics, source control, hemodynamic management, and supportive therapy.

Airway Stabilization

The airway must be stabilized as a priority. Hypoxemia should be addressed by supplemental oxygen or high-flow nasal cannula (HFNC) or noninvasive ventilation, with close supervision. Intubation and mechanical ventilation may be required in children who have an unstable airway or defects in oxygenation and ventilation despite the above measures. Notably, the requirement for vasoactive drug(s) is not the sole indication for mechanical ventilation. Respiratory support minimizes the work of breathing and reduces oxygen consumption, but this can be a high-risk procedure with a risk of peri-intubation collapse.

Antibiotic Selection and Source Control

Focused history and examination are crucial for source detection. Cultures or further diagnostic samples should be considered based on history and clinical findings. If not evident clinically, imaging studies [computed tomography (CT) and ultrasonography] should be considered.

The empiric antibiotic choice depends on the suspected site, likely pathogens, immune status, local epidemiology, and community/nosocomial source.

Source-control measures to eradicate the source of infection and to control microbial proliferation should be addressed wherever possible as foci of undrained infection may not respond to antibiotics.

Hemodynamic Monitoring

Clinical: Invasive arterial blood pressure (BP) monitoring is important to diagnose as well as categorize shock. Mean arterial pressure (MAP) is the upstream pressure for perfusing vital organs. Targeting MAP between 5th and 50th centile is required to optimize macrocirculation, with the higher range preferred for patients with concomitant neurological pathology. Vasodilatory shock is diagnosed by either diastolic BP (DBP) ≤ half systolic BP or a pulse pressure (PP) >40 mm Hg[2] with tachycardia and warm extremities. Narrow PP (<40 mm Hg) with cold peripheries indicates vasoconstrictive shock which is typical in hypovolemic or cardiogenic shock.

Assessing fluid responsiveness (FR): Systolic pressure variation (SPV), pulse pressure variation (PPV), and stroke volume variation (SVV) using pulse contour analysis are currently the most reliable techniques for assessing fluid responsiveness. These are based on heart–lung interactions leading to respiratory variations in stroke volume (SV) that are exacerbated in hypovolemia.[3]

Pulse pressure variation is a reliable and readily available dynamic variable to assess FR, with PPV >12% indicating an FR state ($PPV = PP_{max}\ PP_{min}/PP_{mean} \times 100$). However, the performance of dynamic tests requires rigid criteria: Mechanical ventilation with tidal volumes of at least 8 mL/kg, no spontaneous breathing, and absence of right ventricular (RV) dysfunction, which are infrequent in typical intensive care unit (ICU) patients.

Other tests such as passive leg raise (PLR), although easy to perform even in spontaneously breathing patients, need cardiac output (CO) measurements to demonstrate CO increments.

Noninvasive CO devices are alternative tools to measure hemodynamic variables such as CO, SV, and arterial tone, but lack accuracy.[4]

Functional echocardiography provides comprehensive cardiac assessment including response to therapy.[5] While basic information such as pericardial tamponade, left ventricular (LV) dysfunction, and inferior vena cava (IVC) assessment can help in initial management, a more comprehensive assessment is possible with advanced training, permitting interrogation of RV function, diastolic function as well as SV and systemic vascular resistance index (SVRI) calculations.

Hemodynamic Management (Flowchart 2)

Fluid therapy and vasoactive agents are fundamental hemodynamic interventions in the management of septic shock. As septic shock manifests with variable degrees of altered vascular tones, septic myocardial dysfunction (SMD), and deranged regional blood flow, therapeutic strategies should address the physiological derangements in an individualized manner rather than "one size fits all" approach. Septic shock is predominantly a hyperdynamic state with elevated SV and low SVRI. Hypovolemia may be absolute (intravascular volume lost) and more commonly relative (intravascular volume redistributed). The cardiac function ranges from hyperdynamic to normal or decreased SMD.

Clinical examination, while important to diagnose the shock state, is often unreliable to pinpoint the precise hemodynamic management. For instance, while shock may be readily recognized in a tachycardic patient with cold mottled extremities, this information is insufficient to determine the cause and, consequently, guide precise hemodynamic therapy.

Fluid resuscitation: This typically involves administration of crystalloids in modest volumes of 10–20 mL/kg over 30–60 minutes. Sepsis-induced vasodilatation results in decreased venous return. Repeated fluid boluses (FBs) may exacerbate vasodilation. Additionally, the injured glycocalyx in sepsis contributes to capillary leak resulting in the accumulation of fluids in the interstitial compartment. This process can worsen organ injury including respiratory function. Hence, careful monitoring for signs of fluid intolerance is crucial.

Additionally, with associated SMD and complications of fluid overload, FB after 20 mL/kg should not be instinctive but justified physiologically. Although static indices like central venous pressure (CVP) have several fallacies, the response in CVP to FB may be informative. A post-FB CVP that rises rapidly with no change in cardiac output and/or BP indicates fluid intolerance and cardiac dysfunction. Dynamic tests such as PPV or PLR tests have a sound physiological rationale and can be considered for FB decisions.

The choice of fluid for resuscitation is debatable and crystalloids are preferred to colloids for early resuscitation. Balanced fluids should be considered for large-volume resuscitation. While colloids do not have a mortality benefit compared to crystalloids, their use may be associated with decreased fluid overload, vasopressor requirement, and organ dysfunction scores.[6,7]

Vasoactive agents: Persistent shock despite FBs warrants vasoactive agents. Vasodilatation is a distinctive feature of septic shock; hence, pressors such as norepinephrine are beneficial. Norepinephrine is a potent α-agonist with some β-adrenergic properties which helps not only in improving vascular tone but also in increasing preload by recruiting fluids from expanded venous bed. The introduction of pressors may unveil underlying myocardial dysfunction. Monitoring for new-onset/worsening respiratory distress, hypotension, and serial echocardiographic assessments is essential.[8]

In shock with myocardial dysfunction, with narrow PP, epinephrine can be considered as the initial vasoactive drug. Epinephrine at dose >0.1 μg/kg/min is β-adrenergic and α-agonist. Both norepinephrine and epinephrine can be infused peripherally at a diluted strength as a temporary measure until invasive central access is obtained.

Persistent shock despite both norepinephrine and epinephrine infusions must prompt in-depth assessment of underlying pathology rather than giving more fluids and escalating vasoactive doses. Advanced echocardiographic monitoring and CO monitoring (invasive or noninvasive) can guide therapy. Addressing source control and obstructive pathology is imperative. Assessment of LV systolic and diastolic dysfunction, RV function, and persistent low or high vasomotor tone should be considered to dictate further therapy.[9] Some patients may exhibit shock due to catecholamine excess, and gradual weaning of catecholamine may be helpful with close monitoring. Lusitropic agents such as milrinone should be considered for diastolic dysfunction. If signs of organ hypoperfusion remain despite optimizing BPs, initiating dobutamine or milrinone infusions may improve CO and microcirculation.

De-escalation: Once indicators of clinical perfusion such as BP and other hemodynamic variables are optimized, deresuscitation should be commenced, and weaning of support may be initiated even in the initial 24 hours, provided close monitoring is assured. Diuretics can be considered for oliguria or fluid overload once the BPs are sustained above 5th centile and there is no requirement for escalation of vasoactive drugs. Broad-spectrum antibiotics should be narrowed based on antibiogram.

Supportive Care

- *Ventilator support:* In addition to standard lung-protective strategies (V_T 5–6 mL/kg and plateau pressure < 30 cmH_2O), patients with RV dysfunction may benefit by restricting plateau pressures to <25 cmH_2O, avoiding hypercapnia, hypoxemia, and maintaining pH >7.3.
- *Steroids:* While the addition of low-dose corticosteroids in catecholamine-resistant shock can be beneficial in restoring hemodynamic stability,[9] the evidence for this is not strong. However, early steroids are advocated in patients with chronic corticosteroid exposure, hypothalamic–pituitary–adrenal axis disorders, and congenital adrenal hyperplasia.
- *Blood transfusion:* In children who are hemodynamically unstable with an oxygen deficit, a hemoglobin threshold between 7 and 10 g/dL can be considered along with other measures to optimize oxygen delivery.
- *Nutrition:* Enteral nutrition can be commenced within 48 hours and must be considered after hemodynamic resuscitation in patients who no longer need vasoactive escalation.
- Extracorporeal therapy such as renal replacement therapy (RRT) is indicated in established acute kidney injury (AKI) and also to prevent or treat diuretic-refractory fluid overload. Venoarterial extracorporeal membrane oxygenation (ECMO) is a rescue therapy in children with septic shock refractory to all other treatments.

CONCLUSION

Early recognition of septic shock in children is paramount as clinical signs and symptoms can be nonspecific. Fluid resuscitation and vasoactive drug therapy should be individualized based on hemodynamic derangements, and this strategy also prevents treatment complications. Early appropriate antimicrobial therapy and timely de-escalation along with source control of infection are crucial.

REFERENCES

1. Schlapbach LJ, Watson RS, Sorce LR, Argent AC, Menon K, Hall MW, et al. International Consensus Criteria for Pediatric Sepsis and Septic Shock. JAMA. 2024.
2. Choong K, Bohn D, Fraser DD, Gaboury I, Hutchison JS, Joffe AR, et al. Vasopressin in pediatric vasodilatory shock: A multicenter randomized controlled trial. Am J Respir Crit Care Med. 2009;180:632-9.
3. Marik PE, Cavallazzi R, Vasu T, Hirani A. Dynamic changes in arterial waveform derived variables and fluid responsiveness in mechanically ventilated patients: A systematic review of the literature. Crit Care Med. 2009;37:2642-7.
4. Nguyen LS, Squara P. Non-invasive monitoring of cardiac output in critical care medicine. Front Med (Lausanne). 2017;4:200.
5. EL-Nawawy AA, Abdelmohsen AM, Hassouna HM. Role of echocardiography in reducing shock reversal time in pediatric septic shock: A randomized controlled trial. J Pediatr (Rio J). 2018;94(1):31-9.
6. Kattan E, Castro R, Miralles-Aguiar F, Hernández G, Rola P. The emerging concept of fluid tolerance: A position paper. J Crit Care. 2022;71.
7. The SAFE Study Investigators. A Comparison of Albumin and Saline for Fluid Resuscitation in the Intensive Care Unit. NEngl J Med. 2004;350:2247-56.
8. Annane D, Bellissant E, Bollaert P, Briegel J, Keh D. Corticosteroid treatment for septic shock. Cochrane Database of Systematic Reviews. 2000;2:CD002243.
9. Natraj R, Ranjit S. BESTFIT-T3: A tiered monitoring approach to persistent/recurrent paediatric septic shock–A pilot conceptual report. Indian J Crit Care Med. 2022;26(7):863-70.

Metabolic

33 Diabetic Ketoacidosis in Children

Deepankar Bansal, Jayashree Muralidharan

INTRODUCTION

Diabetic ketoacidosis (DKA) is a life-threatening yet preventable complication of diabetes mellitus. It is also the most common cause of death in children with type 1 diabetes mellitus (T1DM). Worldwide, with an incidence of 3%, TIDM is one of the most common chronic illnesses in children.[1] In the absence of a national registry, the exact prevalence of the disease in India is unknown; however, Diabetes Atlas 2022 reports more than 2.5 lakh children and adolescents with TIDM in India.[2] 15–70% of children with newly diagnosed diabetes mellitus present with DKA compared to 1–10% of children with previously known diabetes mellitus.[3]

DEFINITION

Diabetic ketoacidosis is diagnosed based on the biochemical triad that includes hyperglycemia, metabolic acidosis, and ketosis. All the three criteria are essential for making the diagnosis:[4]

1. *Hyperglycemia:* Blood glucose >200 mg/dL
2. *Acidosis:* Venous pH <7.3 or serum bicarbonate <18 mmol/L
3. Ketonemia (beta-hydroxybutyrate >3 mmol/L) or ketonuria (urine ketones 2+)

Diabetic ketoacidosis without hyperglycemia (euglycemic DKA) can be a rare presentation seen in partially treated cases, those with prolonged fasting, or those with low intake of carbohydrate diet. pH and/or bicarbonate are not only essential for the diagnosis of DKA but also important to monitor improvement and titrate fluid and insulin therapy. Venous pH measurement suffices unless there is a need to assess respiratory function. Three ketone bodies are generated during DKA: Acetone, acetoacetate, and β-hydroxybutyrate (β-OHB). Among these, β-OHB predominately contributes to the metabolic acidosis observed in patients with DKA. During resolution of DKA, β-OHB is converted to acetoacetate which can be detected in urine using a dipstick assay. Consequently, solely relying on urine ketone dipstick assay may incorrectly suggest a lack of improvement. Blood ketone levels using point-of-care meters via capillary finger-prick blood provide a more accurate assessment. This method allows for the direct and precise quantification of β-OHB, facilitating better monitoring and management of children with DKA.[4]

The severity of DKA is categorized based on the degree of acidosis[4] **(Table 1)**:

TABLE 1: Classification of severity of diabetic ketoacidosis (DKA).

Severity	*Mild*	*Moderate*	*Severe*
pH	7.2–7.3	7.1–7.2	<7.1
Bicarbonate (mmol/L)	10–18	5–10	<5
Ketones	Positive	Positive	Positive
Sensorium	Alert	Alert/drowsy	Stupor/coma

PATHOPHYSIOLOGY

Diabetic ketoacidosis results from an absolute or relative deficiency of insulin in the presence of heightened counter-regulatory hormone response incited by intercurrent infections **(Flowchart 1)**. In newly diagnosed T1DM, younger age at diagnosis (<2 years of age), delayed diagnosis, and lower socioeconomic status are risk factors for the initial presentation as DKA. In previously diagnosed cases of T1DM, poor compliance to insulin, adolescent and peripubertal age groups, surgery, intercurrent illness, etc., are known triggers for the precipitation of this metabolic crisis.

Flowchart 1: Pathophysiology of diabetic ketoacidosis.

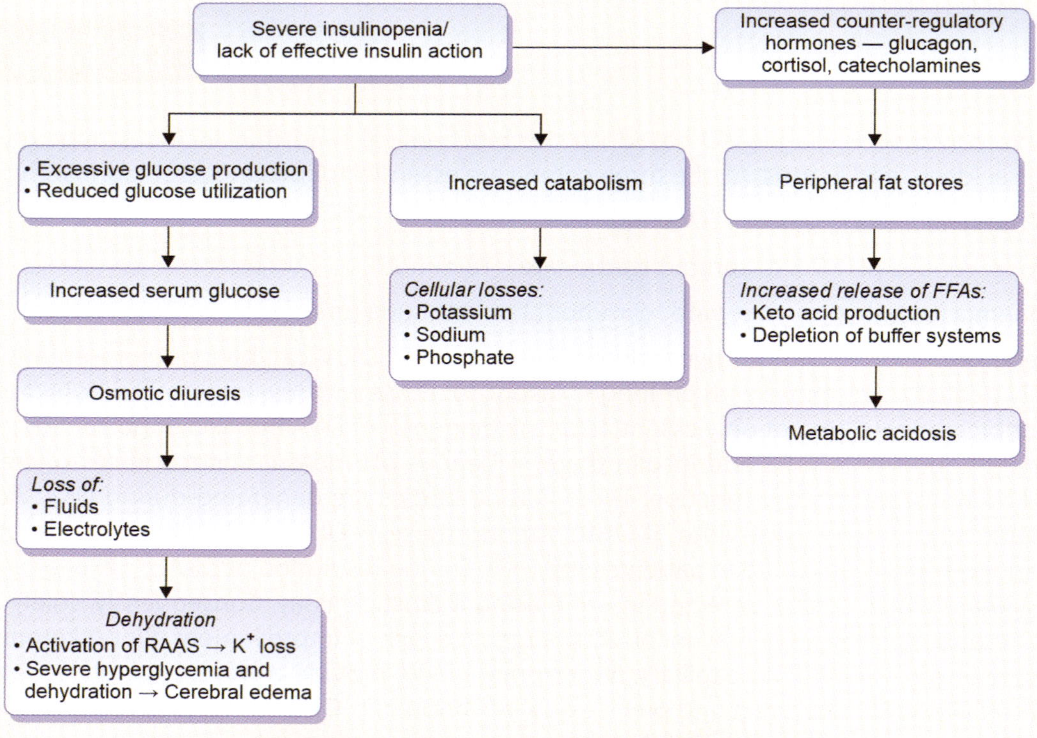

(FFA: free fatty acids; RAAS: renin–angiotensin–aldosterone system)

CLINICAL PRESENTATION

The clinical presentation of DKA may be nonspecific; hence, a high index of suspicion is needed for diagnosis. The common complaints include nausea, vomiting, polyuria, polydipsia, polyphagia, weight loss, and abdominal pain. The mechanism of abdominal pain is not entirely understood and hence is a misleading complaint that can result in missed or delayed diagnosis.

The physical examination findings include signs of dehydration, i.e., tachycardia, loss of skin turgor (tenting of the skin), dry mucosae, prolonged capillary refill time, and cool extremities. Weak peripheral pulses, with or without hypotension, characterize severe dehydration (>10%). Urine output may be preserved due to osmotic diuresis and hence does not serve as a good surrogate of severity of dehydration. Kussmaul breathing, i.e., deep labored and rapid breathing, is an involuntary response to severe acidosis and is a universal finding in a child in DKA. One should not confuse acidotic breathing with tachypnea and breathing patterns associated with airway and/or lung parenchymal diseases. Changes in neurological status are mainly attributed to high serum osmolarity and metabolic acidosis and should progressively improve with therapy. However, suspect cerebral edema if there is deterioration in mental status after initiation of therapy, new-onset neurological symptoms (e.g., cranial nerve palsy), unexplained bradycardia, or other signs of raised intracranial pressure (ICP).

The differential diagnosis of DKA includes hyperglycemic hyperosmolar state, sepsis, acute abdomen, gastroenteritis, asthma/pneumonia, and other causes of high anion gap metabolic acidosis and encephalopathy.

INVESTIGATIONS

- Random blood glucose, blood ketones, and/or urinary ketones
- Serum electrolytes—sodium, potassium, and chloride
- Renal function tests—blood urea nitrogen and creatinine
- Venous blood gas—pH, bicarbonate, lactate, anion gap, serum osmolarity, pCO_2
- HbA1c (glyated hemoglobin)
- Complete blood count
- Calcium, phosphorus, albumin, and magnesium
- Appropriate cultures to rule out infections

MANAGEMENT IN AN EMERGENCY ROOM

- Assessment of airway, breathing, circulation, and level of consciousness
- Oxygen should be started in all children with shock. Intubation is indicated in a comatose/severely obtunded child with absent protective airway reflexes. Drug-assisted intubation should be performed in such cases. The goal of mechanical ventilation in intubated children is to match the baseline CO_2 levels (adaptive physiological ventilation).[5]
- A nasogastric tube should be inserted for gastric decompression and to prevent aspiration.
- Place two peripheral intravenous lines. If the child is in shock, a 20 mL/kg normal saline bolus should be administered over 20–30 minutes. If the child is not in shock but volume depleted, a 10 mL/kg normal saline bolus should be administered over 60 minutes. Reassessment should be done after each bolus. Central line insertion should be avoided due to the high risk of thrombosis.
- Continuous electrocardiogram (ECG) monitoring for tachycardia, arrhythmias, and changes associated with hyperkalemia/hypokalemia
- Measure random blood glucose and blood ketones by a point-of-care bedside glucometer. If ketone strips are unavailable, urinary ketones can be measured to document ketosis. Venous blood gas is used to measure pH, pCO_2, bicarbonate, lactate, anion gap, base deficit, and osmolarity. Baseline serum electrolytes and renal function tests and appropriate cultures (blood, urine, tracheal aspirate, etc.) are done as indicated.

SPECIFIC MANAGEMENT (FLOWCHART 2)

Hydration and insulin therapy, under stringent monitoring of clinical and laboratory parameters, form the basis of the management of DKA. The goals of management include:

- Correction of dehydration and electrolyte imbalances
- Halting ketogenesis and reversing ketoacidosis
- Correction of hyperosmolarity and restoration of blood glucose to near-normal
- Anticipation of treatment-related complications and early intervention
- Identification and treatment of precipitating causes (noncompliance, infections, etc.)

Fluid and Electrolyte Management in Diabetic Ketoacidosis

Fluid therapy aims to restore circulating volume and improve glomerular filtration to enhance renal excretion of ketones and glucose. Fluid resuscitation is the cornerstone of the management of DKA and should always begin before starting insulin therapy.[5]

Flowchart 2: DKA management algorithm.

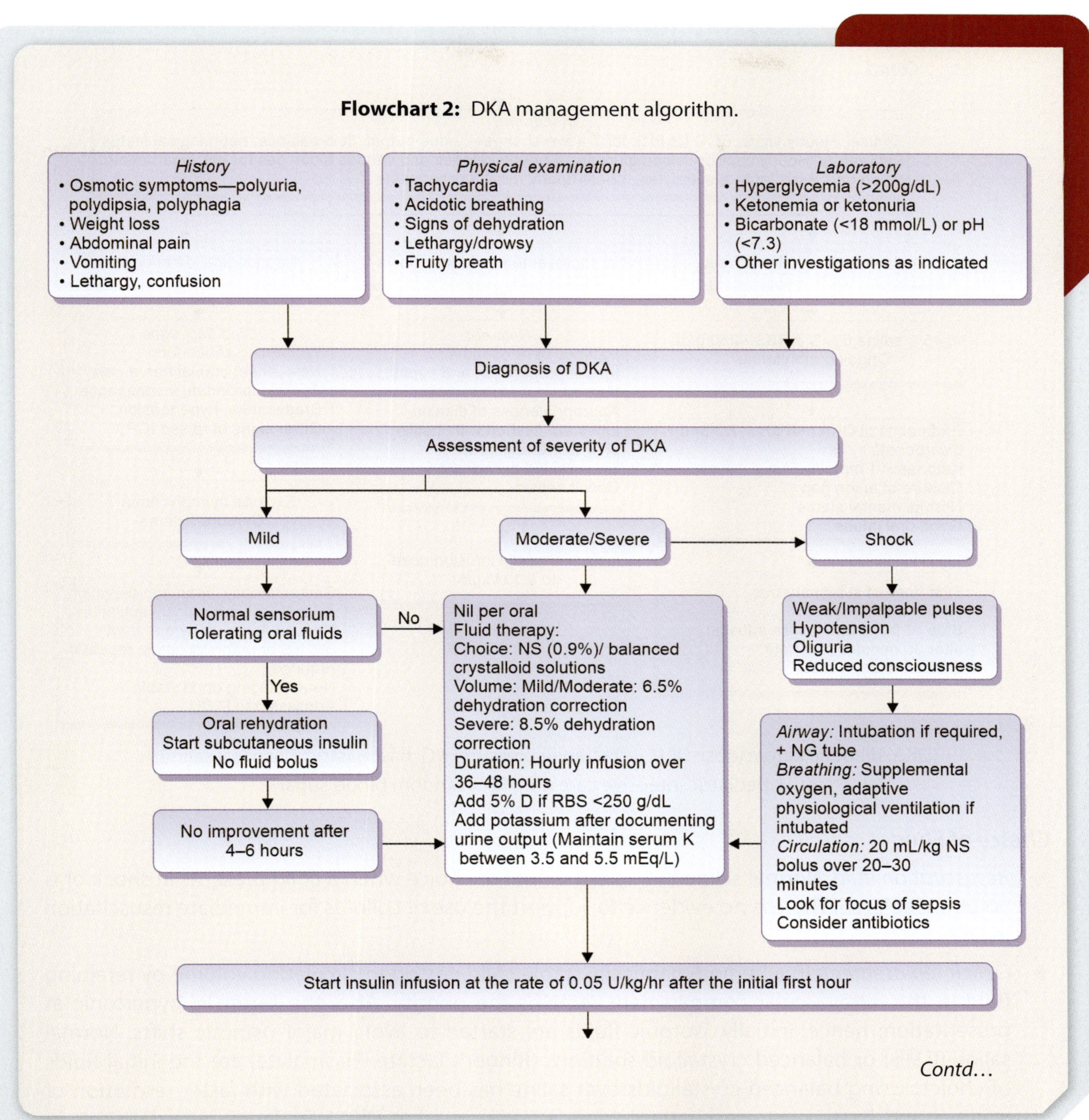

Contd...

Contd...

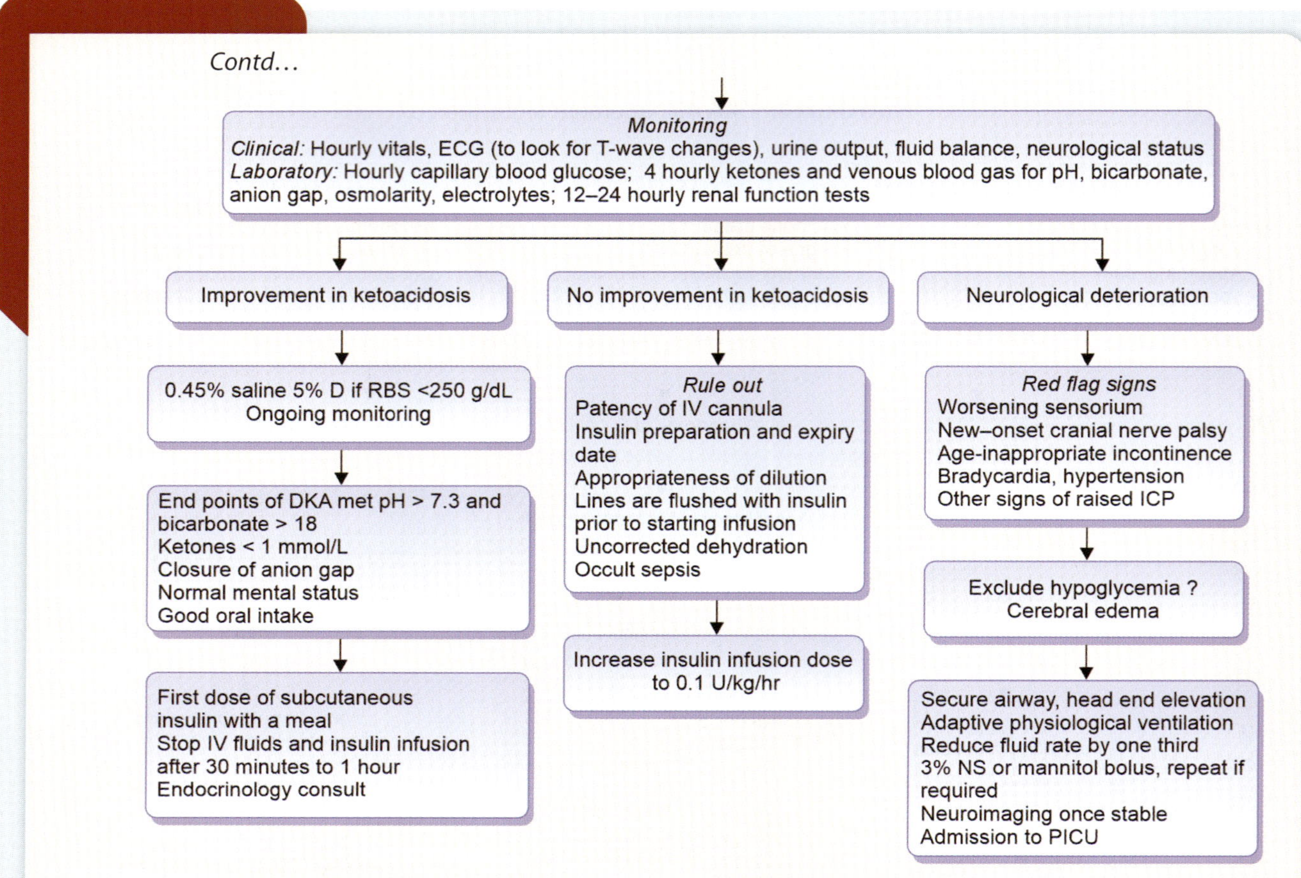

(DKA: diabetic ketoacidosis; ICP: intracranial pressure; NG: nasogastric; NS: nasal saline; PICU: pediatric intensive care unit; RBS: random blood sugar)

Choice of Fluid

- *Resuscitation fluid:* Normal saline (0.9%) is the fluid of choice when a child presents in shock or is volume depleted. There is no evidence to support the use of colloids for immediate resuscitation in DKA.
- *Deficit replacement:* In a hemodynamically stable child, restoring circulating volume by retaining fluid in the intravascular compartment remains the priority. Also, the serum is hypertonic at presentation; hence, initially, isotonic fluids are started to avoid major osmotic shifts. Normal saline (0.9%) or balanced crystalloid solutions (Ringer's lactate, Plasmalyte) are the initial fluids of choice. Using balanced crystalloids over saline has been associated with faster resolution of acidosis and lower postresuscitation chloride levels in adult DKA.[6] Evidence regarding this in pediatric DKA is still evolving. Nevertheless, the latest International Society for Pediatric and Adolescent Diabetes (ISPAD) clinical practice guidelines for pediatric DKA recommend the usage of either normal saline or balanced crystalloids for deficit replacement.[4] After the initial 4–6 hours, while monitoring serum sodium and osmolarity, the tonicity of fluid should be changed to N/2 with addition of 5%D when random blood sugar (RBS) falls to <250 g/dL. In the case of hypoglycemia, 2 mL/kg of 25%D bolus is given, followed by a repeat blood glucose

check after 15 minutes. Potassium is supplemented at 40 mmol/L after ensuring urine output. The indications of phosphate supplementation are cardiogenic shock, respiratory and muscle weakness, or when serum phosphate levels are <1–1.5 mg/dL.

Amount of Fluid

In DKA, clinical estimation of dehydration is not considered accurate. In most cases, fluid deficits range from 5 to 10% and are best correlated with the degree of acidosis and blood urea nitrogen. Hence, a modest correction of 6.5–8.5% is appropriate to avoid over-hydration or under–hydration. Any fluids that were administered before referral should be subtracted. Fluid boluses that are given for resuscitation, however, should not be subtracted.

Duration of Therapy

Rehydration and electrolyte correction should be gradually targeted over 36–48 hours to avoid major osmotic shifts. However, most cases resolve before 24 hours, and oral fluids correct the remaining deficits.

Insulin Therapy

Although fluid therapy alone can partially correct hyperglycemia and ketonemia, insulin therapy is required to normalize blood glucose levels and suppress ketogenesis and lipolysis completely. A low-dose insulin infusion rate (0.05 U/kg/h) is safer and equally effective to the standard dose (0.1 U/kg/h), especially in malnourished children.[6] Insulin infusion is started after 1–2 hours of volume expansion to avoid a precipitous fall in blood glucose. While serum glucose concentrations typically normalize before the complete resolution of ketosis and acidosis, dextrose supplementation in IV fluids are essential to sustain insulin therapy and prevent hypoglycemia. Bolus insulin is not recommended as it increases the risk of cerebral edema. Infusion tubing should be flushed with insulin before connecting to the patient.

Children with mild DKA, i.e., those with normal sensorium and good oral intake, can be managed using oral rehydration protocol and short-acting subcutaneous insulin (lispro, aspart, glulisine) given every 2–4 hours. This lowers the need for infusion pumps, close monitoring, and intensive care unit (ICU) care in such children.[7]

RESOLUTION OF DIABETIC KETOACIDOSIS

The endpoints of DKA resolution include normalization of ketoacidosis (pH >7.3, bicarbonate >18 mmol/L, ketones <1 mmol/L, and closure of anion gap), normal mental status, and good oral intake. After the resolution of DKA, these children are transitioned to a subcutaneous multidose insulin regimen. The insulin infusion is stopped 30 minutes to 1 hour after the first subcutaneous insulin dose.[4]

MONITORING

Monitoring is the most critical part of DKA management. Strict monitoring enables early identification of complications needing early intervention. **Table 2** enlists several variables of clinical and biochemical monitoring in DKA.

TABLE 2: Clinical and biochemical monitoring in DKA.

Monitoring parameter	*Remarks*
Heart rate, respiratory rate, blood pressure, Glasgow Coma Score, pupils	• Hourly • Neurological status improves as dehydration and acidosis improve
Urine output	Hourly
Random blood glucose	• Every hourly until transition to subcutaneous insulin • Desired rate of fall is 50–100 mg/dL/hr
pH, bicarbonate, pCO_2, anion gap, serum osmolarity	• 4 hourly • pH is expected to increase by 0.03/hr
Corrected sodium, potassium, chloride	4 hourly
Blood urea nitrogen and creatinine	• Baseline, 8–12 hourly • Many patients have prerenal AKI at admission, which improves with fluid resuscitation
Serum magnesium and phosphate	Baseline, 8–12 hourly

Complications, broadly, can be prevented if management and monitoring are optimal. The most common complications are hypoglycemia, hypokalemia, hypophosphatemia, hyperchloremic acidosis, acute kidney injury, and infections. Cerebral edema is the most dreaded complication and is seen in 0.5–1% of DKA episodes.[8] The risk factors for developing cerebral edema can be disease-related and treatment-related[9,10] **(Box 1)**. Clinical presentation and management have been discussed in the management algorithm.

BOX 1: Risk factors for developing cerebral edema.

Disease-related	*Treatment-related*
Younger age at presentation	Rapid decline in serum osmolality
Delayed diagnosis of DKA	Use of bicarbonate
Newly diagnosed type 1 diabetes mellitus	Higher volumes of fluids infused within the first 4 hours
Severe acidosis and severe hypocapnia at presentation	Initiation of insulin infusion in the first hour of therapy
	Insulin bolus

(DKA: diabetic ketoacidosis)

Lastly, prevention of DKA is crucial. Improving access to healthcare and day-to-day management of TIDM in individual patients will help in this cause.

KEY LEARNING POINTS

- DKA is a common complication of T1DM in children.
- Clinical features are nonspecific, and a high index of suspicion is required. Clinical symptoms are mainly attributed to dehydration and metabolic acidosis.
- Fluid therapy should always precede insulin therapy.
- Correct dose, rate, technique, and duration of insulin infusion are crucial.
- Stringent monitoring is necessary for favorable outcomes.
- Anticipate and treat complications as and when they occur.
- Equally important is to identify and treat the precipitating trigger.

REFERENCES

1. Vehik K, Hamman R, Lezotte D, Norris J, Klingensmith G, et al. Childhood growth and age at diagnosis with T1D in Colorado young people. Diabet Med J Br Diabet Assoc. 2009;26:961-7.
2. IDF Diabetes Atlas, 10th edition. [online] Available from https://diabetesatlas.org/atlas/tenth-edition/ [Last accessed April, 2024.]
3. Wolfsdorf J, Craig ME, Daneman D, Dunger D, Edge J, Lee W, et al. Diabetic ketoacidosis in children and adolescents with diabetes. Pediatr Diabetes. 2009;10(Suppl 12):118-33.
4. Glaser N, Fritsch M, Priyambada L, Rewers A, Cherubini V, Estrada S, et al. ISPAD clinical practice consensus guidelines 2022: Diabetic ketoacidosis and hyperglycemic hyperosmolar state. Diabetes. 2022;23(7):835-56.
5. Tasker RC, Lutman D, Peters MJ. Hyperventilation in severe diabetic ketoacidosis. Pediatr Crit Care Med. 2005;6(4):405-11.
6. Jayashree M, Williams V, Iyer R. Fluid Therapy For Pediatric Patients With Diabetic Ketoacidosis: Current Perspectives. Diabetes Metab Syndr Obes Targets Ther. 2019;12:2355-61.
7. Self WH, Evans CS, Jenkins CA, Brown RM, Casey JD, Collins SP, et al. Clinical Effects of Balanced Crystalloids vs Saline in Adults With Diabetic Ketoacidosis: A Subgroup Analysis of Cluster Randomized Clinical Trials. JAMA Netw Open. 2020;3(11):e2024596.
8. Nallasamy K, Jayashree M, Singhi S, Bansal A. Low-dose vs standard-dose insulin in pediatric diabetic ketoacidosis: a randomized clinical trial. i2014;168(11):999-1005.
9. Agarwal A, Bansal D, Nallasamy K, Jayashree M, William V. Pediatric Diabetes and Diabetic Ketoacidosis After COVID-19: Challenges Faced and Lessons Learnt. Pediatr Health Med Ther. 2023;14:281-8.
10. Sweney J, Bratton SL. Protecting the Brain During Pediatric DKA Treatment. Pediatrics. 2021;148(3): e2021050611.

34 Acute Kidney Injury

Sasidaran Kandasamy

INTRODUCTION

Acute kidney injury (AKI) is a clinical illness that can present as either isolated kidney disease or a component of multiple organ failure syndrome. It is characterized by an abrupt reduction in kidney function over the course of hours to days. The incidence of AKI in children is reported to range from 2 to 20 per million; higher reporting rates could be a result of early detection and raised awareness over recent years. AKI is multifactorial, particularly in the setting of severe illness; studies have shown that the incidence of AKI in critically ill children varies from 16 to 51%.[1,2] The most effective surrogate measures of glomerular filtration rate (GFR) that are currently available for defining AKI and grading its severity are serum creatinine and urine output.

COURSE OF ACUTE KIDNEY INJURY: CURRENT UNDERSTANDING

Acute kidney injury was formerly believed to be an acute illness with no link to subacute or chronic effects. As we started to understand the relationship between AKI and chronic kidney disease (CKD), interest in "*possible pathways to reverse AKI*" and "*preventing the risk of chronic kidney disease after AKI episode*" rose.[3,4] Determining the "*time zone of best response to therapy*" and "*AKI reversibility*" required an understanding of the disease trajectory. Our implementation of time-sensitive therapeutic interventions is guided by our understanding of the definitions given in **Table 1**.

TABLE 1: Course of AKI and definitions.

AKI	• Increase in creatinine by 50% within 7 days OR • Increase in Serum creatinine by 0.3 mg/dL within 2 days OR • Urine volume <0.5 mL/kg/hr for 6 hours
CKD	GFR <60 mL/min/1.73 m^2 for >3 months
AKD	• AKI OR • GFR <60 mL/min/1.73 m^2 for 3 months OR • Decrease in GFR >35% OR increase in serum creatinine >50% for <3 months
NKD	• GFR >60 mL/min/1.73 m^2 • Stable serum creatinine

(AKD: acute kidney disease; CKD: chronic kidney disease; NKD: no kidney disease)

ACUTE KIDNEY INJURY: SEVERITY GRADING TO GUIDE FURTHER MANAGEMENT

- Given the heterogeneous nature of AKI, a consensus definition is necessary to guarantee consistency in interpretation. The initial step toward definition standardization was the creation of the RIFLE (*r*isk, *i*njury, *f*ailure, sustained *l*oss, *e*nd-stage kidney disease) criteria in 2004, which opened the way for establishment of the pediatric-specific pRIFLE criteria and the Acute Kidney Injury Network (AKIN) criteria.[3,4,5]
- **The Kidney Disease: Improving Global Outcomes (KDIGO)** committee suggested the most recent and widely recognized AKI diagnosis and staging guidelines in 2012.[6] The KDIGO definition categorizes the severity of AKI into three stages based on creatinine and urine output **(Table 2)**. The most important change to the KDIGO guideline is the timeline-based definition, which improves our comprehension of the illness trajectory and acts as a tool for periodic assessments of kidney function status. Differences in the AKI stage between estimates of creatinine and urine output are not unusual. In these situations, it is essential to stage the AKI by giving the severity a higher score (based on serum creatinine or urine output) and to keep assessing often to have a better knowledge of the index child's disease trajectory.

TABLE 2: AKI severity grading (KDIGO 2012).

Stages	*Serum creatinine*	*Urine output*
1	• 1.5–1.9 times increase from baseline creatinine OR • >0.3 mg/dL increase in creatinine	<0.5 mL/kg/hr for 6–12 hours
2	2–2.9 times increase from baseline creatinine OR	<0.5 mL/kg/hr for >12 hours
3	• >3 times baseline creatinine OR • Creatinine >4.0 mg/dL OR • Initiation of renal replacement therapy OR • In patients <18 years age: eCrCl <35 mL/min/1.73 m^2	• <0.3 mL/kg/hr for >24 hours OR • Anuria for >12 hours

(eCrCl: estimated creatinine clearance)
Notes: Creatinine changes should have occurred within 7 days' time period.
Cause of AKI should be identified in each patient whenever possible.

APPROACH TO ACUTE KIDNEY INJURY IN HOSPITALIZED CHILDREN

A methodical approach would enable us to detect problems early and provide the best possible care to assure AKI recovery. Here, we go over a condensed eight-step method that will enable us to accomplish the objectives of AKI management:

1. *AKI risk stratification:*
   - Risk categorization based on Renal Angina Index (RAI) **(Table 3)** (RAI score ≥8—increased risk)
   - "Risk Screening" to identify those with a higher risk of developing AKI **(Table 4)**
   - Institute basic steps to avoid nephrotoxic medication (NTMx) induced AKI **(Table 5)**.

2. Investigative approach in AKI evaluation and cause identification **(Table 6)**
3. Identification of AKI phenotypes for therapeutic decision-making **(Fig. 1)**
4. AKI severity classification based on KDIGO AKI staging **(Table 2)**
5. Pre-KRT (kidney replacement therapy)—AKI support therapy
6. "Frusemide stress test (FST)" and its application in children
7. Context-specific interventions based on primary cause of AKI
8. Initiation of appropriate KRT and other organ support therapies

ACUTE KIDNEY INJURY RISK STRATIFICATION

Risk Screening to Identify those with a Higher Risk of Developing Acute Kidney Injury

- Clinical research studies have shown that AKI is associated with a longer length of stay in the intensive care unit (ICU), mechanical ventilation, and an approximately 6% absolute increase in mortality risk.[7] This sparked curiosity on *"risk factors"* for AKI and *"methods to identify children with higher risk to develop AKI"*.
- One standardized and well-validated scoring system that aids in predicting AKI in pediatric intensive care unit (PICU) population is the RAI **(Table 3)**.[8]
- **Table 4** offers another list of potential risk factors that may be used daily in the PICU as a checklist. It is crucial to realize that this list is neither a standardized scoring system nor a validated list of independent risk variables. Nonetheless, the majority of PICUs employ comparable checklists on daily rounds to identify signals of heightened risk of AKI in a mixed cohort of critically ill children.

TABLE 3: Renal angina index.

RISK		*INJURY: Serum creatinine to baseline*		*Renal angina index*
ICU admission	1	No change	1	Risk × Injury = 1–40 ≥ 8 = POSITIVE
Stem cell/solid organ transplant	3	X 1–1.49 times increase	2	
Mechanical ventilation and/or inotrope use	5	X 1.5–1.99 times increase	4	
		X ≥ 2 times increase	8	

(ICU: intensive care unit)
RAI—validated score-based risk prediction and risk stratification tool.
RAI—maximum score is 40; cutoff value of ≥ 8 is used to predict "increased risk of AKI".

TABLE 4: "Risk Screening Checklist" for assessing risk of AKI in PICU.	
Risk Factor	***Response***
Age group <12 months	Yes/No
Sepsis/septic shock	Yes/No
Renal functional reserve	Likely normal/likely abnormal
>2 NTMx exposure currently	Yes/ No
>1 organ involvement	Yes/ No
>1 vasoactive medication	Yes/No
Postoperative/trauma status	Yes/No
Burn injury/post-transplant	Yes/No
Possible volume depletion	Yes/No
Radiocontrast exposure < 7 days	Yes/No
Obese/overweight	Yes/No

(AKI: acute kidney injury; NTMx: nephrotoxic medications; PICU: pediatric intensive care unit)
Notes: This screening checklist is not equivalent to a "validated score-based risk prediction tool".
Response—no OR likely abnormal to ≥3 risk factors → signal toward a higher risk for AKI.
This can be used in mixed medical/surgical PICU where proportion of transplant patients <20%.

Institute Basic Steps to Avoid Nephrotoxic Medication-induced Acute Kidney Injury

Recording the medications administered by children admitted to the PICU and identifying which ones are nephrotoxic **(Table 5)** are equally important aspects of the AKI preventative care directive. The steps that follow will point us in the direction of the most useful practical strategy:

- Use appropriate diluents in indicated proportions when administering medications.
- Check drug–drug interactions/additive side effects when prescribing polypharmacy.
- Endorse the role of the clinical pharmacist in PICU and conduct pharmacist rounds daily.
- Preoperative renal risk assessment before all complex surgeries in children
- Use NTMx checklist while screening for drug-induced AKI.
- Try to avoid aminoglycosides when drug-level monitoring is not available.
- Try to avoid vancomycin if drug-level monitoring is not feasible.

TABLE 5: Nephrotoxic medications (NTMx) causing AKI in children.[9]			
• Acyclovir	• Enalapril	• Ioxilan	• Polymyxin B
• Amikacin	• Enalaprilat	• Ketorolac	• Sirolimus
• Amphotericin Liposomal	• Foscarnet	• Lisinopril	• Sulfasalazine
• Amphotericin B	• Ganciclovir	• Lithium	• Tacrolimus
• Aspirin	• Gentamicin	• Losartan	• Tenofovir
• Captopril	• Ibuprofen	• Mesalamine	• Ticarcillin–clavulanate
• Carboplatin	• Ifosfamide	• Methotrexate	• Tobramycin
• Celecoxib	• Indomethacin	• Mitomycin	• Topiramate
• Cidofovir	• Iodixanol	• Nafcillin	• Valacyclovir
• Cisplatin	• Iohexol	• Naproxen	• Valganciclovir
• Cyclosporine	• Iopamidol	• Pamidronate	• Valsartan
• Colistimethate	• Iopromide	• Pentamidine	• Vancomycin
• Deferasirox	• Ioversol	• Piperacillin	• Zoledronic acid
• Diatrizoate meglumine	• Ioxaglate meglumine	• Piperacillin–Tazobactam	• Zonisamide
• Diatrizoate sodium	• Ioxaglate sodium		

Notes: The given medication list is adopted from *NINJA* (*N*ephrotoxic *I*njury *N*egated by *J*ust in time *A*ction) study.[9]
It is advisable to create a unit-specific list based on medications used in the specific hospital.

Investigative Approach in Acute Kidney Injury Evaluation and Cause Identification

The etiology-directed investigative workup is listed in **Table 6**. Individualized investigative workups are required, considering the possibility of the disease process and the clinical presentation. For the dynamic evaluation of kidney function status, some tests such as serum creatinine level, pH, bicarbonate, sodium, and potassium may be monitored frequently.

TABLE 6: Laboratory evaluation of acute kidney injury (AKI).		
Test	***Value/ Inference***	
	Prerenal	***Intrinsic AKI***
Urine-specific gravity	>1.020	<1.010
Urine osmolality	>500 mOsm/kg	<350 mOsm/kg
FENa	<1%	>2%
FEUrea	<35%	>35%
BUN/Cr	>20	<20
Glycosuria	Tubular dysfunction/osmotic diuresis	
Red-colored urine	RBC, myoglobin, free hemoglobin	
Proteinuria	Intrinsic AKI, nephrotic syndrome	
Eosinophils in urine	Drug-induced AIN	

Contd...

Contd...

Test	***Value/ Inference***
WBC, WBC cast in urine	UTI, tubulointerstitial cause
RBC, granular cast	Intrinsic AKI
Blood	
Anemia	Dilutional, hemolytic—SLE, HUS, RVT
Leukopenia	SLE
Thrombocytopenia	SLE, HUS, TMA, TAMOF, RVT, DIC
Coagulopathy	HUS, snake bite
Peripheral smear	Fragmented RBCs
Biochemistry	
BUN, Serum creatinine, pH	Increased and acidosis in AKI
Serum K	>6.5—life threatening
Hyponatremia	Dilutional, SIADH
Hypocalcemia	Secondary to hyperphosphatemia
Creatinine kinase	Increased in TLS
LFT	Abnormal in HRS
Serology	
ANA	SLE
Anti-GBM antibody	Goodpasture's disease
ASO	PSGN or IRGN
C3 level	Low in SLE, PIGN, MPGN
Cultures	Relevant cultures to identify infectious etiology
Imaging studies	
CXR	Cardiomegaly, pulmonary edema
Ultrasound KUB	• Loss of corticomedullary differentiation, increased echogenicity • Obstructive pathology, abscess, collection • Any structural issues related to upper or lower urinary tract
CT/MRI	Renal size, structure, and vascularization

(ADH: antidiuretic hormone; AIN: acute interstitial nephritis; ANA: antinuclear antibody; ASO: antistreptolysin O titer; BUN: blood urea nitrogen; CXR: chest X-ray; DIC: disseminated intravascular coagulation; GBM: glomerular basement membrane; HRS: hepatorenal syndrome; HUS: hemolytic uremic syndrome IRGN: infection-related glomerulonephritis; KUB: kidney ureter and bladder; LFT: liver function test; MPGN: membranoproliferative glomerulonephritis; PIGN: pauci-immune glomerulonephritis; PSGN: poststreptococcal glomerulonephritis; RVT: renal vein thrombosis; SLE: systemic lupus erythematosus; SIADH: syndrome of inappropriate ADH secretion; TAMOF: thrombocytopenia-associated multiple organ failure; TLS: tumor lysis syndrome; TMA: thrombotic microangiopathy; UTI: urinary tract infection)

Identification of Acute Kidney Injury Phenotypes for Therapeutic Decision Making

A unified strategy to determine "phenotypic categories" according to drug exposure, current illness state, and predisposition status **(Fig. 1)** may enable us to better develop care strategies and approach pediatric AKI in a methodical manner. It is also essential to acknowledge that determining a single precise etiology for AKI in critically unwell children may not be possible and would imply an oversimplified approach. Therefore, it is wise to take note of the potential that multiple factors contribute to AKI, as this would aid in the multifaceted management of such children.

Example: Applying this on a child with AKI, we may etiologically categorize them as A, B, C, D, or even A + B, A + C + D, etc. When a child presents to an ICU, etiology may fall into more than one category (quadrant). Primary cause-directed therapy is as important as timely KRT. KRT will be decided based on the stage of AKI + anticipated trajectory of primary disease.

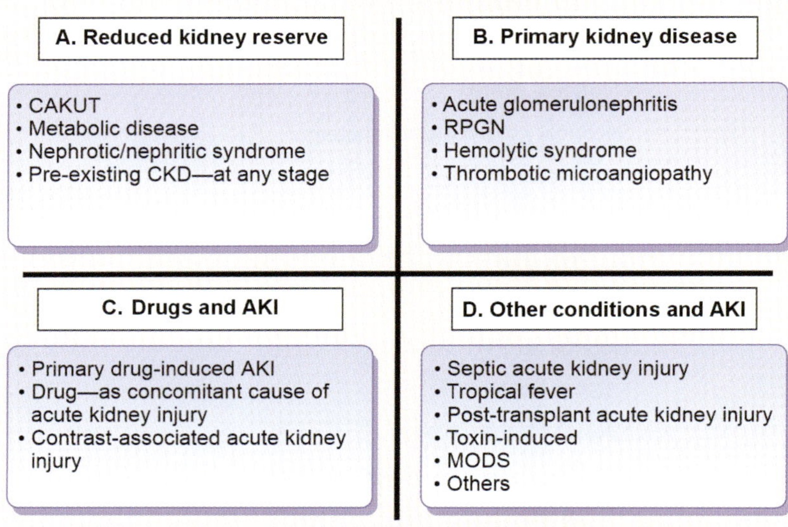

Fig. 1: Schematic diagram depicting therapy-directed AKI grouping in PICU. (AKI: acute kidney injury; CAKUT: congenital anomalies of kidney and urinary tract; CKD: chronic kidney disease; RPGN: rapidly progressive glomerulonephritis; MODS: multiorgan dysfunction syndrome; PICU: pediatric intensive care unit)

Acute Kidney Injury Severity Classification-based on KDIGO-AKI Staging

According to KDIGO 2012 staging, as we previously discussed, all children with AKI must be staged according to severity grade (refer to **Table 2**). It is vital to remember that the severity grading is dynamic and bidirectional with respect to time.

AKI Support Optimization Prior to KRT Initiation

The optimization of pre-KRT therapy converges on several preventive actions in the management of AKI. The careful implementation of preventative interventions is essential in improving the outcome of AKI in critically sick children, particularly in light of the limited access to KRT in low- to middle-income countries (LMIC). KRT outcome can also be improved by good para-KRT medical management of these children.

The following are *steps in the preventive approach* to AKI management:

1. Optimize effective circulatory volume and preload status in the index child.
2. Optimize mean arterial pressure (MAP) to restore renal perfusion—add vasoactive as per need.
3. Correct hemoglobin to optimize oxygen-carrying capacity [use Transfusion and Anemia Expertise Initiative (TAXI) guidelines].
4. Monitor and maintain electrolyte (sodium, calcium, potassium) homeostasis.
5. Remove all nonessential/avoidable nephrotoxic medications (i.e., ionic contrast).
6. Appropriate therapeutic drug dose modification and drug-level monitoring
7. Monitor "other organ function" in parallel and optimize support (i.e., liver, lung, brain).
8. Consider context-specific interventions based on the primary disease.
9. Administer FST only when clinically indicated.
10. Monitor and avoid fluid overload (target FO% <2%—diuretics if needed)
    - In the ICU, precise fluid balance measurement necessitates rigorous hourly intake–output monitoring.
    - Volume of *obligatory fluids* such as drug dilutions, vasoactive infusions, electrolyte adjustments, and blood components need to be accounted appropriately.
    - FO%, a standardized measuring and monitoring tool, was presented in this context as a surrogate for fluid status monitoring.
    - FO% is the percentage of "All Ins in L" minus "All Outs in L" expressed in percentage. If the FO% is >2%, it is time to relook at our fluid prescription.
    - If a critically ill child's FO% creeps up to more than 10% on any given day of their hospital stay, it may be necessary to consider KRT.[10]

Frusemide Stress Test and its Application in Children

The use of the FST in critical care practice is limited. Over the past 20 years, there have been significant changes to the FST approach in oligoanuric AKI in both adults and children.[11] When administering the FST, the following considerations must be made:

- FST response assessment is a "continuous process"; a transient response needs to be differentiated from sustained response.
- "Anticipated disease trajectory" and the index child's "primary disease" will be the basis for administering the FST and evaluating the response.
- The sole goal of frusemide is to increase urine output; renal function is not supposed to be enhanced by it.
- FST can be attempted only in those hyper/euvolemic by clinical assessment and serum albumin level >2 g/dL.

Frusemide Stress Test

Urine output response is assessed after 1 mg/kg frusemide bolus dose OR 0.4 mg/kg frusemide bolus followed by 0.1–0.4 mg/kg/hr infusion of 6–8 hours. Since an infusive dosage may cause a slow response pattern, the assessment duration was also correspondingly extended to 6–8 hours rather than the 2 hours that bolus frusemide administration required. The choice to forego KRT might be more dependent on factors such as FO%, the kind of AKI, the volume of fluids or blood products to be administered over the course of the next 12 hours, etc., even if urine output >1 mL/kg/hr is typically thought of as a response to FST.

Context-specific Interventions-based on the Primary Cause of Acute Kidney Injury

Sepsis and AKI

Apart from KRT and preventive principles-based support therapy, *targeted anti-infective therapy*, *source control* and *other organ function optimization* are of paramount importance in salvaging kidney function.

AKI after Cardiopulmonary Bypass

Acute kidney injury after cardiopulmonary bypass (CPB) is predominantly caused by hemodynamic changes and unfavorable renal perfusion status due to nonpulsatile flow of CPB. Further, systemic inflammatory response syndrome (SIRS) is triggered by surgical trauma, contact with CPB surface, and free hemoglobin. *CPB-related rheological injury can be minimized by modified ultrafiltration methods.*

AKI in Stem Cell Transplant

Acute kidney injury in SCT is usually culmination of multiple factors like prior kidney reserve, chemotherapy exposure, myeloablative medications used for conditioning, large volume of fluids and diluents used in therapy, sinusoidal obstruction syndrome, sepsis, other nephrotoxic medications, etc. A preventive approach may be more ideal in these circumstances; *treating the primary cause of AKI by antibiotics or immunomodulatory medications* may need to be decided simultaneously.

Hemolytic Uremic Syndrome and Thrombotic Microangiopathies

Targeted therapy toward the primary disease—*steroids, immunoglobulin, plasma exchange, KRT* in different combinations—may need to be decided based on primary etiology and disease trajectory assessment. Detailed discussion on hemolytic uremic syndrome (HUS) is beyond the scope of this guideline.

Pigment Nephropathy

Acute kidney injury induced by hemoglobinuria and/or myoglobinuria is classified as "pigmenturia-associated nephropathy". This may be due to myriad of causes like drug induced, traumatic muscle injury, hyperpyrexia, vascular occlusion, intravascular hemolysis, primary muscle disease, carbon monoxide poisoning, and prolonged seizure. Apart from early initiation of KRT, *therapy targeting to stop the process of hemoglobinuria or myoglobinuria* becomes very important in successful renal recovery.

Hepatorenal Syndrome

Hepatorenal syndrome (HRS) is initiated by stress factors such as gastrointestinal bleed, sepsis, paracentesis, or surgical procedure in a patient with pre-existing liver disease. Reduction in GFR occurs because of intense vasoconstriction. *Medication therapy for HRS is to be initiated once it is confirmed.*

Initiation of Appropriate Kidney Replacement Therapy and Other Organ Support Therapies

Indications for KRT in AKI

- Hyperkalemia—K >6.5 mEq/L OR rapidly rising OR refractory to treatment
- Metabolic acidosis—pH <7.15
- BUN >101 mg/dL
- Urine output <0.3 mL/kg/hr for 24 hours OR anuria >12 hours
- Pulmonary edema not responding to diuretics defined by all of the following:
  - 10% Fluid accumulation (FO% >10%)
  - Urine output <0.5 mL/kg/hr for 12 hours
  - Severely impaired oxygenation (P/F <200)

KRT Planning for a Specific Patient

In KRT, it is always recommended to adhere to a charted strategy that consists of targets, assessment techniques, and indications (replacement or supporting indications). Though we think that the cause of AKI influences modality choice, in reality, the "assessment methods" and "Targets" given in **Table 7** and the unit's experience with a specific therapy approach (CKRT vs. PIRRT vs. PD) determine the choice of modality. Since there is no evidence to support one modality over the other, the decision to use blood-based or peritoneal dialysis depends on several factors, including availability, expertise, unit comfort, child size, coagulation requirement, vascular cannulation abilities, required dosage of dialysis, hemodynamic condition of the child, etc.

TABLE 7: KRT planning.

KRT Indications:	*Assessment methods:*
• Hyperkalemia • Acidemia • Pulmonary edema • Uremic complications • Solute control • Fluid removal	• Hemodynamic status and vasoactive support • Primary disease and anticipated pathway • Recent abdominal surgery +/– • Raised intracranial pressure +/– • Active bleeds +/– • Vascular access difficulty +/– • MODS and other organ supports +/– • Weight of the child • FO % at beginning • Need of middle molecule removal • Need of cytokine removal
KST Indications: • Volume control • Drug/blood products delivery • Nutrition delivery • Solute modulation • Other organ support	*Targets:* • UF target in 24 hours • Initial 6 hours strategy [Fluid removal, vasoactive etc.,] • Intracranial pressure at beginning • Anticoagulation possibility and choice

(KRT: kidney replacement therapy; KST: kidney supportive therapy)
Index patient may have more than one indication for KRT/KST, enlisting this will guide us to decide the therapeutic targets in the beginning and weaning plan later.

Timing of KRT Initiation in Pediatric AKI

Early KRT commencement is thought to increase critically ill children's chances of renal recovery. Determining the right timing to start KRT continued to be contentious. Studies on adult KRT that aimed to compare the effectiveness of early versus late or conventional versus accelerated KRT commencement did not demonstrate any therapeutic advantage for early or accelerated initiation. Considering this, developing clinical management guidelines based on information borrowed from adult literature might not be suitable, particularly in the case of AKI as the comorbid illnesses and associated status of CKD in children vary greatly from adults. The primary disease trajectory is currently used to determine the "*accelerated or conventional KRT initiation timeline*" for pediatric AKI, rather than solely kidney function status.

ACUTE KIDNEY INJURY OUTCOME AND PROGNOSIS

Recovery from functional AKI may be dramatic but not in the case of established AKI. Recovery from intrinsic or established AKI may pass through phases of high urine output, poor tubular function, and poor urinary concentration. It is increasingly recognized that children with AKI requiring KRT may need a long-term follow-up even if the creatinine values get normalized at the time of discharge. Extended monitoring is crucial since a child's normal creatinine level does not rule out a partial recovery of AKI.

KEY POINTS

- Special effort to identify 'children with high risk for AKI' may help improving outcome.
- Maintaining adequate effective circulatory volume is vital to maintain renal perfusion.
- Monitoring renal function and FO% in PICU helps in early initiation of support.
- Overzealous fluid therapy leads to fluid overload and worse AKI outcome.
- Avoid nephrotoxic medications to preserve functional kidney status in PICU children.
- Dose modification of medications excreted by kidney and therapeutic drug monitoring of specific medications are helpful while treating children with AKI.
- Time-sensitive initiation of KRT based on disease trajectory is important.

REFERENCES

1. Selewski DT, Cornell TT, Heung M, Troost JP, Ehrmann BJ, Lombel RM, et al. Validation of the KDIGO acute kidney injury criteria in a pediatric critical care population. Intensive Care Med. 2014;40(10):1481-8.
2. Sutherland SM, Byrnes JJ, Kothari M, Longhurst CA, Dutta S, Garcia P, et al. AKI in hospitalized children: comparing the pRIFLE, AKIN, and KDIGO definitions. Clin J Am Soc Nephrol. 2015;10(4):554-61.
3. Sigurjonsdottir VK, Chaturvedi S, Mammen C, Sutherland SM. Paediatric acute kidney injury and subsequent risk of CKD – Is there a harm? Pediatr Nephrol. 2018;33(11):2047-55.
4. Chawla LS, Bellomo R, Bihorac A, Goldstein SL, Siew ED, Bagshaw SM, et al. Acute kidney disease and renal recovery: consensus report of the Acute Disease Quality Initiative (ADQI) 16 Workgroup. Nat Rev Nephrol. 2017;13(4):241-57.
5. Thomas ME, Blaine C, Dawney A, Devonald MAJ, Ftouh S, Laing C, et al. The definition of acute kidney injury and its use in practice. Kidney Int. 2015;87(1):62-73.
6. Palevsky PM, Liu KD, Brophy PD, Chawla LS, Parikh CR, Thakar CV, et al. KDOQI US commentary on the 2012 KDIGO clinical practice guideline for acute kidney injury. Am J Kidney Dis. 2013;61(5):649-72.
7. Mehta P, Sinha A, Sami A, Hari P, Kalaivani M, Gulati A, et al. Incidence of acute kidney injury in hospitalized children. Indian Pediatr. 2012;49:537-42.
8. Abbasi A, Rabori PM, Farajollahi R, Ali KM, Ataei N, Yousefifard M, et al. Discriminatory Precision of Renal Angina Index in Predicting Acute Kidney Injury in Children; a Systematic review and meta-analysis. Arch Acad Emerg Med. 2020;8(1):e39.
9. Goldstein SL, Dahale D, Kirkendall ES, Mottes T, Kaplan H, Muething S et al. A prospective multi-center quality improvement initiative (NINJA) indicates a reduction in nephrotoxic acute kidney injury in hospitalized children Kidney Int. 2020;97(3):580-8.
10. Alobaidi R, Morgan C, Basu RK, Stenson E, Featherstone R, Majumdar SR, et al. Association Between Fluid Balance and Outcomes in Critically Ill Children: A Systematic Review and Meta-analysis. JAMA Pediatr. 2018; 172(3):257-68.
11. Chawla LS, Davison DL, Mitchell EB, Koyner JL, Arthur JM, Shaw AD, et al. Development and standardization of a furosemide stress test to predict the severity of acute kidney injury. Crit Care. 2013;17(5):R207.

Toxicology–I: Environmental Hazards/Bites

35 Chest Injuries

Indumathy Santhanam, Sharada Sathishkumar

INTRODUCTION

The incidence of pediatric chest injuries is 4–8% of all trauma patients. Blunt chest trauma is the most common (85%) mechanism of injury. Penetrating chest injuries are less frequent but more dangerous as they cause organ damage. High mortality (30%) is related to associated injury to other organs. Early recognition and stabilization in the emergency department (ED) improve outcomes in pediatric chest trauma.

TERMINOLOGIES AND DEFINITIONS

- *Blunt thoracic trauma:* Nonpenetrating traumatic injury to the chest wall.
- *Penetrating thoracic trauma:* An injury caused by sharp objects puncturing through the chest wall and damaging the internal organs.
- *Pulmonary contusion:* Bruising of the lung parenchyma secondary to blunt trauma to the chest.
- *Rib fractures:* Fracture of one or more ribs. Significant force is necessary to cause rib fracture.
- *Pneumothorax:* Air leak into the pleural cavity leading to collapse of the lung; open or closed.
- *Open pneumothorax:* Penetrating chest wall trauma causes direct communication between the atmosphere and the pleura resulting in accumulation of air in the pleural cavity.
- *Closed pneumothorax:* Accumulation of air within the pleura due to a communication between the lung parenchyma and bronchi.
- *Hemothorax:* Accumulation of blood in the pleural space.
- *Diaphragm rupture:* Tear in the hemidiaphragm can cause herniation of abdominal organs into the thorax.

- *Flail chest:* Paradoxical movement of the affected segment occurs when three or more adjacent ribs are fractured in at least two different sites
- *Cardiac tamponade:* Accumulation of fluid/blood leading to poor cardiac output and obstructive shock
- *Myocardial contusion:* Focal damage to the myocardium of heart due to blunt cardiac injury resulting in life-threatening arrhythmia and cardiac failure
- *Tracheobronchial injury:* Injury occurring anywhere in the tracheobronchial tree due to penetrating or blunt injury to neck/chest

ETIOPATHOLOGY

- *Blunt thoracic trauma:* Road traffic accidents (runover/hit and run by vehicles), heavy vehicle clashes, bicycle injuries, stampedes. It is usually seen in association with head injury and abdominal injury. Isolated chest trauma occurrence is rare.
- *Penetrating thoracic trauma:* Stab or gunshot, accidental fall over sharp objects, or being gored by animals.

ANATOMIC AND PHYSIOLOGIC CONSIDERATIONS IN CHILDREN

- Children have greater pliability of the ribs than adults. Hence, more kinetic injury is transmitted to the underlying organs. Blunt trauma manifests as abrasion, laceration, and ecchymosis, in addition to respiratory symptoms.
- Lung contusion may occur in the absence of fracture ribs in children.
- The immature cartilaginous bone structure responsible for more compliant chest wall is protective as significant force is needed to cause rib fracture.
- Injury of airway and great vessels is relatively less due to mobility of mediastinum.
- The metabolic demands are high in growing children leading to rapid deterioration.

Emergency Assessment

- Immediately assess the airway, breathing and circulation.
- Identify life-threatening thoracic injury as follows:
  - *Tension pneumothorax:* Severe hypoxia, severe respiratory distress, refractory shock, altered level of consciousness, shift in mediastinum or trachea to the contralateral side, absent or decreased breath sounds bilaterally, hyper-resonance to percussion.
  - *Open pneumothorax:* Secondary to penetrating injury. Negative pressure generated during inspiration leads to preferential influx of air in pleural space if wound is more than two-third diameter of trachea.
  - *Flail chest:* It is rare in children. Clinical features are "paradoxical movement"—the flail segment, respiratory distress, subcutaneous emphysema.
  - *Massive hemothorax:* Rapid and large volume accumulation. There is potential to lose 40% blood volume in each hemithorax. Clinically, it is presented with severe respiratory distress, diminished chest movement, decreased air entry, and dullness on percussion.
  - *Cardiac tamponade:* The origin of blood may be from cardiac chamber, a great vessel, or from the myocardium. The patient may present with severe hypotension, pulsus paradoxus, elevated jugular venous pressure (JVP) in older children, narrow pulse pressure, soft heart sounds, refractory shock, respiratory distress.

Emergency Care

- Interrupt, intervene, and stabilize life-threatening airway, breathing, circulation, and disability (ABCD) issues as depicted in **Flowchart 1**.

Flowchart 1: Emergency care.

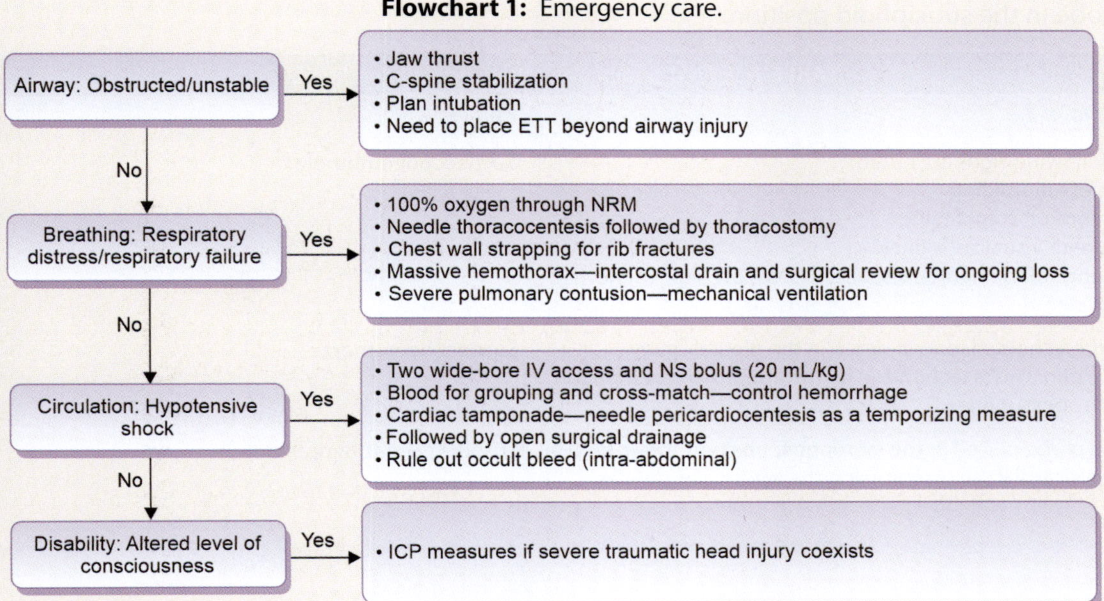

(ETT: endotracheal tube; NRM: nonrebreathing mask; NS: normal saline)

Emergency thoracotomy: It is indicated in a periarrest scenario by a cardiothoracic/pediatric surgeon.

CLINICAL FEATURES

Presentation of thoracic injuries ranges from chest wall injuries (rib fracture, abrasion, ecchymosis, pneumothorax), injury to the lung (contusion and laceration), injury to the heart (myocardial contusion), and injury to the mediastinum (tracheobronchial tree, aorta, esophagus) and the diaphragm. Mortality in a pediatric chest injury is determined by the nature of other associated organ injuries, i.e., polytrauma.

INVESTIGATION

Chest X-ray

Chest X-ray is diagnostic for tension pneumothorax, cardiac tamponade, flail chest, hemothorax, lung contusion, and rib fractures.

Point-of-care Ultrasound (POCUS)

The ultrasound is an additional tool in the evaluation of chest trauma. FAST (Focused Assessment with Sonography in Trauma) is used to identify fluid (blood in the chest). It is also useful to visualize the pericardial, perihepatic, perisplenic, and pelvic space.

Extended FAST helps to look into the anterior and lateral pleural spaces (thoracic view) for pneumothorax or hemothorax **(Table 1)**. The need for pericardiocentesis can be decided by placing the probe in the subxiphoid position.

TABLE 1: E-FAST findings and their relevant condition.

E-FAST findings	*Condition*
If the following signs are noted: • Loss of lung sliding • Absence of "comet tail" • Failure to visualize "A-lines" • Absence of the normal visualized "seashore sign" in the M mode	Suspect pneumothorax
• If hyperechoic shadow is noted in the pleural cavity • *Spine sign:* This is recognized by the abnormal continuation of the spinous line	Suspect hemothorax
• If the probe placed in the subxiphoid position shows fluid in the pericardial sac compressing the ventricular cavities	Suspect cardiac tamponade

Plain CT Scan

This modality is the gold standard for evaluation of blunt trauma chest in a hemodynamically stable child.

Contrast-enhanced CT Scan

This is indicated if penetrating lung injury has occurred. It aids to delineate vascular structures. Add a sentence "The clinical presentation decides the need of specific investigations **(Table 2)**.

TABLE 2: Clinical features and investigations for different types of thoracic trauma.

Type of thoracic trauma	*Clinical Features*	*Investigations*
Chest wall contusion	Palpable chest discomfort	
Pneumothorax	• Breathlessness • Chest pain • Decreased chest wall movement ipsilateral side • Decreased air entry • Ipsilateral hyper-resonance to percussion	• Chest X-ray (CXR) • Ultrasound—absent or diminished pleural movement, absent B lines, presence of lung points. Bar code sign in M mode
Hemothorax	• Diminished breath sounds in the basilar segment • Dullness to percussion • Respiratory distress	• CXR • USG—nearly as sensitive as CT
Lung contusion	• Chest pain • Hypoxia • Respiratory distress • Tachycardia	• CXR—patchy consolidation • Changes evolve over 14–72 hours • CT—more sensitive to detect minor injury
Rib fracture	• Chest wall bruising/abrasion • Breathlessness • Worsening chest wall pain on inspiration • Crepitus and subcutaneous emphysema *Note:* The possibility of nonaccidental trauma must be considered in children presenting with rib fractures	CXR—fracture and consolidation
Cardiac tamponade	• Hypotension • Pulsus paradoxus • Elevated jugular venous pressure (JVP) in older children • Respiratory distress • Narrow pulse pressure • Soft heart sounds • Refractory shock	Ultrasound—point-of-care ultrasound (POCUS
Diaphragm rupture	• Chest and abdominal pain • Increased respiratory effort • Abdominal tenderness • Contusion/abrasion (commonly left sided) • Decreased chest wall movement • Decreased air entry on left with potential for bowel sounds in chest • Mediastinal shift may occur	• CXR—obliteration of diaphragm outline, abdominal contents in hemithorax, tip of nasogastric tube (NGT) in chest • Contrast study—better delineation
Tracheobronchial injury	• Asymptomatic • Respiratory distress • Hemoptysis • Pneumothorax (fails to resolve after tube thoracostomy) • Hemothorax • Pneumomediastinum • Subcutaneous emphysema	Fiberoptic bronchoscopy
Myocardial contusion	• Hypotension • Arrhythmias	Cardiac MRI

SPECIFIC MANAGEMENT

- *Rib fractures:* IV analgesics and transcutaneous analgesic patches are useful intervention to manage pain.
- *Hemothorax:*
  - Intercostal chest drainage (ICD) aids relief of hemothorax.
  - Whole blood/packed red blood cells (PRBC) transfusion is indicated with massive hemothorax.
  - If ICD fails to evacuate within 1 week, surgical exploration and evacuation are warranted.
- *Tension pneumothorax:* Urgent needle thoracocentesis followed by ICD insertion.
- *Lung contusions*:
  - Minor cases require supportive care with supplemental oxygen and fluid restriction.
  - Severe contusions need to be managed with mechanical ventilation.
- *Traumatic pneumatoceles:*
  - Monitor if the pneumatoceles is small.
  - Plan surgical evacuation if the pneumatocele is big or it is causing respiratory compromise.
- *Tracheobronchial injury:* Consider urgent bronchoscopy. If more than one-third of the tracheal diameter is injured, consider surgical management.
- *Aortic rupture:* Widened mediastinum on chest radiograph warrants emergent surgical correction.
- *Diaphragmatic injury:*
  - *Urgent operative repair:* Successful trauma outcomes are dependent on timely identification and intervention by the emergency team. A pediatric surgeon is necessary on arrival. Post stabilization, referral to a higher center is dependent on the specialist availability (cardiothoracic surgeon).

LEARNING POINTS

- Blunt trauma is the most common presentation in pediatric chest trauma.
- Thoracic POCUS/E-FAST is useful to identify thoracic injury when the chest radiograph appears normal.
- Thoracic trauma is managed by a combination of oxygen administration, analgesia, chest drain placement, and IV fluids/blood product transfusion.
- Indications for surgical intervention include massive hemothorax, cardiac tamponade, and aortic and diaphragmatic injuries.

SUGGESTED READING

1. Alemayehu H, Aguayo P. Pediatric Blunt Thoracic Trauma. J Pediatric Intensive Care. 2015;4(1):35-9.
2. ATLS Subcommittee; American College of Surgeons' Committee on Trauma; International ATLS working group. Advanced trauma life support (ATLS®): the ninth edition. J Trauma Acute Care Surg. 2013;74(5): 1363-6.
3. Cooper A. Early assessment and management in trauma. In: Holcomb GW, Murphy JP (Eds). Ashcraft's Pediatric Surgery. Philadelphia, PA: Elsevier; 2008. pp. 167-81.
4. The Royal Children's Hospital Melbourne. Chest injury. [online] Available from https://www.rch.org.au/trauma-service/manual/chest-injury [Last accessed March, 2024].

High-Altitude-Associated Illness

Ashish Simalti, Sheikh Minhaj Ahmed

INTRODUCTION

- High-altitude-related illness (HARI) is a peculiar type of illness that affects people who usually live in lower altitudes but ascend without acclimatization.
- With increase in tourism, it has become common for people to go to high altitudes with children either for religious reasons or for recreational purposes.
- Lack of preparedness and awareness is primary reason for this illness.

TERMINOLOGIES AND DEFINITIONS

High altitude is classified according to the height above sea level. Three categories include:

1. High altitude (1,500–3,500 meters)
2. Very high altitude (3,500–5,500 meters)
3. Extremely high altitude (above 5,500 meters)

Impaired physical performance can be noticed at the height of 2,500 m (8,200 feet) and beyond, but severe HARI occurs above 3,500 m, hence it is very important to acclimatize before climbing these heights.[1]

High-altitude-related illness is of three types:

1. Acute mountain sickness (AMS)
2. High-altitude cerebral edema (HACE)
3. High-altitude pulmonary edema (HAPE)

ETIOPATHOLOGY

As one goes higher, atmospheric pressure reduces, which leads to proportionate fall in partial pressure of oxygen leading to hypoxia, which is the primary cause of HARI. Humidity, cold weather, and increased radiation (ultraviolet) are other factors hypothesized as stressors. From host's point of view, lack of acclimatization is the most important risk factor. With acclimatization, respiratory system, cardiovascular system, and hemoglobin levels change to adapt to new conditions. Other risk factors include history of previous illness related to high altitude suggesting genetic susceptibility. Physical exertion and preexisting viral illness are other common risk factors. AMS is more common among children than adults. AMS is usually self-limiting but HACE and HAPE can be fatal. There seems no gender predilection for AMS, but more severe forms of cerebral and pulmonary edema may be more common among males. Preexisting pulmonary arterial hypertension, coagulopathies, and congenital heart diseases associated with increased pulmonary flow predispose to HARI. Alcohol, barbiturates, and opioids can suppress ventilation and precipitate AMS.[2]

CLINICAL FEATURES

Acute mountain sickness is a self-limiting condition but it can deteriorate into cerebral edema if not managed in time. The Lake Louise questionnaire can be used to diagnose AMS, which uses four symptoms and grades disease severity.[3] These symptoms are (1) headache, (2) gastrointestinal symptoms, (3) fatigue, and (4) dizziness **(Table 1)**. To diagnose AMS, headache must be present and onset should be within days of onset.

TABLE 1: Lake Louise questionnaire for grading acute mountain sickness (AMS).

Symptom	*0*	*1*	*2*	*3*
Headache	None	A mild headache	Moderate headache	Severe headache, incapacitating
Gastrointestinal symptoms	Good appetite	Poor appetite or nausea	Moderate nausea or vomiting	Severe nausea and vomiting, incapacitating
Fatigue and/or weakness	Not tired or weak	Mild fatigue/weakness	Moderate fatigue/ weakness	Severe fatigue/weakness, incapacitating

High-altitude cerebral edema is most severe form of AMS and is life-threatening. Its incidence increases with increasing altitude and usually, it happens after ascent beyond 2,750 m (9,022 ft). Altered sensorium is main presenting feature and ataxia, particularly, truncal ataxia is considered typical of HACE. Clinical findings include retinal hemorrhages, papilledema, cranial nerve palsy, and abnormal reflexes. Focal neurological deficits are not very common. Coma is followed by cerebral herniation leading to death **(Box 1)**.

BOX 1: Signs and symptoms of high-altitude cerebral edema (HACE).

Symptoms of HACE:
- Confusion
- Lethargy
- Ataxia
- Coma

Signs of HACE:
- Truncal ataxia
- Papilledema
- Retinal hemorrhages
- Cranial nerve palsy
- Abnormal reflexes
- Focal neurological deficits

High-altitude pulmonary edema presents with breathing difficulty, chest tightness, and crackles on auscultation. Increased pulmonary arterial pressure secondary to hypoxia-induced pulmonary vasoconstriction leads to pulmonary edema. Onset is with dry cough and reduced effort tolerance, which may be ignored by patient. It usually occurs above 2,440 m (8,000 ft) with rate of progression also depending on physical activity and ambient temperature. Dry cough worsens to pink frothy sputum characteristic of pulmonary edema along with severe breathlessness even at rest. Onset is within first 72 hours, hence if respiratory issues begin after days, other possibilities like pneumonia should be considered. At least two signs and two symptoms are required to make diagnosis of HAPE **(Box 2)**.

BOX 2: Signs and symptoms of high-altitude pulmonary edema (HAPE).

Symptoms of HAPE:
- Dyspnea
- Cough
- Asthenia
- Reduced physical performance
- Chest tightness
- Congestion

Signs of HAPE:
- Crackles
- Whistles
- Tachypnea
- Tachycardia

EVALUATION

Evaluation of a child should follow pediatric advanced life support (PALS) guidelines, which is primary assessment focusing on airway, breathing, circulation, disability, and exposure followed by detailed inquiry of signs and symptoms. Respiratory distress and neurological status are the most common areas needing intervention for HARI. Diagnosing HARI is usually straightforward based on history. Most important risk factor is lack of acclimatization. Onset of AMS, HACE, and HAPE is within 72 hours of arriving at high altitude. **Table 1** and **Boxes 1 and 2** provide clinical features for evaluation of HARI.[4]

Algorithm for evaluation of a child with suspected HARI is given in **Flowchart 1**.

Flowchart 1: Evaluation of a child with suspected high-altitude-related illness.

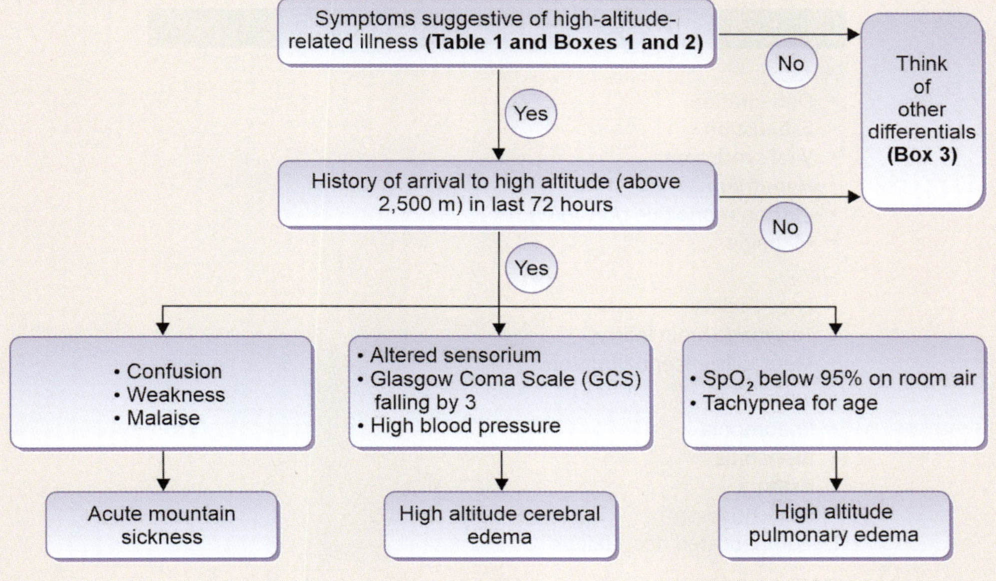

DIFFERENTIALS

It is very important not to miss other critical conditions with presentations similar to HACE or HAPE. Most important differentiating feature is timing of onset. The onset of HARI is usually within 72 hours of arriving at high altitude. So, if symptoms appear after 3 days, other possibilities should be kept in mind. Common complaints that can be confused with AMS include dehydration, exhaustion, viral syndrome, hypothermia, carbon monoxide poisoning, and migraine. In case of adolescents, one must keep in mind issues like alcohol hangover, substance abuse, or caffeine withdrawal. Meningoencephalitis may also initially present as AMS but can be differentiated with clinical examination. HACE should be differentiated from other causes of raised intracranial pressure (ICP) like encephalitis, traumatic brain injury, and metabolic encephalopathies. HAPE should be differentiated from other causes of respiratory distress like pneumonia, bronchitis, asthma, bronchospasm, and cardiac conditions like decompensated heart failure **(Box 3)**.

BOX 3: Differential diagnoses for HARI.

AMS:
- Dehydration
- Exhaustion
- Viral syndrome
- Hypothermia
- Carbon monoxide poisoning
- Migraine

HACE:
- Encephalitis
- Traumatic brain injury
- Metabolic encephalopathies

HAPE:
- Pneumonia
- Bronchitis
- Asthma
- Bronchospasm

Decompensated heart failure

(AMS: acute mountain sickness; HACE: high-altitude cerebral edema; HAPE: high-altitude pulmonary edema)

EMERGENCY CARE

Management of HARI depends on severity of illness. For mild AMS, only bedrest, nonsteroidal anti-inflammatory drugs (NSAIDs), and antiemetics are sufficient. For more severe cases, the first priority should be to shift patients to lower altitudes (rapid descent) while monitoring vital parameters on the way. Treatment includes oxygen therapy, descent to lower altitudes, and if patient is unstable, measures to reduce cerebral or pulmonary edema. Hyperbaric oxygen chambers, if available, should be used to reduce cerebral blood flow by causing cerebral vasoconstriction and reduce pulmonary hypertension by causing pulmonary vasodilatation. For most cases of HACE, treatment focuses on reducing cerebral edema by bedrest, keeping head elevated at 30° and in the midline while preparing for shifting patient to lower altitudes. For HAPE, primary treatment consists of reliving respiratory distress for which oxygen therapy is primary mode. If available, oxygen can be given through high-flow or pressure-generating devices like heated humidified high-flow nasal cannula (HHHFNC), bilevel positive airway pressure (biPAP), or continuous positive airway pressure (CPAP).

Algorithm for emergency care in cases with HARI is given in **Flowchart 2**.

Flowchart 2: Emergency care in cases with high-altitude-related-illness.

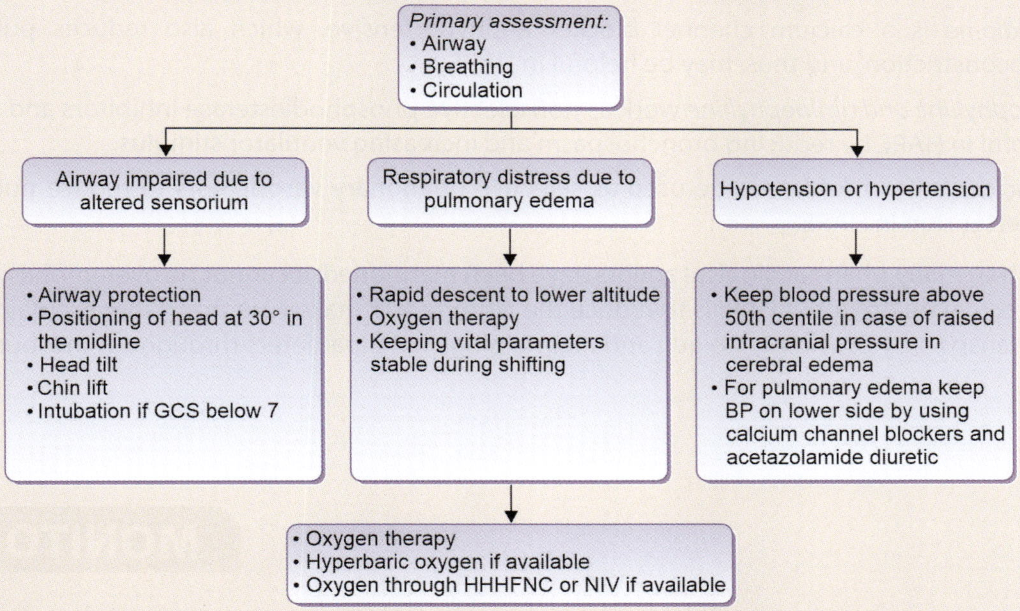

Primary assessment:
- Airway
- Breathing
- Circulation

→ **Airway impaired due to altered sensorium**
- Airway protection
- Positioning of head at 30° in the midline
- Head tilt
- Chin lift
- Intubation if GCS below 7

→ **Respiratory distress due to pulmonary edema**
- Rapid descent to lower altitude
- Oxygen therapy
- Keeping vital parameters stable during shifting

→ **Hypotension or hypertension**
- Keep blood pressure above 50th centile in case of raised intracranial pressure in cerebral edema
- For pulmonary edema keep BP on lower side by using calcium channel blockers and acetazolamide diuretic

→
- Oxygen therapy
- Hyperbaric oxygen if available
- Oxygen through HHHFNC or NIV if available

(BP: blood pressure; GCS: Glasgow Coma Scale; HHHFNC: heated humidified high-flow nasal cannula; NIV: noninvasive ventilation)

SPECIFIC MANAGEMENT

Besides shifting patient to lower altitude and oxygen therapy, there are few therapeutic agents that can be used for HACE and HAPE. These drugs have only supportive role in the management of HARI:

- *Acetazolamide* acts on proximal tubules of kidneys by inhibiting carbonic anhydrase. It leads to diuresis by excretion of carbonic acid and metabolic acidosis. Acetazolamide has prophylactic role as it reduces cerebral fluid formation and also causes pulmonary vasodilatation.[5]
- *Corticosteroids* have a role in preventing edema by reducing endothelial damage and thus, cerebral and pulmonary edema. One steroid, medroxyprogesterone, also acts as ventilator stimulant.
- *NSAIDs* like aspirin, paracetamol, and ibuprofen also reduce cerebral vascular permeability by inhibiting prostaglandin synthesis.
- *Sumatriptan* is a selective 5-hydroxytryptamine receptor inhibitor and is used for migraine. It has selective cerebral vasoconstrictor property and also reduced cerebral vascular permeability.
- *Gabapentin* is an anticonvulsant, which also has analgesic property and can be used in AMS and HACE.
- *Nifedipine* is a calcium channel blocker antihypertensive, which also reduces pulmonary vasoconstriction, and thus, may be helpful in HAPE.
- *Theophylline and aminophylline* work as nonselective phosphodiesterase inhibitors and they are helpful in HAPE by reducing bronchospasm and increasing ventilator stimulus.
- *Nitric oxide* if available can be used as selective pulmonary vasodilators to reduce pulmonary hypertension in HAPE.

Although so many pharmacological agents have been mentioned, it cannot be overemphasized that most effective treatment of HARI is to reduce the altitude and make sure that patient remains stable during transport by providing oxygen and maintaining vital parameters throughout the journey.

MONITORING

Monitoring would include monitoring vital parameters and sensorium. In cases of HACE, worsening sensorium would suggest increasing ICP, which if unabated, may lead to herniation and death. For HAPE, respiratory rate and oxygen saturation are the two main parameters of concern. Temperature monitoring is also important as hypothermia worsens HARI and fever also should be avoided.

PREVENTION

High-altitude-related illness is preventable by acclimatization. It is recommended that ascent should not be faster than 600 m in a day and there should be 1 day of rest for altitude gain of 600–1,200 m. If there is past history of HARI, ascent should be even slower at 300 m/day. Acetazolamide can be taken prophylactically 2 days prior to ascent and should be continued 2 days after reaching maximum height. One must know that physical fitness does not protect against HARI and exercise may even precipitate this.

KEY LEARNING POINTS

- HARI is a group of disorders related to rapid ascent to high altitude and includes three distinct disease entities—AMS, HACE, and HAPE.
- Environmental hypoxia is primary etiology, which leads to inappropriate cerebral vasodilatation and pulmonary vasoconstriction leading to HACE and HAPE, respectively.
- HARI is a preventable disease by ensuring that ascent to high altitude is slow and individual takes adequate rest during altitude gain.
- Physical fitness does not protect against HARI and exercise may even precipitate this.
- AMS can be confused with viral fever, general weakness, and hangover.
- HACE is associated with raised ICP and can be fatal.
- HAPE is pulmonary edema without cardiac dysfunction. It is the most common cause of death among HARI.
- Rapid descent and oxygen therapy are two most effective modalities of management for HAPE and HACE.
- Hyperbaric oxygen if available should be given as hypoxia is the primary culprit.
- Acetazolamide can be used as prophylaxis at least 2 days prior to onset of ascent. Other pharmacological agents have only adjuvant role.

REFERENCES

1. Savioli G, Ceresa IF, Gori G, Fumoso F, Gri N, Floris V, et al. Pathophysiology and therapy of high-altitude sickness: Practical approach in emergency and critical care. J Clin Med. 2022;11(14):3937.
2. Richalet JPS, Lhuissier FJ. Aging, tolerance to high altitude, and cardiorespiratory response to hypoxia. High Alt Med Biol. 2015;16:117-24.
3. Roach RC, Hackett PH, Oelz O, Bärtsch P, Luks AM, MacInnis MJ, et al.; Lake Louise AMS Score Consensus Committee. The 2018 Lake Louise acute mountain sickness score. High Alt Med Biol 2018;19(1):4-6.
4. Roeggla G, Roeggla M, Podolsky A, Wagner A, Laggner AN. How can acute mountain sickness be quantified at moderate altitude? J R Soc Med. 1996:89;141-3
5. Wright A, Brearey S, Imray C. High hopes at high altitudes: Pharmacotherapy for acute mountain sickness and high-altitude cerebral and pulmonary oedema. Expert Opin. Pharmacother. 2008;9:119-27.

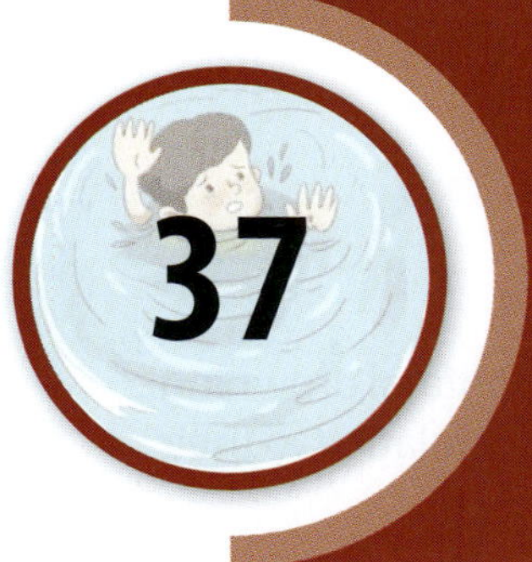

Drowning and Submersion Injuries

Arun Bansal

INCIDENCE

The World Health Organization (WHO) reports that drowning is a preventable public health issue, claiming about 40 lives every hour throughout the day. Over 90% of these deaths occur in low- and middle-income countries, making it the third most significant cause of unintentional injuries worldwide.[1] International data significantly underestimates drowning mortality rates in high-income nations, while survey data from low- and middle-income countries suggests rates four to five times the WHO calculated rate.[1]

DEFINITION

Drowning is the process of experiencing respiratory impairment from submersion or immersion in liquid.[2] If there is no breathing impairment, this is a rescue rather than a drowning.

TYPES

Nonfatal drowning occurs when the victim is rescued at any juncture, thereby interrupting the progression of the drowning process.

Fatal drowning: Losing the victim at any moment constitutes a fatal drowning.

The usage of phrases such as "dry or wet drowning," "near-drowning," and "secondary drowning" is incorrect. The Utstein template is a standardized method for documenting data about drowning resuscitation cases.[3]

Nonfatal Drowning Categorization Framework

The WHO has classified the severity of respiratory impairment and morbidity in nonfatal drowning as given in **Table 1**. Morbidity is a reduction in the individual's functional capacity relative to their predrowning state.

TABLE 1: Nonfatal drowning categorization framework (NDCF).

The severity of respiratory impairment after the drowning process stopped		
Mild impairment	Moderate impairment	Severe impairment
• Breathing • Involuntary distressed coughing[a] And • Fully alert	• Difficulty breathing And • Disoriented but conscious	• Not breathing And • Unconscious
Morbidity category (based on any decline from previous functional capacity[b]) at the time of measurement		
A. No morbidity	B. Some morbidity	C. Severe morbidity
No decline	Some decline	Severe decline

[a]*Involuntary distressed coughing:* Coughing up liquid/moving liquid out of the airway; in water, in distress and coughing; sustained coughing.

[b]*Previous functional capacity:* It includes the person's cognitive, motor, and psychological capacity.

PATHOPHYSIOLOGY

Aspirating water into the airways causes coughing as a reflex response. Less than 2% of cases may exhibit laryngospasm, which is immediately terminated by the onset of hypoxia. Continuing aspiration of water can cause hypoxemia, leading to loss of consciousness and apnea within seconds to minutes if not rescued. Hypoxic cardiac arrest typically follows bradycardia and pulseless electrical activity, not ventricular fibrillation or tachycardia.

Water in alveoli destroys and washes out surfactant, leading to acute lung injury. It also disrupts alveolar–capillary membrane integrity, increases permeability, and worsens fluid, plasma, and electrolyte changes. A clinical picture of localized or widespread pulmonary edema is manifested, affecting the alveolar exchange of oxygen and carbon dioxide. Water aspiration of 1–3 mL/kg can significantly disrupt pulmonary gas exchange and reduce compliance by 10–40%. Lung fluid, surfactant loss, and increased capillary–alveolar permeability can cause reduced compliance, increased right-to-left shunting, atelectasis, and alveolitis, leading to noncardiogenic pulmonary edema.

MANAGEMENT IN THE EMERGENCY ROOM

The key to successful resuscitation of a drowning patient is effective rewarming and following advanced life support (ALS) guidelines with correction of hypoxemia and acidosis. The detailed management in ER is as per **Table 2**.

TABLE 2: Management of a child with drowning.

Basic management	• Careful history and examination • Continuous vital sign monitoring • Record temperature • C-spine stabilization • Dry the chest before using defibrillator • Look for any external or internal injury	*Passive rewarming:* • Remove wet clothes • Dry the patient • Warm blanket • Warm environment	*Active rewarming (if core temperature <30°C):* • Warm IV fluids (39°C) • Warm saline (42°C) gastric or bladder lavage
Child is conscious with no respiratory distress	Basic management	Consider ECG	Discharge with safety advise
Child is conscious with respiratory distress	• Basic management • Oxygen • Ventilatory support (invasive or noninvasive) • IV fluid (warm) • Rewarming (active or passive as per need) • Hemodynamic support (as per need)	• CXR • ECG • CBC • LFT • Electrolytes • Blood gas	Needs admission in ER/ Ward/PICU
Child is unconscious or having cardiac arrest	• Intubate and ventilate • Nasogastric tube • IV/ IO access • Treat shock with fluids • IV fluid (warm) • Rewarming (active and passive)	• CXR • ECG • CBC • LFT • Electrolytes • Blood gas • Blood glucose • Consider CT head	Shift to PICU

(CBC: complete blood count; CXR: chest X-ray; ER: emergency room; ECG: electrocardiogram; IO: intraosseus; IV: intravenous; LFT: liver function test; PICU: pediatric intensive care unit)

Ventilation

- In a conscious child with no distress, low-flow oxygen through a nasal cannula or face mask may be sufficient.

- A child with distress may require high-flow nasal cannula (HFNC) or noninvasive ventilation (NIV) support.
- An unconscious child will need intubation and mechanical ventilation:
  - Lung protective ventilation strategy
  - Low tidal volume
  - High positive end-expiratory pressure (PEEP) may be required.

Fluids

- If shock is present, give IV saline at 10 mL/kg.
- Continuous hemodynamic monitoring
- Use echocardiography to monitor fluids and inotropes as early myocardial dysfunction is known in hypothermia.

Correction of Metabolic and Electrolyte Abnormalities

- Correction of hypoxemia and fluid status will improve acidosis.
- There is no benefit of using sodium bicarbonate to correct acidosis.
- Monitor electrolytes and correct any electrolyte disturbances.

Antibiotics

Routine use of prophylactic antibiotics is not recommended.

Steroids

Routine use of steroids is not recommended.

Surfactant

There is no evidence to support the use of surfactant.

Correction of Hypothermia

Gradual rewarming is essential. The aim is to raise body temperature by 0.5°C/h till a target of 35°C is reached.

Changes in ALS Guidelines in Hypothermia

- If the core temperature is <30°C
    - Defibrillation is less effective in hypothermic myocardium. Limit the number of defibrillation shocks to less than three shocks.
    - Do not use inotropes or antiarrhythmic agents, as they may precipitate arrhythmias.
- If the core temperature is 30–35°C
    - Double the dose interval of inotropic or antiarrhythmic drugs (e.g., epinephrine or norepinephrine)

Associated Injuries

Complete physical examination and skeletal survey are important poststabilization.

Extracorporeal Membrane Oxygenation (ECMO)

It is helpful in cases of severe hypothermia and cardiac arrest. If facilities are available, early ECMO should be initiated.

PROGNOSIS

Children who are conscious when they arrive at the emergency room (ER) have a very excellent prognosis. It is difficult to determine the prognosis in unconscious children. Evidence suggests that children who are submerged for <6 minutes have a better outcome than those who are submerged for >25 minutes.

DISCHARGE AND DISPOSITION

Normal and conscious children with no distress can be discharged after an observation period of 8 hours. A child requiring ventilatory or hemodynamic support will need further care and monitoring and need to be shifted to an intensive care unit (ICU).

REFERENCES

1. Bloomberg LP, World Health Organization, (Eds.). Global Report on Drowning: Preventing a Leading Killer. Geneva: World Health Organization; 2014.
2. van Beeck EF, Branche CM, Szpilman D, Modell JH, Bierens JJLM. A new definition of drowning: towards documentation and prevention of a global public health problem. Bull World Health Organ. 2005;83(11):853-6.
3. Idris AH, Bierens JJLM, Perkins GD, Wenzel V, Nadkarni V, Morley P, et al. 2015 Revised Utstein-style recommended guidelines for uniform reporting of data from drowning-related resuscitation: an ILCOR Advisory Statement. Circ Cardiovasc Qual Outcomes. 2017;10(7):e000024.

38 Snake Envenomation

Gomathy Srividya V, Thangavelu S

INTRODUCTION

Snake envenomation is a preventable cause of death in children in rural and forest areas. With the availability of antisnake venom (ASV) and intensive care support, survival has improved. About 300 species of snakes exist in India, among which the big four—common krait (*Bungarus caeruleus*), Indian cobra (*Naja naja*), saw-scaled viper (*Echis carinatus*), and Russell's viper (*Daboia russelii*)—are the common snakes in India. They are responsible for 95% of snakebite deaths. It is estimated that India had 1.2 million snakebite deaths (average 58,000/year) from 2000 to 2019.[1]

ETIOPATHOGENESIS

The complex mixture of enzymes and proteins present in snake venom leads to complications as mentioned in **Table 1**.

TABLE 1: Clinical manifestation of different envenomations.[2]

Features	*Cobra*	*Krait*	*Russell's viper*	*Saw-scaled viper*	*Hump-nosed viper*
Local pain/tissue damage	Yes	No	Yes	Yes	Yes
Ptosis/neurological signs	Yes	Yes	Yes*	No	No
Hemostatic abnormalities	No	No	Yes	Yes	Yes
Renal complications	No	No	Yes	No	Yes
Response to neostigmine	Yes	No	No	No	No

*South Indian and Sri Lankan Russell's Viper.

Note: Usually, the clinical features of envenomation will evolve over 24 hours and rarely up to 36 hours.

EVALUATION

History

The questions given in **Box 1** will help to bring out key information in the history.[3]

BOX 1: Important questions for history taking.

- What is the site of the bite? Any fang marks visible? Bite felt, snake witnessed? Painful or painless? (krait bite may be painless or felt as a thorn prick)
- Any bleeding tendency? (viper)
- Is there any difficulty in breathing, dysphagia, double vision, drooping of eyelids, inability to stand up or walk, seizures, head lag, and/or perioral numbness? (krait or cobra)
- Are there any anxiety, fear, sweating, and emotional disturbances? (difficult to differentiate from envenomation)
- Are there any early features of envenomation such as nausea, vomiting, abdominal pain?
- Is any first aid such as alcohol or tourniquet given?
- When was the last voiding of urine? What was the color?
- Krait bites are known to occur at night without pain or fang marks, and sometimes pediatricians will consider the possibility of envenomation based on clinical findings and decide to start antisnake venom (ASV)

Examination

- Initial IAP advanced life support (ALS) guidelines based examination is essential to plan the resuscitation **(Fig. 1)**.

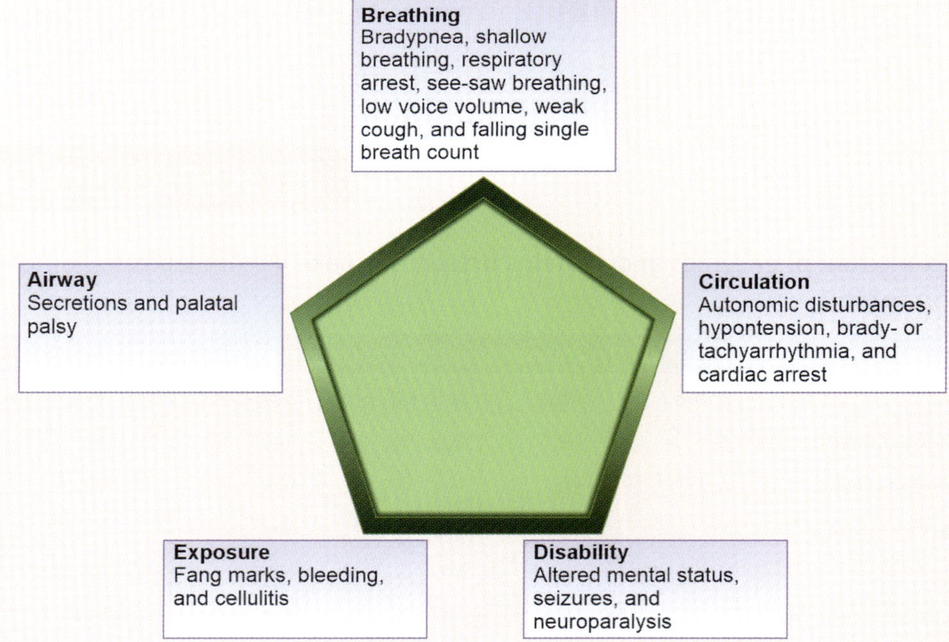

Fig. 1: Initial IAP ALS (Indian Academy of Pediatrics-advanced life support) based assessment.

- A focused examination will be helpful, which is listed in **Box 2**.

BOX 2: Focused examination.

Signs may evolve over time and hence need repeated examination:

- Fang marks, seen as two puncture wounds or two parallel short lines. In krait bite, fang marks may not be easily detectable with no necrosis or pain and may be felt as a thorn prick **(Fig. 2A)**
- Local cellulitis such as erythema, swelling, blistering, ecchymosis, persistent oozing of blood from the bite site, compartment syndrome, gangrene in delayed presentation, and tender regional lymph node enlargement (in viper bite) **(Figs. 2B and C)**
- Measurement of limb circumference and marking the limit of swelling will be useful to track the trend of worsening which can occur even in a few hours
- Muscle tenderness, weakness, and dark urine may suggest the diagnosis of rhabdomyolysis
- Acute compartment syndrome should be suspected based on the presence of 5Ps (pain on passive stretching, paresthesia, pulselessness, pallor, and paralysis)
- *Neuroparalytic manifestations **(Fig. 2D)**:* Six Ds (diplopia, dilated pupils, dysarthria, dysphonia, dyspnea, and dysphagia) and two Ps (ptosis and paralysis of limbs and respiratory muscle) may be observed

  In addition, loss of extraocular movements, palatal weakness, pooling of secretions, and drooping of jaws may be present. Dilated nonreactive pupil with complete weakness of limbs can be a presentation mimicking brain death (krait and cobra)
- *Locked-in syndrome:* Dilated pupils, quadriplegia, and anarthria may mimic brain death even though there is consciousness. Vertical eye movements are retained and are a way to identify nonverbal communication

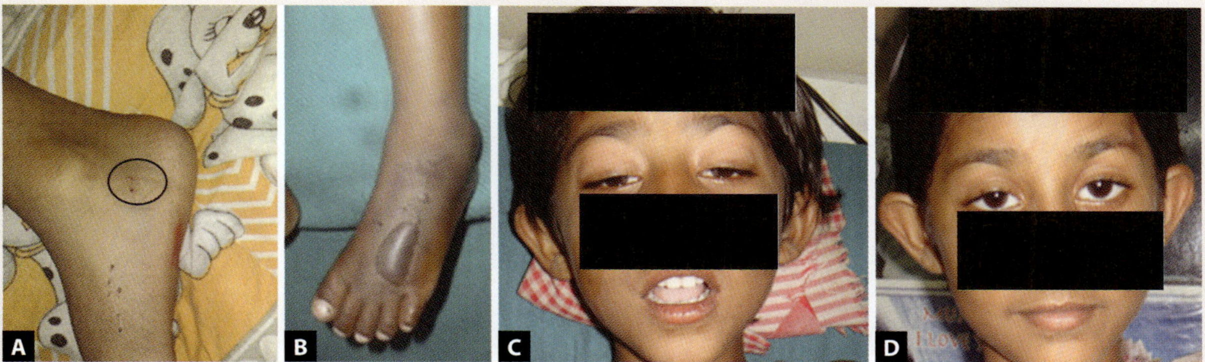

Figs. 2A to D: (A) Fang marks; (B) Blister formation; (C) Drooping of eyes and jaw; (D) Drooping resolved after antisnake venom (ASV).

Courtesy: Dr Balaji, Associate Professor, Government Dharmapuri Medical College, Tamil Nadu, and Dr S Thangavelu.

LABORATORY INVESTIGATIONS

- *20-minute whole blood clotting test (20WBCT):* It is a useful bedside screening test indicating failure of the blood to clot in a clean glass tube after 20 minutes. Prolonged 20WBCT is an indication for ASV, but a negative result cannot rule out the need when other clinical findings of coagulopathy are present.

  Procedure:[5] 2 mL of freshly sampled venous blood is placed in a small, new, dry glass test tube. The test tube should be left undisturbed for 20 minutes at ambient temperature and tilted after 20 minutes. Do not use unclean or coated test tube, injection vials, or detergent-cleaned tubes. If the blood is still liquid (unclotted) and runs out at the end of 20 minutes, it is considered as prolonged because of venom-induced consumption coagulopathy **(Figs. 3A to C)**. Prolonged 20WBCT warrants ASV therapy. If the test is negative in suspected envenomation, it should be repeated hourly for the first 3 hours and then 6 hourly for 24 hours.
- *Further coagulation workup (if available):* Prothrombin time (PT), activated partial thromboplastin time (aPTT), international normalized ratio (INR), platelet count, fibrin degradation products (FDP), D-dimer, complete blood count (CBC), peripheral smear, reticulocyte count, lactate dehydrogenase (LDH), and serum creatinine
- *Tests for rhabdomyolysis:* Rapid urine dipstick for blood and/or myoglobin, red blood cells (RBCs), serum creatine kinase, electrolytes, calcium, phosphate, uric acid, blood urea nitrogen, and creatinine
- *Tests for renal involvement:* Raised creatinine, hyperkalemia, hyperphosphatemia, hyperuricemia, and hypocalcemia
- *ECG: To identify hyperkalemia and cardiac arrhythmias*

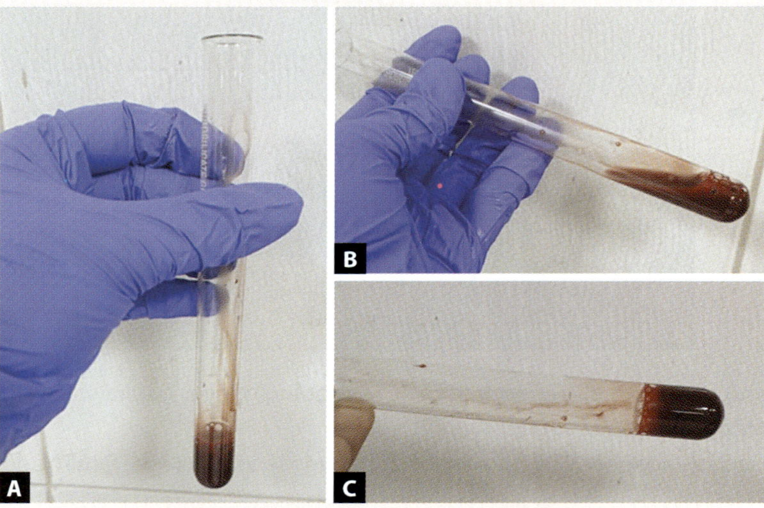

Figs. 3A to C: 20WBCT. (A) Sample collected; (B) Tilting after 20 minutes—blood not clotted; (C) Blood clotted. (20WBCT: 20-minute whole blood clotting test)
Courtesy: Dr Gomathy Srividya V.

DIFFERENTIAL DIAGNOSIS

In any child with an unknown bite, snakebite should be considered if signs of envenomation are present with or without bite mark. Rarely, scorpion sting may be confused with snakebite. But the presence of fang marks, local necrosis, bleeding tendency, and neurotoxicity will strongly favor the snakebite.

MANAGEMENT

Prehospital First Aid[6] (Do it RIGHT)

- **R:** Reassure the patient as 70% of all snakebites are nonvenomous, and only 50% of bites by venomous species envenomate.
- **I:** Immobilize the limb in the same way as a fractured limb **(Fig. 4)**. (Use bandages or cloth to hold the splints; do not block the blood supply or apply pressure. Do not apply any compression in the form of tight ligatures as they do not work and can be dangerous. Do not encourage walking.)
- **GH:** Get to hospital immediately. Traditional remedies have no proven benefit.
- **T:** Tell the doctor of any systemic symptoms such as ptosis.

Incision, suction, electric shock, cryotherapy, and washing the wound are contraindicated.

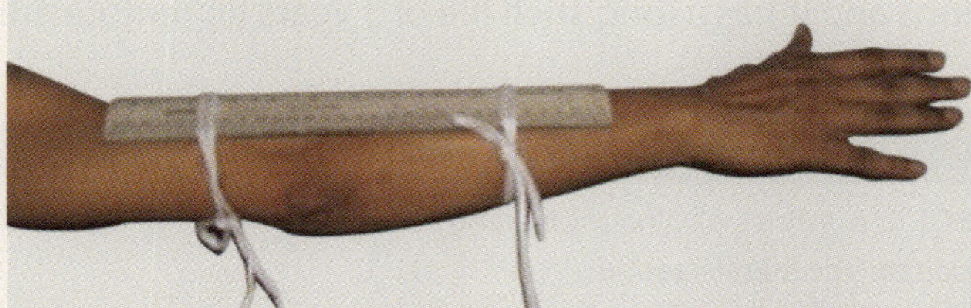

Fig. 4: Limb immobilization.
Source: Standard Treatment Guidelines (2016).

Resuscitation

When the child is received in the emergency department (ED), the objective of the management is to resuscitate the child.[7]

- If the child is received late in cardiac arrest, cardiopulmonary resuscitation (CPR) should be started without any delay. Snake envenomation is one of the reasons for prolonging the duration of CPR beyond 20–30 minutes.

- *Airway stabilization:* The presence of palatal weakness, weak cough reflex, inability to clear the secretions, and poor respiratory effort warrant intubation and ventilatory support. Ketamine is used for analgesia, with atropine premedication, to reduce the secretions. Muscle relaxants should be avoided, and the intubation procedure should be gentle as bleeding can occur.
- *Shock:* It should be managed with crystalloids, vasoactive agents, and blood transfusion (if the shock is due to blood loss).
- In a comatose child, check and treat for common causes like hypoglycemia.
- *Imaging:* It may be needed after stabilization to recognize trauma or bleeding. Snake venom can cause pupillary dilatation; hence the patient should not be considered as brain dead.
- If a child is referred with pressure immobilization, he/she should be released only after stabilization and ASV administration. Massive release of the venom may lead to life-threatening complications including cardiac arrest.

SPECIFIC MANAGEMENT

Indian ASV is polyvalent against all the four (big four) common snakes causing envenomation. It is available as 10-mL vials, liquid and lyophilized forms, requiring reconstitution. For liquid ASV, a reliable cold chain is needed and its shelf life is short (2 years). But lyophilized ASV requires to be kept only under cool conditions and it has a long shelf life of 5 years (in remote areas). Indications for ASV are given in **Box 3**.

BOX 3: Indications for ASV.[8]

- Prolonged 20WBCT or presence of clinical bleeding
- Evidence of neuroparalytic manifestations
- Local symptoms such as rapidly progressive swelling across a joint or local tissue necrosis in the absence of a tourniquet. When a tourniquet is applied, if the swelling persists for 1 hour after removal of the tourniquet, it should be attributed to venom

Shock in the presence of snake envenomation

Antisnake Venom Doses and Administration[7,8]

- The initial dose is 10 vials. The lyophilized preparation is dissolved in the diluent given, which is further diluted in 5–10 mL/kg body weight (BW) by normal saline and administered as intravenous (IV) infusion for over 30–60 minutes at a constant rate with careful monitoring, with the physician sitting at the bedside during the initial period. ASV test dose is not indicated. ASV must never be given by the intramuscular (IM) or subcutaneous route. Administration of ASV can lead to anaphylaxis and has to be monitored throughout infusion.

- *Signs of response to ASV:* Cessation of bleeding, clotting observed in 20WBCT, improvement in ptosis, eye, or limb movements. Local swelling may take some time to improve.
- *Repeat dose of ASV:* In hemotoxic envenomation, repeat dose is given 6 hours after the first dose if bleeding persists or 20WBCT remains abnormal. In neurotoxic envenomation, if paralysis persists 1 hour after the first dose of ASV and neostigmine therapy, repeat another 10 vials. The maximum dose is 20 vials, but in viper bites, it can be up to 30 vials, if needed.

If a child is received in a peripheral center with serious signs of envenomation, he/she can be referred to a tertiary care hospital where mechanical ventilator and dialysis facilities are available after stabilization of airway, breathing, and circulation (ABC) and completion of ASV.

No ASV is needed for sea snakebite or pit viper bite (provided they are identified correctly) as the currently available ASV does not contain antibodies against them. Management of snake envenomation and related complications, in addition to ASV, is given in **Table 2**.

TABLE 2: Management of envenomation and related complications, in addition to antisnake venom (ASV).[10,11]

Problem	*Management*
ASV anaphylaxis (sudden dry cough, dyspnea, fall of BP, shock, swelling of face, and conjunctiva)	• Close bedside monitoring and keeping adrenaline loaded in the syringe • When signs of reaction are noted, stop ASV. Adrenaline 0.01 mg/kg IM (deltoid or thigh) followed by antihistamine IM and hydrocortisone/dexamethasone IV, O_2, NS bolus, if needed • Once there are signs of recovery, ASV is restarted at a slower rate and gradually increased to the usual rate, under close monitoring
Neuroparalytic envenomation (krait and cobra)	• In the presence of shallow breathing, priority is intubation or LMA insertion and ventilation • In all cases of neuroparalytic envenomation, a trial of AN therapy is warranted following ASV – Injection of atropine 0.5 mg/kg followed by injection of neostigmine 0.04 mg /kg as initial dose – Repeat doses, atropine 0.05 mg/kg and neostigmine 0.01 mg/kg to be given every 30 minutes in five doses and stop after three doses, if no response is seen – Bradycardia and excessive secretions are managed with suction • Response to neostigmine will be seen in envenomation with postsynaptic block as in cobra bites. Positive response to "AN" trial is measured as 50% or more recovery of the ptosis in 1 hour • If there is no improvement after three doses of AN trial, this indicates probable krait bite, which affects presynaptic fibers where calcium ion acts as a neurotransmitter. Hence, inj. calcium gluconate 1–2 mL/kg to a maximum of 10 mL (1:1 dilution) slowly over 20 minutes every 6 hourly is given and continued till neuroparalysis recovers.[3]
Hemotoxic envenomation	• After 6 hours, if 20WBCT is abnormal or bleeding persists, a second dose of ASV, further 10 vials, can be given (time taken for the liver to regenerate clotting factors). If normal, ASV need not be repeated. Blood products are considered only after completion of ASV therapy. The maximum dose is 30 vials
Acute kidney injury (AKI) (Russell's Viper) caused by hemolysis, direct toxicity, hypotension, and rhabdomyolysis	• Serial monitoring of BP, urine output, urea, creatinine, and electrolytes • Control of hypertension, fluid management, and referral to higher centers • Appropriate ASV therapy, giving blood products after ASV to correct coagulopathy, is safer before dialysis catheter insertion • *RRT:* PD or HD

...Contd.

Contd...

Problem	*Management*
Compartment syndrome (viper and sometimes in cobra bite)	• Suspected in the presence of 5 Ps with significant swelling in limb: Pain on passive stretching, paresthesia, pulselessness, pallor, and paralysis • Swelling due to tourniquet can be differentiated by improvement after removal • Doppler studies to study distal flow and intracompartmental pressure measurement are useful • Fasciotomy after completion of ASV and correction of coagulopathy unless there is an impending vascular compromise
Venom-induced consumption coagulopathy (VICC)	• It is due to procoagulant toxins present in the snake venom. Coagulopathy appears within hours and usually resolves spontaneously or after ASV in 24–48 hours • Prolonged prothrombin time, elevated D-dimer, and low fibrinogen are commonly seen • ASV should be administered as early as possible once coagulopathy is detected. Other therapies like heparin, warfarin, FFP, and cryoprecipitate are not helpful and may worsen the coagulopathy
Rhabdomyolysis	• Associated with viper bite, and usual features are raised CPK, hyperkalemia, and AKI. It is managed with fluid resuscitation, correction of electrolyte imbalance, and dialysis for AKI
Thrombotic micro-angiopathy (TMA)	• It is characterized by thrombocytopenia, AKI, and features of microangiopathic hemolytic anemia. Supportive care, ASV, blood products, and dialysis are recommended

(AN: atropine neostigmine; ASV: antisnake venom; CPK: creatine phosphokinase; FFP: fresh frozen plasma; HD: hemodialysis; IM: intramuscular; IV: intravenous; LMA: laryngeal mask airway; NS: normal saline; PD: peritoneal dialysis; RRT: renal replacement therapy; WBCT: whole blood clotting test)

Practical Questions About Antisnake Venom

- **If the patient is brought late after few days after snakebite, up to what day ASV can be considered?**

  If there are signs of venom activity such as bleeding, prolonged 20WBCT, or neuroparalytic signs, ASV can be administered, otherwise there is no need.

- **What are the responsibilities of the referring doctor?**

  He/she should communicate to the receiving center about the current status of the child and the prehospital treatment provided. The child should be transported by an ambulance accompanied by medical or paramedical personnel. If possible, complete the ASV infusion and transfer to a place where ventilation, blood products, and dialysis facilities are available.

- **If the patient does not show any signs of envenomation on arrival, does he/she still need hospitalization?**

  Even if asymptomatic after a snakebite, the child should be monitored in the hospital for 24–48 hours and administered ASV when there is an indication.

- **What is occult snakebite?**

  Occult snakebite is a situation where the patient is unaware of snakebite, and the physician does not see any distinct fang mark, but acute neuroparalysis or acute-onset spreading cellulitis is observed (in a rural, forest, or bushy park area environment). Here, a physician can strongly suspect snakebite and initiate ASV.

- **Does accident register (AR) entry needed for snakebite?**

  In some states, medicolegal (AR) entry is mandatory, because compensation is given in a rural accident.

OTHER SUPPORTIVE MANAGEMENT

- Antibiotics, if there is local tissue necrosis
- Tetanus prophylaxis is needed in children. Tetanus toxoid (TT) and tetanus immunoglobulin should be given after correction of coagulopathy.
- *Analgesia:* Ketamine, fentanyl, or paracetamol is preferred. Avoid nonsteroidal anti-inflammatory drugs (NSAIDs).
- Using blood products without neutralizing the toxins is not preferable and can be used only in life-threatening situations.
- Surgical consultation should be done when compartment syndrome is suspected.

Equipping a Hospital or Peripheral Center for the Management of Snake Envenomation

Antisnake venom, emergency drugs like adrenaline, antihistamine, hydrocortisone, and IV fluids are adequately stocked. Mechanical ventilatory support, blood products, and dialysis facilities in higher centers should be available. A standard protocol should be available in the ED and pediatric intensive care unit (PICU).

Prevention of Snakebite

- Avoid places where the snakes are likely to live and hide.
- Attempting to catch, frighten, or attack a snake is dangerous.
- Simple measures such as using torchlights, sticks, wearing long boots, and avoiding barefoot walk and walking in the darkness can prevent snakebites.
- Precautions should be taken while cutting grass, or picking fruit or vegetables, or clearing the base of trees.
- Sleeping on the ground is to be avoided in the field. Using a bamboo cot and mosquito net can prevent snakebites.
- Picking up a snake, even if it appears to be dead, is dangerous.
- Do not keep livestock, especially chickens, in the house, as snakes may come to hunt them.

APPROACH

The approach to the management of snake envenomation is illustrated in **Flowchart 1**.

Flowchart 1: Approach to the management of a child with snake envenomation.

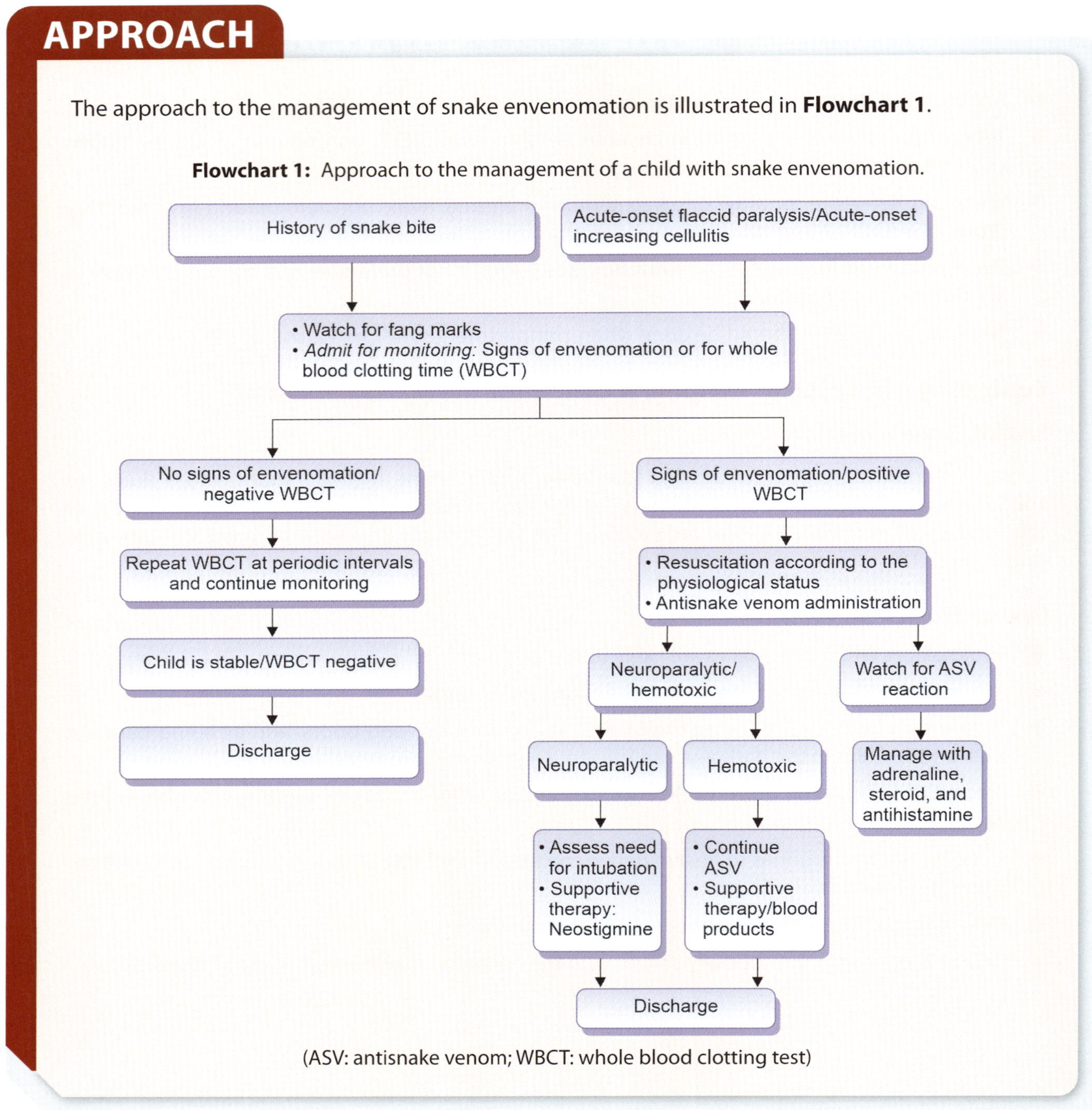

(ASV: antisnake venom; WBCT: whole blood clotting test)

KEY LEARNING POINTS

- History and focused examination are helpful to initiate the treatment.
- All children with snakebites should be admitted in high dependency units (HDU)/PICU.
- Absence of history of snakebite does not exclude envenomation, and a high degree of suspicion to recognize signs of envenomation is needed in rural areas.
- ASV and written protocols on snakebite management must be available in every primary care setting and referral centers.
- Signs of brain death, such as dilated pupils, and absent cough reflex during suction will be seen in snakebite; hence, brain death certification should not be undertaken without expert consultation.

ACKNOWLEDGMENTS

I extend my profuse thanks and gratitude to Professor V Poovazhagi, PICU, ICH, Madras Medical College, Dr Sheeja Sugunan, Associate Professor, SAT Hospital, Govt Medical College Thiruvananthapuram and Dr Anjana Chari, DNB Resident, Mehta Multispeciality Hospitals, Chennai, for assistance.

REFERENCES

1. Suraweera W, Warrell D, Whitaker R, Menon G, Rodrigues R, Fu SH, et al. Trends in snakebite deaths in India from 2000 to 2019 in a nationally representative mortality study. elife. 2020;9:e54076.
2. Ministry of Health & Family Welfare Government of India. (2016). Management of Snake Bite: Quick Reference Guide. p. 12. [online] Available from https://nhm.gov.in/images/pdf/guidelines/nrhm-guidelines/stg/Snakebite_QRG.pdf [Last accessed January, 2024].
3. Mehta SR, Sashindran VK. Clinical features and management of snake bite. Med J Armed Forces India. 2002;58(3):247-9.
4. Isbister GK, Maduwage K, Shahmy S, Mohamed F, Abeysinghe C, Karunathilake H, et al. Diagnostic 20-min whole blood clotting test in Russell's viper envenoming delays antivenom administration. QJM. 2013;106(10):925-32.
5. Warrel D (Ed). Guidelines for the Management of Snakebites, 2nd edition. Geneva: World Health Organization; 2016. [online] Available from https://www.who.int/publications/i/item/9789290225300 [Last accessed January, 2024].

6. Simpson ID. The pediatric management of snakebite: The national protocol. Indian Pediatr. 2007;44:173-6.
7. Le Geyt J, Pach S, Gutiérrez JM, Habib AG, Maduwage KP, Hardcastle TC, et al. Paediatric snakebite envenoming: Recognition and management of cases. Arch Dis Child. 2021;106(1):14-9.
8. Kumar R, Mahadeven S. Snake envenomation in children. In Pediatric Intensive Care Unit Protocols. Indian J Pract Pediatr. 2021; 571-80.
9. White J. (2023). Snakebites Worldwide: Management. In: Ruha M, Danzl DF (Eds). [online] Available from https://medilib.ir/uptodate/show/93182 [Last accessed January, 2024].
10. Rajakumar PS, Singaravelu M, Nakate D. Snakebite. Standard Treatment Guidelines 2022. Mumbai: Indian Academy of Pediatrics. [online] Available from https://iapindia.org/pdf/Ch-102-Snakebite.pdf [Last accessed January, 2024].

Scorpion Envenomation

Sivamurukan Palanisamy, Narayanan Parameswaran

INTRODUCTION

Scorpions are arthropods belonging to the class Arachnida, which are primarily seen in tropical and subtropical regions with hot and dry temperatures. Only around 25 species have venom which can harm humans. The usual habitat of scorpions includes cracks in houses, burrows beneath logs, rice husks, and sugarcane fields. Since scorpions hide in the cracks of buildings during the day and only come out at night, the majority of stings are reported at night.[1]

Scorpion sting is a common life-threatening and time-limiting medical emergency seen among children in rural areas of India. Although scorpion sting envenomation is seen throughout the country, its incidence is higher in the southern states like Tamil Nadu, Puducherry, Maharashtra, and Karnataka along with fewer northern states like Madhya Pradesh and West Bengal. The pediatric age group has reported mortality rates of 7.07 per 1,000,000 in infants and 3.78 per 1,000,000 in children between 1 and 4 years of age.[2] This is attributed to their smaller body surface area making the dose per surface area higher in them during envenomation. The mortality of scorpion sting among the pediatric age group in the preprazosin era was up to 30 %; however, post introduction of prazosin, the mortality had reduced to <1–3%.[3,4] But still, death due to scorpion envenomation does occur, bringing to fore the importance of early identification and appropriate interventions to prevent scorpion sting-related mortality.

ETIOPATHOGENESIS

Though there are multiple species of scorpions seen in India, *Hottentotta tamulus*, (previously known as *Mesobuthus tamulus*) (Indian red scorpion, most poisonous) is the most common species to cause significant clinical manifestations and toxicity. Stings from this scorpion present predominantly with autonomic hyperstimulation (autonomic storm), pulmonary edema, and cardiac effects. The other common scorpion found in India is *Palamnaeus swammerdami* (black scorpion).

Scorpion venom is a complex compound with various toxins of which the most clinically relevant compound is scorpion alpha toxin. This alpha toxin binds to voltage-gated sodium channels and prevents them from inactivation causing hyperpolarization and persistent autonomic excitation (autonomic storm).[5]

The autonomic storm starts as an initial transient cholinergic storm (parasympathetic excess phase) followed by a prolonged adrenergic storm (sympathetic excess phase) with an overlap of symptoms while transition.[6] Myocardial dysfunction sets in due to vasospasm and increased myocardial demand during the adrenergic storm. Subsequently, there may be a catecholamine-depletion phase in some children leading to vasoplegic shock. The entire course usually settles in within 48 hours post scorpion sting.

CLINICAL FEATURES

The clinical manifestations and severity of scorpion envenomation depend on multiple factors such as scorpion species, size of the child, dose of venom injected, timing of presentation since sting, and timing of prazosin administration after the sting.

Children with scorpion envenomation (especially Indian red scorpion) can present with any of the following phenotypes **(Flowchart 1)**:

- Asymptomatic
- *Local symptoms:* Severe pain, tap sign (tapping at the sting site causes severe pain.)
- *Autonomic storm*:
  - *Cholinergic phase (parasympathetic excess phase):* Projectile vomiting, profuse sweating (skin diarrhea), miosis, excessive salivation, bronchial secretions (noncardiogenic pulmonary edema), priapism in boys, urinary incontinence, bradycardia, arrhythmias, and hypotension.
  - *Adrenergic phase (sympathetic excess phase):* Hyperglycemia, mydriasis, cold extremities (vasoconstriction), hypertension, tachycardia, and arrhythmias
  - Stage of catecholamine depletion leading to vasoplegic shock
- *Myocardial dysfunction:* Congestive cardiac failure, cardiogenic pulmonary edema, and cardiogenic shock

There may be an overlap between parasympathetic excess and sympathetic excess phases; hence, it is necessary to closely monitor the child, which is essential in deciding the management.

Scorpion envenomation by certain species can cause neuromuscular manifestations like muscle jerks, fasciculations, paralysis, abnormal oculomotor movements, visual disturbances, and vasospasm leading to stroke, dysphagia, and dysphonia. Rarely neurological manifestations may be severe enough to cause respiratory compromise.[7]

Other rare manifestations like skin necrosis, hemolysis, disseminated intravascular coagulation, and renal failure are also reported in the literature.[8]

Flowchart 1: Timeline of scorpion envenomation and its symptomatology.

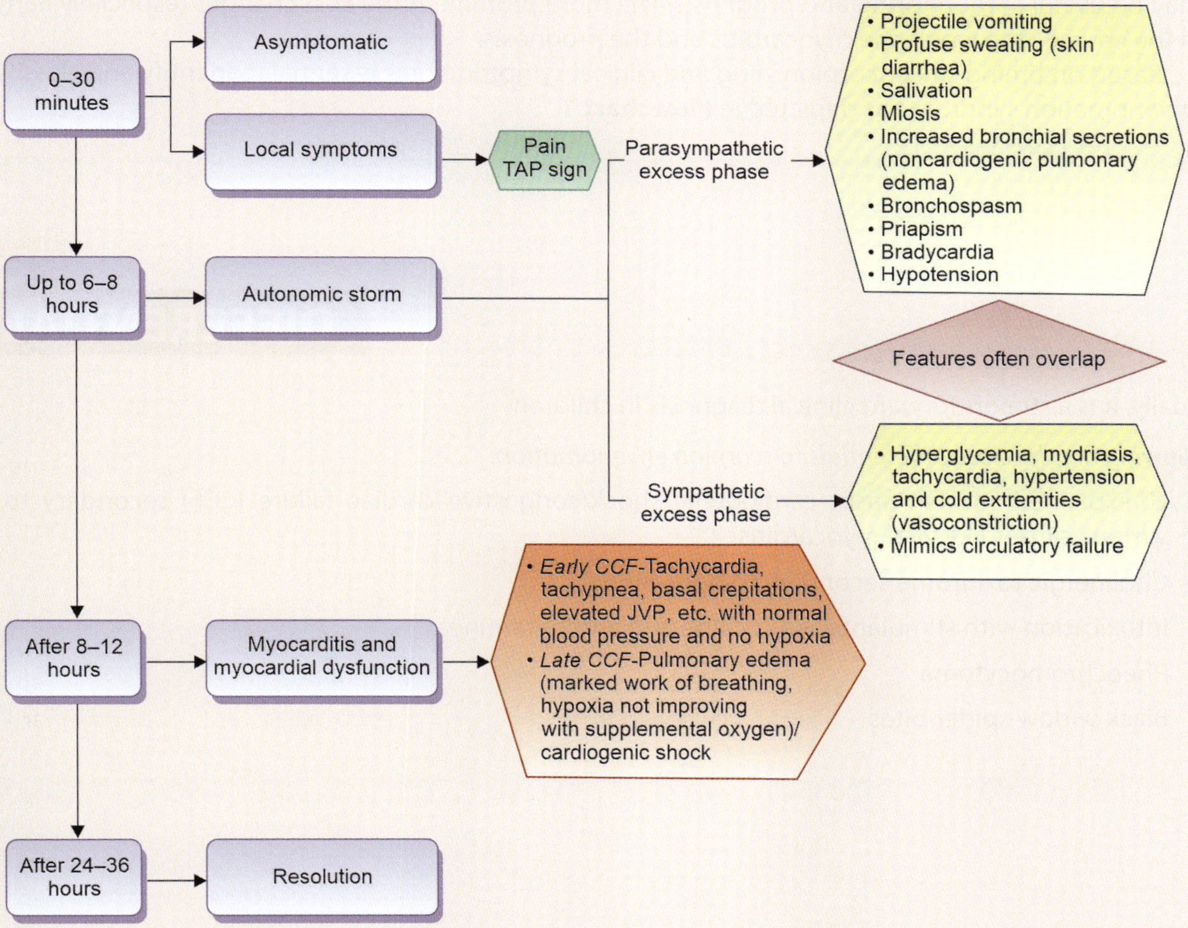

0–30 minutes → Asymptomatic
0–30 minutes → Local symptoms → Pain TAP sign

Up to 6–8 hours → Autonomic storm

Autonomic storm / Pain TAP sign → Parasympathetic excess phase →
- Projectile vomiting
- Profuse sweating (skin diarrhea)
- Salivation
- Miosis
- Increased bronchial secretions (noncardiogenic pulmonary edema)
- Bronchospasm
- Priapism
- Bradycardia
- Hypotension

Features often overlap

Autonomic storm → Sympathetic excess phase →
- Hyperglycemia, mydriasis, tachycardia, hypertension and cold extremities (vasoconstriction)
- Mimics circulatory failure

After 8–12 hours → Myocarditis and myocardial dysfunction →
- *Early CCF*-Tachycardia, tachypnea, basal crepitations, elevated JVP, etc. with normal blood pressure and no hypoxia
- *Late CCF*-Pulmonary edema (marked work of breathing, hypoxia not improving with supplemental oxygen)/ cardiogenic shock

After 24–36 hours → Resolution

(CCF: congestive cardiac failure; JVP: jugular venous pulse)

EVALUATION

A thorough clinical assessment (history and examination) along with a 12-lead electrocardiography (ECG) and chest X-ray would suffice for optimal management of scorpion envenomation in most settings. In the setting of a tertiary care pediatric intensive care unit (PICU), availability of bedside echocardiography (ECHO) may be used as an additional tool in evaluating cardiac function. In critically ill children requiring PICU, additional investigations like hemogram, renal function test, and electrolytes will aid in providing optimal care.

In ECG, features like low voltage, wide QRS complex, peaked T waves, hemiblock, and ST-segment elevation/depression are reported. ECG changes can also vary over time and serial ECG recordings may be useful in monitoring and prognosis. The more prominent the ECG changes (especially early in the course), the worse the myocarditis and the prognosis.

Based on timing since scorpion sting and clinical symptoms, it is essential to identify and classify envenomation syndrome as depicted in **Flowchart 1**.

DIFFERENTIALS

Usually, it is a straightforward clinical diagnosis in children.

Following are the close differentials to scorpion envenomation:

- Unexplained sudden-onset cardiogenic shock/congestive cardiac failure (CCF) secondary to various causes like viral myocarditis
- Cholinergic toxidrome secondary to poisonings
- Intoxication with stimulants like cocaine and amphetamines
- Pheochromocytoma
- Black widow spider bites

EMERGENCY CARE

Initial assessment and stabilization should be as per pediatric advanced life support (PALS) guidelines.

Management of children with scorpion sting depends on the type of envenomation syndrome **(refer to Flowchart 1)** identified based on clinical manifestation at the time of presentation. The clinical picture can change over time too (e.g., from autonomic storm with hypertension to pure cardiogenic shock over few hours).

Symptom-specific management of scorpion sting is classified into five groups based on *physiological hemodynamic patterns* as given below.

1. *Asymptomatic children:* Require close monitoring of vitals for 24 hours
2. *In children with local pain and no systemic features:* Administer oral paracetamol (15 mg/kg). Avoid lignocaine injections and steroids.
3. *In children with evidence of autonomic storm and/or features of myocarditis [like persistent unexplained tachycardia, third heart sound (S3) gallop, etc.] with no evidence of CCF:* Start them on oral prazosin (dose and tablet strength) and consider repeating every 6 hourly till resolution of autonomic storm (return of warm extremities is a useful sign at bedside). Ensure adequate oral intake and if oral intake is poor, start them of full-maintenance intravenous fluids in the initial 6 hours (during autonomic storm, fluid deficit is more common due to diaphoresis, profuse sweating, vomiting, and poor oral intake) and subsequently fluid intake can be adjusted based on bedside assessment of urine output and intravascular volume status. Misdiagnosing a child with autonomic storm (cold peripheries and tachycardia due to sympathetic overactivity) as having myocarditis and cardiogenic shock can lead to unnecessary overuse of catecholamines (dobutamine, etc.) early in the course which can worsen the autonomic storm. Hence, careful bedside evaluation looking for evidence of autonomic overactivity involving both sympathetic (hypertension, mydriasis, cold extremities, etc.) and parasympathetic (miosis, priapism in a boy, profuse sweating, diaphoresis, bradycardia alternating with tachycardia, etc.) will help in classifying the child accurately.
4. *In children with features of myocarditis and CCF:* Classify them into early CCF [tachycardia, tachypnea, basal crepitations, elevated jugular venous pulse (JVP), etc., with normal blood pressure (BP) and no hypoxia] and late CCF (early CCF features plus pulmonary edema as evidenced by marked work of breathing, worsening hypoxia not improving with supplemental oxygen, pink frothy sputum, coarse crepitations over lung fields, etc., and/or cardiogenic shock) based on their severity of clinical manifestations.

- *Management of children with early CCF:*
  - Start on dobutamine infusion at 4–6 µg/kg/min and titrate up to 10–15 µg/kg/min. Target normal peripheral perfusion and decrease in heart rate rather than normalization of BP as it may not increase to 50th centile with dobutamine. Accept 5th centile BP if perfusion is adequate.

- Transfer to PICU, if possible.
- Avoid furosemide in the initial 12 hours, until the intravascular volume deficit caused by profuse sweating, vomiting, etc. is corrected.
- It is preferable not to use inotropes with longer half-life (e.g., milrinone and levosimendan) as first-line agents, as the clinical status can rapidly change over time.
- Avoid adrenaline and noradrenaline infusions unless hypotension is refractive to dobutamine and optimization of intravascular volume.
- Avoid opioids like morphine early in the course.
- Be cautious with oral prazosin, if a child is on dobutamine infusion and has a BP on the lower side of normal (close to 5th centile).

◈ *Management of children with late CCF (pulmonary edema and cardiogenic shock):*

- Transfer to PICU, if not already done.
- Provide noninvasive ventilation (NIV), and if not improving within 1 hour, intubate and mechanically ventilate with adequate positive end-expiratory pressure (PEEP) (to improve lung compliance and to decrease left ventricular afterload). For sedation and analgesia, use drugs like ketamine with least impact on hemodynamics along with short-acting paralytic agents peri-intubation.
- Continue dobutamine at maximum tolerated dose (maximum 15 µg/kg/min).
- If pulmonary edema and hypoxia persist even after positive-pressure ventilation, start intravenous sodium nitroprusside (SNP) infusion at 0.5–1 µg/kg/min and titrate up to achieve improvement in oxygenation parameters and lung compliance (maximum up to 5 µg/kg/min). Avoid SNP if hypotensive (BP <5th centile) with poor perfusion.
- In children who are hypotensive (BP <5th centile) with poor perfusion, the preferred vasodilator for pulmonary edema is intravenous nitroglycerine infusion (1–5 µg/kg/min).[9]
- Avoid oral prazosin if a child is on intravenous vasodilators.
- Adrenaline infusion can be tried as a desperate measure in a child with refractive hypotension and poor perfusion.

◈ In both early and late phases of CCF, all the supportive measures should be continued for at least 24 hours before attempting withdrawal. Taper and stop the vasodilator first, followed by dobutamine.

5. Rarely children may present with *atypical features* like central nervous system (CNS) manifestations with seizures/encephalopathy. In this scenario, management is purely supportive. Benzodiazepines are the first-line agents for controlling seizures followed by phenobarbitone or levetiracetam. Avoid phenytoin as the risk of cardiac arrhythmias is high.

SPECIFIC MANAGEMENT

Do's and don'ts in the management of scorpion sting envenomation are given in **Table 1**.

TABLE 1: Do's and don'ts in scorpion sting envenomation.	
Do's	***Don'ts***
• Report to a hospital immediately • Observe for 24 hours minimum • Prazosin must be given at the first sign of autonomic storm as soon as possible[10]	• Use of tourniquet • Incision and drainage • Prophylactic antibiotics • Morphine (increases the risk of arrhythmia) • Steroids • Lytic cocktail

Table 2 shows scorpion antidotes, their mechanism of action, dose, and indications.

TABLE 2: Scorpion antidotes.				
Antidote	***Mechanism of action***	***Dose***	***Indications***	***Comments***
Prazosin[11] (pharmacological and physiological antidote)	*Alpha 1 blocker:* Reduces the preload and left ventricular afterload	• 30 µg/kg/dose • Every 4–6 hourly interval	• Autonomic storm • Myocarditis without cardiogenic shock	• No prophylactic role • Watch for first-dose hypotension • Caution in cardiogenic shock • Photosensitive (so store away from light)
Indian scorpion antivenom (SAV) (monovalent)	• Neutralizes red scorpion venom • 1 mL neutralizes 1 mg of red scorpion venom	• 3 vials of SAV (30 mL) + 70 mL NS 100 mL over 1 hour as slow infusion (1 vial of SAV diluted in 10 mL sterile water)	• May be given if patient presents within 6 hours of sting with autonomic storm	• No survival benefit over prazosin, except for early resolution of symptoms[12-14] • Reports of life-threatening anaphylaxis and death

MONITORING

Monitoring sheet for scorpion envenomation during the initial 24–48 hours.

Time									
Heart rate									
Peripheral perfusion									
Blood pressure									
Respiration rate									
SpO_2									
Basal crepitations									
Urine output (mL/kg/hr)									
Blood sugar									
Clinical syndrome*									
Prazosin dose (30 µg/kg/dose)									
Oxygen									
Positive-pressure ventilation									
Dobutamine									

*Asymptomatic/local symptoms/autonomic storm/myocarditis.

KEY LEARNING POINTS

- In scorpion sting envenomation, the autonomic storm predominates in the initial 4–6 hours, which is often followed by myocarditis by 8–12 hours with some overlap in between 6 and 12 hours phase.
- Diuretics should be avoided in the initial 12 hours, even if there is pulmonary edema, as the intravascular volume is likely to be low.
- In the initial autonomic storm phase, prazosin and adequate fluids are the mainstay of therapy. Prazosin can be given even if BPs are borderline, provided the intravascular volume is preserved.
- In myocarditis, prazosin is still continued, but it acts mainly as a vasodilator (decreases afterload) and aids in the management of cardiac failure. If the child is already on inotropes, then easily titratable vasodilators like nitroglycerin (NTG) and SNP (short acting agents) are preferred over prazosin.
- Morphine should be avoided (when given for initial pain), as it increases the chance of arrhythmia.
- Bedside ECG recording, available in all settings, is a very good indicator of the severity of myocardial injury and useful for prognosis.
- Inotropes should be tapered based on the trends of clinical assessment of perfusion rather than actual BP or serial ECHO.

REFERENCES

1. Mahadevan S. Scorpion sting. Indian Pediatr. 2000;37(5):504-14.
2. Celis A, Gaxiola-Robles R, Sevilla-Godínez E, Orozco Valerio Mde J, Armas J. [Trends in mortality from scorpion stings in Mexico, 1979-2003]. Rev Panam Salud Publica. 2007;21(6):373-80.
3. Bahloul M, Chabchoub I, Chaari A, Chtara K, Kallel H, Dammak H, et al. Scorpion Envenomation Among Children: Clinical Manifestations and Outcome (Analysis of 685 Cases). Am J Trop Med Hyg. 2010;83(5): 1084-92.
4. Bawaskar HS, Bawaskar PH. Severe envenoming by the Indian red scorpion Mesobuthus tamulus: The use of prazosin therapy. QJM. 1996;89(9):701-4.
5. Isbister GK, Bawaskar HS. Scorpion Envenomation. N Engl J Med. 2014;371(5):457-63.
6. Bawaskar HS, Bawaskar PH. Scorpion sting: Update. J Assoc Physicians India. 2012;60:46-55.
7. Godoy DA, Badenes R, Seifi S, Salehi S, Seifi A. Neurological and Systemic Manifestations of Severe Scorpion Envenomation. Cureus. 13(4):e14715.

8. Sagheb MM, Sharifian M, Moini M, Sharifian AH. Scorpion bite prevalence and complications: Report from a referral centre in southern Iran. Trop Doct. 2012;42(2):90-1.
9. Narayanan P, Mahadevan S, Serane VT. Nitroglycerine in scorpion sting with decompensated shock. Indian Pediatr. 2006;43(7):613-7.
10. Bawaskar HS, Bawaskar PH. Clinical profile of severe scorpion envenomation in children at rural setting. Indian Pediatr. 2003;40(11):1072-5.
11. Bawaskar HS, Bawaskar PH. Prazosin in management of cardiovascular manifestations of scorpion sting. Lancet. 1986;1(8479):510-1.
12. Rodrigo C, Gnanathasan A. Management of scorpion envenoming: A systematic review and meta-analysis of controlled clinical trials. Syst Rev. 2017;6(1):74.
13. Pandi K, Krishnamurthy S, Srinivasaraghavan R, Mahadevan S. Efficacy of scorpion antivenom plus prazosin versus prazosin alone for Mesobuthus tamulus scorpion sting envenomation in children: A randomised controlled trial. Arch Dis Child. 2014;99(6):575-80.
14. Abimannane A, Rameshkumar R, Satheesh P, Mahadevan S. Second dose of scorpion antivenom in children with Indian red scorpion (Mesobuthus tamulus) sting envenomation. Indian Pediatr. 201815;55(4):315-8.

40

Wasp and Honeybee Stings

Rashna Dass Hazarika, Devajit K Sharma

INTRODUCTION

Wasps and bees fall under the family Hymenoptera which also includes hornets, yellow jackets, and ants. These are social creatures and use the sting as a defense mechanism when they feel threatened. Victims can have variable presentations depending on the amount of envenomation, and treatment is usually supportive. Anaphylaxis following wasp and bee stings can be life-threatening and require immediate management.

TERMINOLOGIES AND DEFINITIONS

- *Hymenoptera:* Order of arthropods composed of bees, wasps, ants, hornets, yellow jackets
- *Major subgroups:* Vespids (yellow jacket, hornet, and wasp) and Apids (honey bee and bumble bee)
- *Venom:* Composed mostly of proteins along with peptides, amino acids, carbohydrates, lipids, and enzymes. The toxicity results from the presence of low-molecular-weight substances such as bradykinin, acetylcholine, dopamine, histamine, and serotonin. Antigenic substances present in wasp and bee stings result in hypersensitivity and anaphylaxis. One bee sting can release up to 140 µg of venom and 3 µg of venom per wasp sting.

ETIOPATHOLOGY

Both the wasps and the bees have similar ways of delivering the venom. The females have modified barbed ovipositors on the undersurface of the abdomen which acts like a hypodermic needle to deliver the venom, and this action pulls the stinger from the bee's body and thus kills it. The wasps on the other hand have unbarbed stinger which can inflict multiple stings without dying. The stinger of bee remains embedded in the skin and continues to release a huge amount of venom into the victim's circulation causing more reactions. Once stung, the components of the venom, especially the low-molecular-weight substances, initiate a reaction from the human body. The main target organs are the skin and vascular and respiratory systems. The reactions are similar to immunoglobulin E (IgE)-mediated allergic reactions. There is a release of basophils and mast cells resulting in urticaria, vasodilatation, angioedema, laryngospasm, and progressive respiratory distress. Reports of multiorgan dysfunction are there after multiple wasp stings.

CLINICAL FEATURES

Four types of reactions can take place:

1. Local reaction
2. Anaphylaxis
3. Unusual sting reactions
4. Systemic intoxication (after a large number of stings)

Local Reactions

The most common effect is severe pain at the site of sting followed by local tenderness, swelling, redness, and itching. It is usually <10 cm in diameter and improves significantly within 24 hours. The local area swelling can involve a large area and may be confused with cellulitis in severe local reactions. Here, the area of involvement is >10 cm and this may resolve spontaneously in a few hours or persists for days.

Anaphylaxis

Anaphylaxis occurs in about 1.2–3.5% of all people with wasp or bee stings. This is a typical immediate type of allergic reaction and it occurs from 10 to 30 minutes of the sting. IgE-mediated reactions can occur from a few minutes up to 1 week of the sting and may cause the victim to have features of anaphylaxis such as generalized swelling including edema of the upper airways, urticaria, Ring and

Messmer's grading of the severity of allergic reactions, coughing, respiratory difficulty, wheezing, hypotension, and coma. The severity of the sting is classified based on the clinical manifestations **(Table 1)**.

TABLE 1: Ring and Messmer's grading of the severity of allergic reactions.[1]

Grade	*Skin*	*Abdomen*	*Respiratory*	*Cardiovascular*
1.	• Itching • Flushes • Urticaria • Angioedema	–	–	–
2.	• Itching • Flushes • Urticaria • Angioedema	• Nausea • Abdominal cramps	• Rhinorrhea • Hoarseness • Dyspnea	• Tachycardia (rise ≥ 20/min) • Hypotension (≥20 mm Hg drop in SBP) • Arrhythmia
3.	• Itching • Flushes • Urticaria • Angioedema	• Vomiting • Defecation	• Laryngeal edema • Bronchospasm • Cyanosis	Shock
4.	• Itching • Flushes • Urticaria • Angioedema	• Vomiting • Defecation	Respiratory arrest	Circulatory arrest

(SBP: systolic blood pressure)

Unusual Sting Reactions

Unusual sting reactions are rare presentations and can manifest as serum sickness, vasculitis, thrombocytopenic purpura, neurologic, and renal and cardiovascular diseases.

Systemic Reactions

Multiple stings can result in multiorgan involvement and lead to rhabdomyolysis, hemolysis, cerebral disturbances, and hepatic and renal involvement. Patients have serious reactions within the first 30 minutes. The local pain and swelling can take 2–3 days to subside and the delayed hypersensitivity reactions may take 1 week to 10 days to subside.

EVALUATION

The victim is examined for the effects at the site of sting, presence of any stinger, and any systemic side effects. Vital parameters at admission are noted. The victim has to be assessed for A—airway patency, B—breathing difficulties and bronchospasm, C—heart rate and blood pressure, D—urticaria, flushing, multiorgan involvement, sensorium. No specific investigations are needed unless the victim has severe envenomation. In sick cases, multiorgan involvement may need to be ruled out by doing renal function tests, liver function tests, coagulation parameters, urine analysis, hemoglobin with peripheral blood smear examination, and reticulocyte count to look for hemolysis **(Flowchart 1)**.[2] A history of the nature of sting can be assessed by asking the circumstances of the sting. If the sting occurred near a beehive, then it is probably due to bee sting but if it occurred in an open area, it may be due to a wasp sting.

Flowchart 1: Clinical approach to wasp/bee sting.

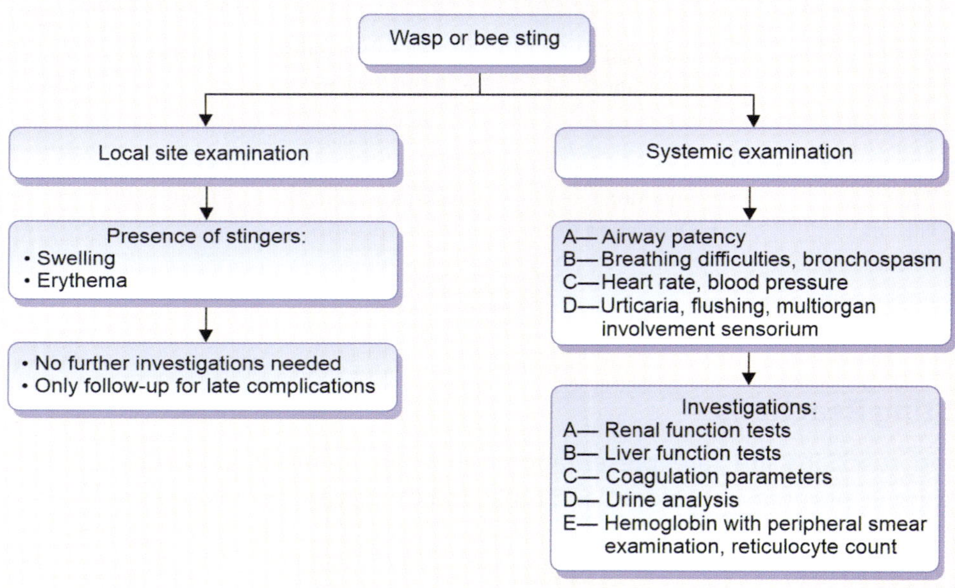

Risk Assessment

Risk assessment is important for individuals who are frequently exposed to insects or are at a higher risk for severe anaphylactic reactions. About 3–5% victims with insect venom anaphylaxis have systemic mastocytosis and 10% have high baseline tryptase levels. These victims are at a very high risk for severe anaphylaxis. The individuals at high risk are outlined in **Table 2**.

TABLE 2: Risk factors for Hymenoptera venom-induced anaphylaxis.[1]	
Type of risk	***Individuals at risk***
Risk of frequent exposure	• Beekeepers, their families and neighbors • Other professions, including persons who sell fruit or baked goods, foresters, gardeners, firefighters, farmers, construction workers, truck drivers • Intense outdoor activity
Elevated risk of severe anaphylaxis	• Prior episode(s) of severe sting anaphylaxis (grade III or IV, or grade II with significant airway obstruction) • Age (from about 40 years of onward) • Cardiovascular disease • Asthma • Certain drugs including beta-blockers (eye drops as well), ACE inhibitors, nonsteroidal anti-inflammatory drugs • Physical and mental stress • Basal serum tryptase concentration >11.4 µg/L (mastocytosis is not rare in such cases) • Cutaneous or systemic mastocytosis

(ACE: angiotensin-converting enzyme)

DIFFERENTIALS

The wasp and bee stings can be confused with similar presentations in children secondary to:

- Angioedema
- Snake envenomation
- Scorpion stings
- Cellulitis
- Drug or food allergies
- Hereditary angioedema

EMERGENCY CARE[3,4]

No specific antivenin exists for wasp and bee stings. Local reactions require local wound care and supportive measures such as cold compress. Immediate treatment is required for victims with anaphylactic reactions as this is life-threatening. In mild cases, oral diphenhydramine or oral steroids may be needed sometimes. Adrenaline in repeated doses or in infusion and hydrocortisone are used in severe anaphylactic reactions. Oral H1 blockers may be used up to four times the normal dose. The algorithm for management is outlined in **Flowchart 2**.

Flowchart 2: Management of wasp/bee stings.

Wasp/bee stings
↓
Immediate action
↓
I. Remove stinger(s)
II. Be careful not to squeeze the sac to prevent release of more venom
III. Simultaneous assessment of ABCD

→ Local reactions
- I. Apply cold compress
- II. Analgesics if required
- III. Oral antihistaminics if the local reaction persists or spreads
- IV. Oral steroids for 2–3 days—in extensive lesions
- V. H1 blocker (Ranitidine) for severe reactions

→ Systemic reactions
- I. Administer inj adrenaline IM
- II. High-flow O_2

→ Assess airway
- Partial obstruction
  1. Repeat inj adrenaline every 5 minutes
  2. If needed adrenaline infusion
  3. Inform PICU
- Complete obstruction
  1. Intubation
  2. Bag and mask ventilation
  3. Adrenaline IM every 5 minutes
  4. If required adrenaline infusion
  5. Inj hydrocortisone if needed
  6. Inform ICU

→ Assess breathing
- Apnea or wheeze
  1. Repeat adrenaline every 5 minutes
  2. If required adrenaline infusion
  3. Nebulized salbutamol
  4. Inform PICU

→ Assess circulation
- No pulse
  1. Basic and advanced life support
  2. Shift to PICU
- Shock
  1. Repeat adrenaline every 5 minutes
  2. If required adrenaline infusion
  3. NS bolus
  4. Nebulized salbutamol
  5. Inform PICU

↓
Reassess ABC and investigate for multiorgan involvement

Doses of drug and route of administration:

- *Inj. Adrenaline:* 1:1000 solution—dose is 0.01 mL/kg IM
- *Adrenaline infusion:* 0.05–5 µg/kg/min IV
- *Inj. Hydrocortisone:* 5–10 mg/kg every 4–6 hours in severe cases IV
- *Diphenhydramine:* 1.25 mg/kg up to 10 mg orally
- *Ranitidine:* 1 mg/kg/dose 8 hourly (oral or IV)
- *Oral prednisolone:* 0.5–1 mg/kg/day
- *Nebulized salbutamol:* 0.15 mg/kg per dose
- *Normal saline:* 20 mL/kg in first hour IV and repeat if needed

Monitoring

Patients need to be monitored in hospital for any deterioration and development of complications. It is advisable to keep patients with severe reactions in the hospital. Anaphylaxis can appear anytime and up to 1 week of the sting.

Prophylaxis

Children who have suffered from a wasp or bee sting need prophylaxis. They are advised to wear long-sleeved clothes and full pants to avoid being stung. Secondly, they should always carry life-saving drugs like Inj. Adrenaline and H1 blockers. In severe cases of anaphylaxis, further testing and venom immunotherapy might help.

KEY LEARNING POINTS

- Allergic reactions to wasp or bee stings are common. Most have mild local reactions.
- Multiple stings predispose the individual to severe reactions.
- Removal of the stinger and immediate local treatment are essential.
- Severe reactions require aggressive management to prevent deaths.
- The most important steps in severe anaphylaxis are to call for help, aggressive resuscitation for grade 4 reactions, and epinephrine for all grade 2 reactions and above.
- Prophylaxis is important to prevent future severe reactions.

REFERENCES

1. Przybilla B, Ruëff F. Insect stings. Clinical features and management. Dtsch Arztebl Int. 2012;109(13):238-48.
2. Shanto P, Sushmita B. Wasp stings with multisystem dysfunction. Indian Pediatr. 2007;44:788-90.
3. Singhi S. Scorpion and insect stings. In: Singhi S, Surpure JS (Eds). Synopsis of Pediatric Emergency Care, 2nd edition. New Delhi: Peepee Publishers; 2010. pp. 539-40.
4. Nagaraju K. Anaphylaxis. In: Major Nagaraju K (Ed). Manual of Pediatric Allergy, 2nd edition. New Delhi: Jaypee Brothers Medical Publishers; 2021. pp. 143-57.

41

Electrical Burns

Sheikh Minhaj Ahmed, Rajeev Redkar

INTRODUCTION

Electrical burns in children are serious life-threatening injuries. Electrical burns result from thermal energy that is produced as an electrical current pass through the body. The amount of thermal energy produced is directly proportional to the degree of the electric current. Children younger than 6 years are likely to encounter low-voltage outlets or electric cords electrical injuries. Older children have an increased incidence of high-voltage injuries because of their increased mobility and adventurousness. An electrical injury represents a peculiar burn injury that requires additional considerations from other burn injuries. These include cardiac arrhythmias, and evaluation and treatment of the injured extremities. Late complications of high-voltage injuries, include cataract development, progressive nerve degeneration and cognitive or psychological ramifications.

PATHOPHYSIOLOGY

- Three forms of electrical injury include low voltage injuries (<440 V), high-voltage injuries (>1000 V), and ultra-high voltage (lightning: 300,000 A; 100,000,000 V). Electrical burns are caused by 3 different mechanisms:
  1. Precipitation of cytoplasmic proteins under the influence of electrical charges
  2. Tissue heat generated by the passage of current
  3. Collateral flames burn caused by ignited clothes or electrical flash (arc), which is superheated ionized air that flashes from the high voltage electrical source.
- The factors determining the electrical burn severity are, child susceptibility, contact point resistance, contact duration, current flow pathway, current type (direct or alternate), amperage and voltage.
- As nerves, muscles, and blood vessels offer low electrical resistance, electric current preferentially flow through these structures and cause maximum damage to them. Vascular thrombosis caused by passage of current through blood vessels will result in extensive gangrene of dependent tissues.
- Simultaneous tetanic muscle contraction of flexors and extensors of forearm can lead to "No let-go" phenomenon, caused by the alternate current.
- Additionally, electric current can also produce a variety of other direct and indirect injuries. Direct damage is caused when the electric current passes through excitable tissues such as heart (arrhythmia or sudden cardiac arrest), nerves (seizures) or muscles (tetanic spasms, fractures). Indirect injury is commonly from muscle contractions that can cause falls or even asphyxia from tetanic contraction of the respiratory muscles.

CLASSIFICATION OF ELECTRICAL BURNS

From a clinical point of view, there are four varieties of electrical burns:

1. The true electrical burn caused by the flow of current
2. An arc burn resulting from the electric arc generated as the current passes from the source to an object
3. Flame burn caused by the ignition of clothing or surroundings
4. Lightning strikes. Electricity arcs at temperatures up to 4000°C and causes a flash-type burn without actual current flow through the body.

CARE ELECTRICAL BURN

Three issues are required to be addressed in the "golden hour" are:

1. Which patients require cardiac monitoring
2. Which patients are at risk for compartment syndrome and may need emergency surgical intervention
3. How fluid resuscitation should proceed with deep tissue injury that may not be appreciated on physical examination, particularly in the presence of pigmented urine.

CARDIAC MONITORING

Cardiac dysrhythmia, cardiac arrest and myocardial damage can occur postelectrical injuries requiring cardiac evaluation and monitoring. Children with electrical injuries should have ECG evaluation performed; and children with documented dysrhythmias, cardiac ischemia or history of loss of consciousness should be hospitalized for monitoring and care.

SURGICAL INTERVENTIONS

- Three clinical conditions necessitate emergency surgery for a patient with electrical burn:
    1. Evidence of compartment syndrome
    2. Evidence of nerve or vessel compression due to edematous compartment
    3. Ongoing rhabdomyolysis with myoglobinuria that threatens kidney failure. For circumferential 3rd degree thermal burn with evidence of tissue compression and neurovascular compromise escharotomy is indicated.
- Fasciotomies is reserved for patients with compartment syndrome and ongoing myonecrosis or neurovascular compromise.

FLUID THERAPY

Resuscitation fluids should be based on the extent of burn visible plus the estimated daily needs of the patient, adjusted according to the patient's response. Though, the optimal fluid and rate of repletion are unclear, aggressive intravenous (IV) fluid replacement is recommended in a patient with soft tissue injuries from electrical burn, especially if there are signs of muscle necrosis. Begin initial fluid resuscitation with isotonic saline. Avoid IV fluids containing potassium due to potential risk of hyperkalemia. Monitor heart rate, blood pressure, and urine output for guiding fluid therapy. Urine output of 1.5 to 2 mL/kg per hour is reasonable to minimize intratubular cast formation.

MYOGLOBINURIA

The presence of darker than light pink urine in a patient with an electrical burn indicates significant muscle damage, leading to myoglobinuria and/or hemoglobinuria secondary to rhabdomyolysis, present a risk of acute renal failure. This has been reported to be associated with poor outcomes, hence must be identified early and treated promptly. Fluid therapy is titrated to maintain the urine output double the goal rate of standard burn patient, which is continued till the urine appears clear. Failure to clear pigment from the urine is generally an indication of significant muscle necrosis or ongoing ischemia, can often be considered as an indication for operative intervention for decompression versus debridement.

COMPLICATIONS OF ELECTRICAL BURNS

Cataract formation is a common complication reported in 5–20% of electrical injury patients. Cataract can develop within a few weeks or may present years after the electrical injury with an average time till presentation of 6 months. Early ophthalmology evaluation as well as postdischarge follow-up is advised for these patients. Neurological complications as sequelae of high voltage electrical injuries are common and range from paralysis to Guillain-Barré, paresis, and transverse myelitis. Central manifestations include cognitive and emotional changes.

CONCLUSION

- Depending on the current pathway, different organs can get affected by the electrical burn. In high voltage electrical injury, ventricular fibrillation, myocardial damage and cardiac standstill is the common causes of mortality.
- "No let-go" phenomenon, caused by the alternate current may cause violent muscle contractions and fractures of long bones.
- Compartment syndrome is caused by deep tissues electrical burns, require early identification and surgical intervention/s as fasciotomy and/or early debridement for affected extremity salvage.
- Age-appropriate electric burn prevention measures as, electric outlet safety covers, keeping the electric appliances beyond the child's reach and not using the electric gadgets in bath or shower should be in place.

SUGGESTED READING

1. Arnoldo B, Klein M, Gibran NS. Practice guidelines for the management of electrical injuries. J Burn Care Res. 2006; 27:439–47.
2. Eileen Bernal, Brett D. Arnoldo. Electrical Injuries. In: Total Burn Care; Edited by: David N. Herndon. 5th edition, Elsevier; 2018; pp. 394–402.
3. Jonathan Friedstat, David A. Brown, Benjamin Levi. Chemical, Electrical, and Radiation Injuries. Clin Plastic Surg 44; 2017; 657–69.
4. Nicole Gibran. Electrical Injuries. In: Burn Care for General Surgeons and General Practitioners; Edited by: David G. Greenhalgh. Springer; 2016; pp.193–200.
5. Ten Duis HJ. Acute electrical burns. Semin Neurol. 1995;15(4):381–6.

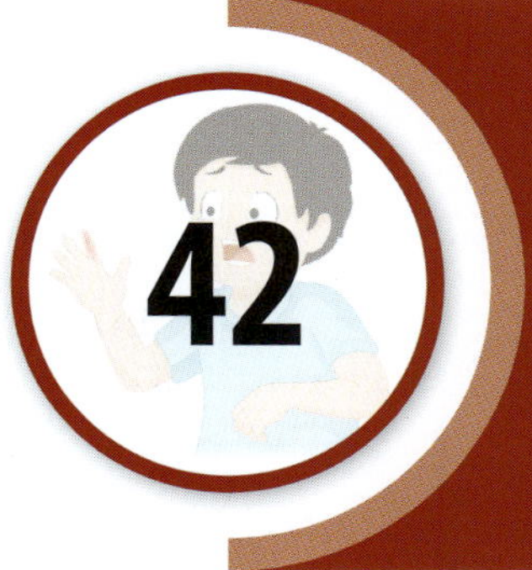

Burns and Scalds

K Sathishkumar, Manjula Anand

INTRODUCTION

Burns and scalds are acute injuries to the skin and underlying tissues caused by heat, friction, electrical discharge, chemicals, or radiation. Burns are a global health problem accounting for 1.8 lakh deaths annually. Ten lakh people are affected every year in India, and childhood burns contribute a significant proportion. Burns are the fifth most common cause of nonfatal childhood injuries. Most burns in children especially <5 years happen in kitchens due to spillage of hot liquids in utensils. Global burn registry data reveals >50% of children sustain major burns [≥15% total body surface area (TBSA)].

BURN CLASSIFICATION

Burns are classified based on the depth of injury and the percentage body surface of burns and are related to the outcome.

Burn classification			
Depth	*Appearance*	*Sensation*	*Healing*
Superficial	Dry, red, and blanches	Painful	3–6 days
Superficial partial thickness	Blisters, red, and blanches	Painful	7–21 days
Deep partial thickness	• Pink to white color • Sluggish blanching	Less painful	• >21 days • Usually needs surgery
Full thickness	• Waxy white to charred and black • No blanching	Not painful to touch	Does not heal without surgical treatment

TYPES OF THERMAL BURNS

Thermal burns are the most common type of burns in children and can result from:

- *Scalds:* Contact with hot liquids
- *Contact:* Hot solid objects
- *Flame:* From fire

PATHOPHYSIOLOGY

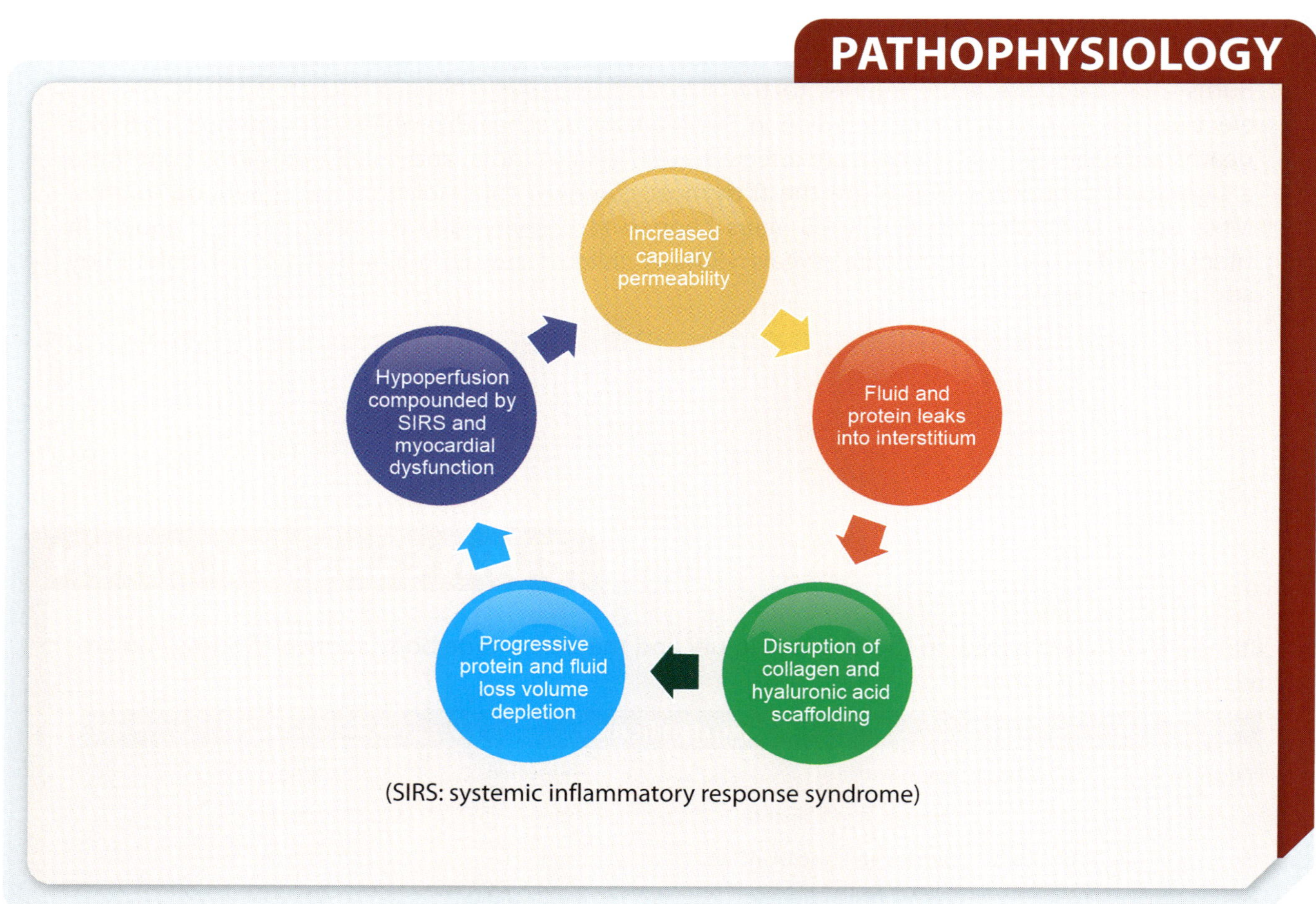

(SIRS: systemic inflammatory response syndrome)

ACUTE MANAGEMENT

- Do not be distracted by the dramatic nature of the burns. Treat any child with burns as trauma.
- *Focus on ABCDE (airway, breathing, circulation, disability, and exposure) approach to trauma. Correct issues with ABCDE first.*
- Start with cervical spine immobilization

ABCDE approach			
	Look for	***Concern***	***Intervention***
Airway	Stridor, hoarse voice, singed facial/nasal hair, soot at mouth or nose, and significant facial/neck burns/swelling	Airway obstruction from edema and respiratory collapse	• Early intubation if airway concerns • Consider difficult intubation Succinylcholine can be used until 48 hours
Breathing	• Burns in closed space respiratory distress and or hypoxemia (SpO_2 <94%) • Chest wall and abdominal burns, especially circumferential	• Carbon monoxide (CO) and cyanide poisoning • Smoke inhalational injury • Restriction of chest wall movements	• 100% oxygen • Hydroxocobalamin 70 mg/kg • O_2/nebulization, ventilatory support • Early escharotomy
Circulation	• Shock/profound hypovolemia is not a normal initial response to a burn • Look for absent/weak peripheral pulses	• *Shock at admission:* Look for blood loss (head, chest, abdomen, pelvis, and long bones) • *Cardiac dysfunction:* Cyanide poisoning/pneumothorax • Circumferential limb burn	• Blood products • Surgical consultation • Early escharotomy
Disability	• Hypoxemia • Shock • Head/spine injuries	Consider CO/Cyanide poisoning	Treat underlying cause
Exposure	• Check temperature • Other traumatic injuries	Hypothermia is invisible to the naked eye, unlike a burn injury	• Temperature control of room • Remove burnt clothing • Give warm intravenous (IV) fluids • Increase room temperature to 28–32°C • Remove constricting jewelry
Consider child abuse	• History inconsistent/not compatible with injury pattern • Delay in seeking treatment • Straight line of demarcation • Glove and stocking distribution • Child unusually passive • Burns of different ages		

INITIAL MANAGEMENT

- Remove hot burned clothing; copious irrigation with saline
- Cover open burns with dry sterile dressings. Do not break or aspirate intact blisters.
- Topical antibiotics—silver sulfadiazine (avoid near eyes and mouth), bacitracin can be used
- Consider early transfer to the burn center if:
  - Third-degree burns
  - Partial thickness burns >10%
  - Any burns involving the face, hands, feet, perineum, and genitalia
  - Electrical burns, chemical burns, and inhalational burns
  - Concomitant trauma or underlying comorbidities

FLUID RESUSCITATION

- Indications for resuscitation include >15% TBSA burnt, partial thickness (blistered), and full-thickness burns. In cases of <15–20 % burn area, start with 150% maintenance fluids.
- Crystalloids are the first choice, Ringer's lactate (RL) is used commonly. Isotonic crystalloids with 5% dextrose maintenance should be administered to infants and young children.

BURN SURFACE AREA CALCULATION

- *For older children >14 years:* Can use rule of nines
- *For young children:* Use age-appropriate charts like Lund–Browder chart or Shriners hospital chart.

Shriners Hospital Chart

Area	*Newborn (Area in %)*	*3 years (Area in %)*	*6 years (Area in %)*	*12 years (Area in %)*
Head	18	15	12	6
Trunk	40	40	40	38
Arms	16	16	16	18
Legs	26	29	32	38

INITIAL FLUID REQUIREMENT

Parkland formula: 4 mL × weight in kg × % body surface area (BSA) burnt (1/2 over first 8 hours from time of burn and 1/2 over next 16 hours) + maintenance fluids

- Formulas provide only a rough approximation of actual requirements. Careful tracking of response and adjustment of infusions are indicated.
- Urine output is easily monitored and is a sensitive indicator in the acute stage. Target >1 mL/kg for young children and >0.5 mL/kg for older children and adolescents.
- Combine urine output with monitoring of vital signs, sensorium, pulse volume, blood pressure, and metabolic acidosis to decide on increasing or decreasing the fluids.
- Use a multimodal approach [arterial blood pressure (BP) and echocardiogram) to assess the adequacy of resuscitation, especially in >40% body surface area (BSA) burns].

Be aware of increased fluid requirements in: Inhalational injury, electrical injury, delay in resuscitation, and concomitant trauma

ROLE OF COLLOIDS

Large-volume crystalloids lead to edema, compartment syndrome, airway edema, and acute respiratory distress syndrome (ARDS). 5% Albumin can be considered after 8–12 hours in burns with > 40% TBSA burns or high crystalloid requirement as evidenced by:

- The Ivy index of >250 mL/kg
- Total (or predicted total) resuscitation volume of 6 mL/kg/% TBSA

COMPREHENSIVE BURN MANAGEMENT

- *Pain:* Adequate pain control with intravenous (IV) fentanyl or morphine infusions or bolus. Procedural pain will need additional analgesia including fentanyl/ketamine.
- *Nutrition:* Burns cause a hypermetabolic response with protein and fat catabolism. Provide early enteral feeds within the first 24 hours if possible. Calories at 150% of basal metabolic rate (BMR) with 3–4 g/kg of protein are suggested for patients with burns. Early excision and grafting, adequate pain control, and temperature control reduce this catabolic response.
- *Immunization:* Tetanus immunization is indicated for burns >10%.
- *Antibiotics:* Empirical antibiotics are not routinely needed.
- *Infection prevention:* Surgical burn wound management and prevention of infection are important in improving outcomes. Children with >30% burns need to be managed in isolation units to prevent cross-infection and for temperature control.

SUGGESTED READING

1. Antoon AY. Burn injuries. In: Kliegman RM, Stanton BF, Schor NF, St. Geme JW, Behrman RE (Eds). Nelson Textbook of Pediatrics, volume 1, 21st edition. Philadelphia: Elsevier; 2021.
2. Bittner EA, Shank E, Woodson L, Martyn JA. Acute and perioperative care of burn injured patient. Anaesthesiology. 2015;122(2):448-64.
3. Duran C, Sheridan RL: Current concepts in the medical management of the pediatric burn patient. Curr Trauma Rep. 2016;2:202-9.
4. Jordan KC, Di Gennaro JL, von Saint André-von Arnim A, Stewart BT. Global trends in pediatric burn injuries and care capacity from the World Health Organization Global Burn Registry. Front Pediatr. 2022;10:954995.
5. Pruitt BA Jr. Protection from excessive resuscitation: "Pushing the pendulum back". J Trauma. 2000;49(3):567-8.
6. Romanowski KS, Palmieri TL. Pediatric burn resuscitation: Past, present, and future. Burns Trauma. 2017;5:26.
7. Rousseau AF, Massion PB, Laungani A, Nizet JL, Damas P, Ledoux D. Towards targeted early burn care: Lessons from a European survey. J Burn Care Res. 2014;35(4):e234-9.
8. Sheridan RL. Burn care for children. Pediatr Rev. 2018;39(6):273-86.
9. World Health Organization. (2013). Burns. [online] Available from https://www.who.int/news-room/fact-sheets/detail/burns [Last accessed March, 2024].

9 Section

Toxicology–II: Poisoning

Button Battery Ingestion in Children

Namrata Das, GV Basavaraja

INTRODUCTION

Button batteries (BBs) are found in common household items and when ingested, can lead to significant morbidity and mortality in the pediatric population.

They are disc-shaped metallic objects that look similar to coins and can get lodged in the pediatric esophagus, leading to significant injury. They are available in different unique sizes, shapes, and chemical properties.

Why is there a sudden increase in the incidence and morbidity?

The cause behind this rapid increase in morbidity and mortality seems to be due to a few specific changes in the market through that time period—change to lithium cells and increase in the size:

- *Change to lithium cells:* Lithium became the preferred cell type because of its longer shelf-life capacity, better stability at cool temperatures, lighter weight, and ability to carry twice the voltage of previously used mercuric oxide, manganese dioxide, and zinc-air cells.
- *Increase in size:* The larger diameter results in increased likelihood of esophageal impaction, whereas the lithium composition results in increased voltage delivery.
- More use of lithium batteries in remote control toys, watches, games, hearing aids, television (TV) remotes, etc.

TERMINOLOGIES AND DEFINITION

Some terminologies and definitions are as follows:

- *Parts of a button battery:* Lithium-ion batteries have *positive* electrode, *negative* electrode, battery separator, spacer, spring, and electrolyte. They are named according to their size and thickness.
- *Isothermic reaction:* An isothermic reaction is a type of thermodynamic process in which the temperature (T) of a system remains constant—$\Delta T = 0$.

- *Imprint:* The imprint on a button battery is a code that identifies the battery's chemical composition and size. The side of the imprint is the positive electrode and without the imprint is the negative electrode, which is important for a clinician to know to anticipate the severity and type of injury. For example, CR: lithium; LR: alkaline; SR: silver oxide; and 2032: where 20 mm is diameter and 32 mm is thickness.

ETIOPATHOLOGY

There are three mechanisms of how BBs cause tissue damage:

1. *Electrolysis and production of hydroxide ions* (most important mechanism)
2. Leakage of cell contents
3. Pressure injury

The main mechanism of injury by BB ingestion has been depicted in **Flowchart 1**.

Flowchart 1: The main mechanism of injury by button battery ingestion.

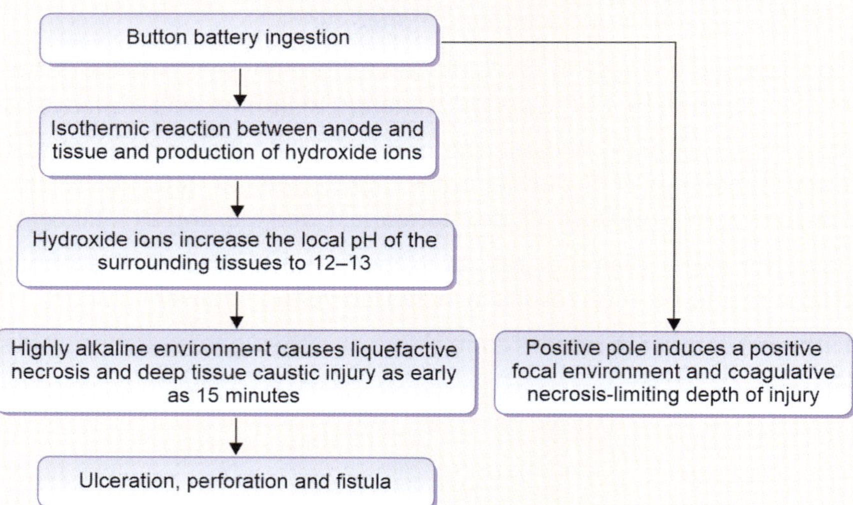

- Any battery over 1.2 V can cause injury hence even "dead" or "spent" BB unable to power electronics have enough retained capacitance to cause significant injury.
- Smaller BBs are less likely to cause injury as they pass through to the stomach but are implicated in cases of insertions into orifices (ear, nose, eyelid, and vagina) and should not be overlooked.

WHY ESOPHAGUS?

Button battery ingestion causes the most damage to the esophagus because:

- Esophagus contains anatomically narrowed regions where a large BB can get stuck.
- Electrolyte-rich esophageal environment facilitates BB current/injury.
- Rapid injury occurs with lithium batteries, whereas alkaline and zinc oxide take a few more hours to cause similar injury.
- Injury can even progress postremoval of BB causing delayed esophageal perforation and fistula.

Locations in esophagus:

- Upper esophageal sphincter (70%)
- Aortic crossover and mid bronchus (20%)
- Lower esophageal sphincter (10%)

The extent and type of injury has been illustrated in **Table 1**.

TABLE 1: Extent and type of injury.

Esophageal location	
Acute	• Extensive tissue damage leading to ulceration and perforation (<2 hours) • Esophageal stenosis, stricture, and perforation • Mediastinitis • Vocal cord injury (paresis and paralysis) • *Fistula:* Tracheoesophageal fistula and aortoesophageal fistula • Aspiration (rare)
Delayed	• Stricture, stenosis, and fistula • Spondylodiscitis (can take weeks or months to develop) • Recurrent laryngeal nerve injury
• Stomach • Intestine	• Ulceration, necrosis, and rarely perforation

After the esophagus, BB usually passes the remaining gastrointestinal (GI) tract successfully. Only 7 and 1.3% of overall complications occur in the stomach and small bowel, respectively as electrolysis does not occur there.

Even if the BB is not impacted in the esophagus and has passed lower down into the stomach, one cannot exclude esophageal injury, especially in unwitnessed ingestions when the total time of BB exposure is unknown.

Furthermore, the coingestion of a magnet may lead to entrapment in the stomach or intestinal wall with the battery and magnet causing necrosis. Children can present with an acute abdomen (stomach/intestinal perforation) to the emergency department.

RISK FACTORS FOR SEVERITY

Risk factors include:

- Esophageal location and orientation of the BB's negative pole (more necrosis at the side of negative pole)
- The estimated duration of impaction
- The properties of the specific battery:
  - *Metal:* Lithium
  - *Voltage:* 3 V
  - *Size:* >20 mm
- *Age of the child:* <6 years
- Magnet coingestion
- Presence of esophageal pathology (stenosis, stricture, and past surgery)

The presence of any of the above factors can be predictor of severe injury and need immediate attention and intervention.

CLINICAL FEATURES

The clinical features are given in **Table 2.**

TABLE 2: Clinical features.

Symptomatic	*Asymptomatic*
• Nausea, vomiting, drooling, chest discomfort • Difficulty swallowing, choking, gagging, refusal to eat • Fever, coughing, stridor, decreased appetite, fast breathing (may mimic a bacterial/viral illness) • Older children may give history of ingestion • Hematemesis, malena, epistaxis, poor sensorium suggests a severe injury—GI hemorrhage due to an aortoesophageal fistula	• Most of the children will be asymptomatic and have unwitnessed ingestion • Most complications occur after unwitnessed ingestions, as symptoms are variable and nonspecific, leading to delayed diagnosis • A high index of clinical suspicion of foreign body ingestion is very necessary in a toddler with nonspecific clinical presentation

EVALUATION

The evaluation of BB ingestion has been illustrated in **Flowchart 2**.

Flowchart 2: Evaluation of button battery ingestion.

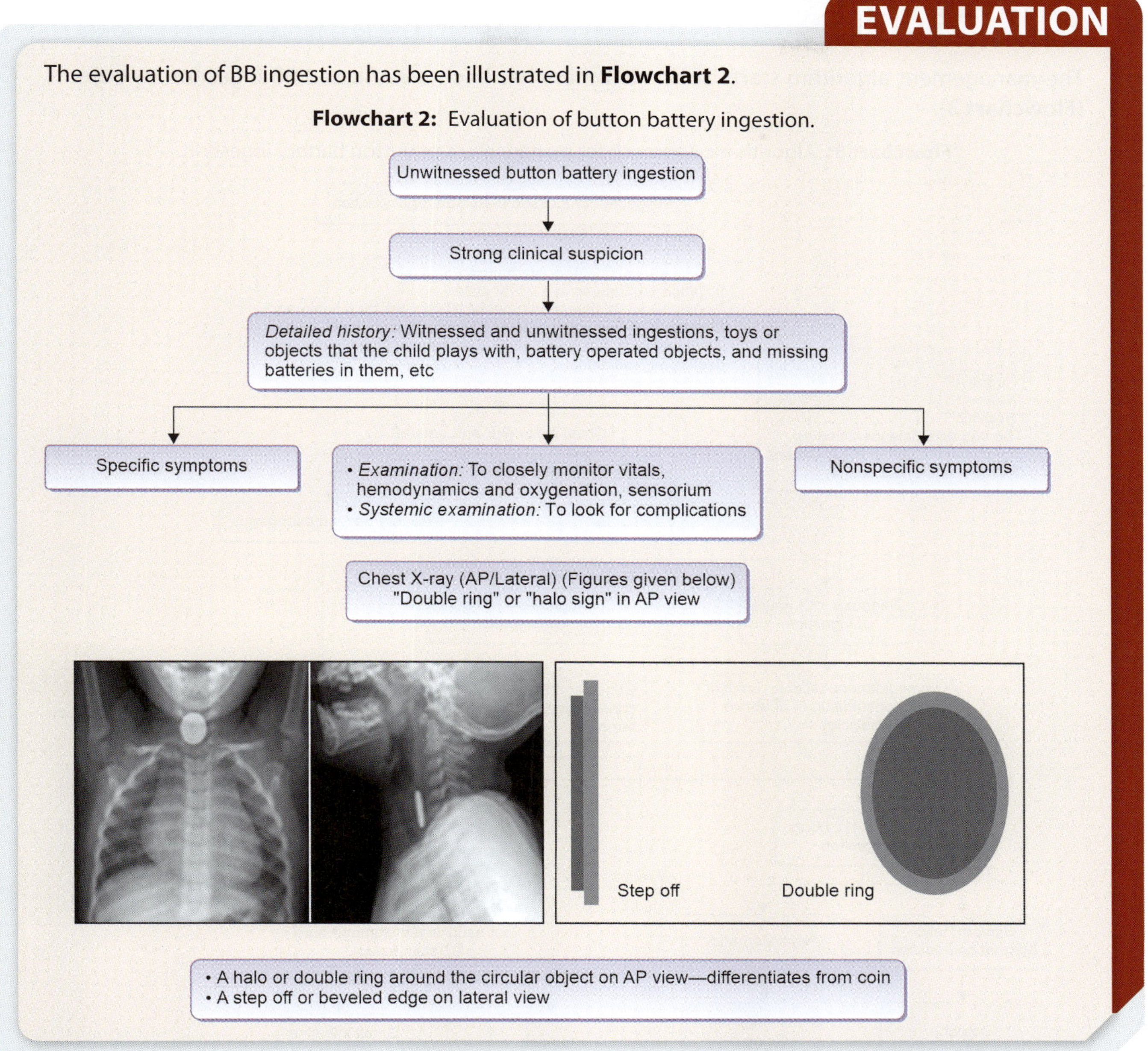

MANAGEMENT

The management algorithm starts at home if there has been a witnessed BB ingestion by parents **(Flowchart 3)**.

Flowchart 3: Algorithmic approach for management of button battery ingestion.

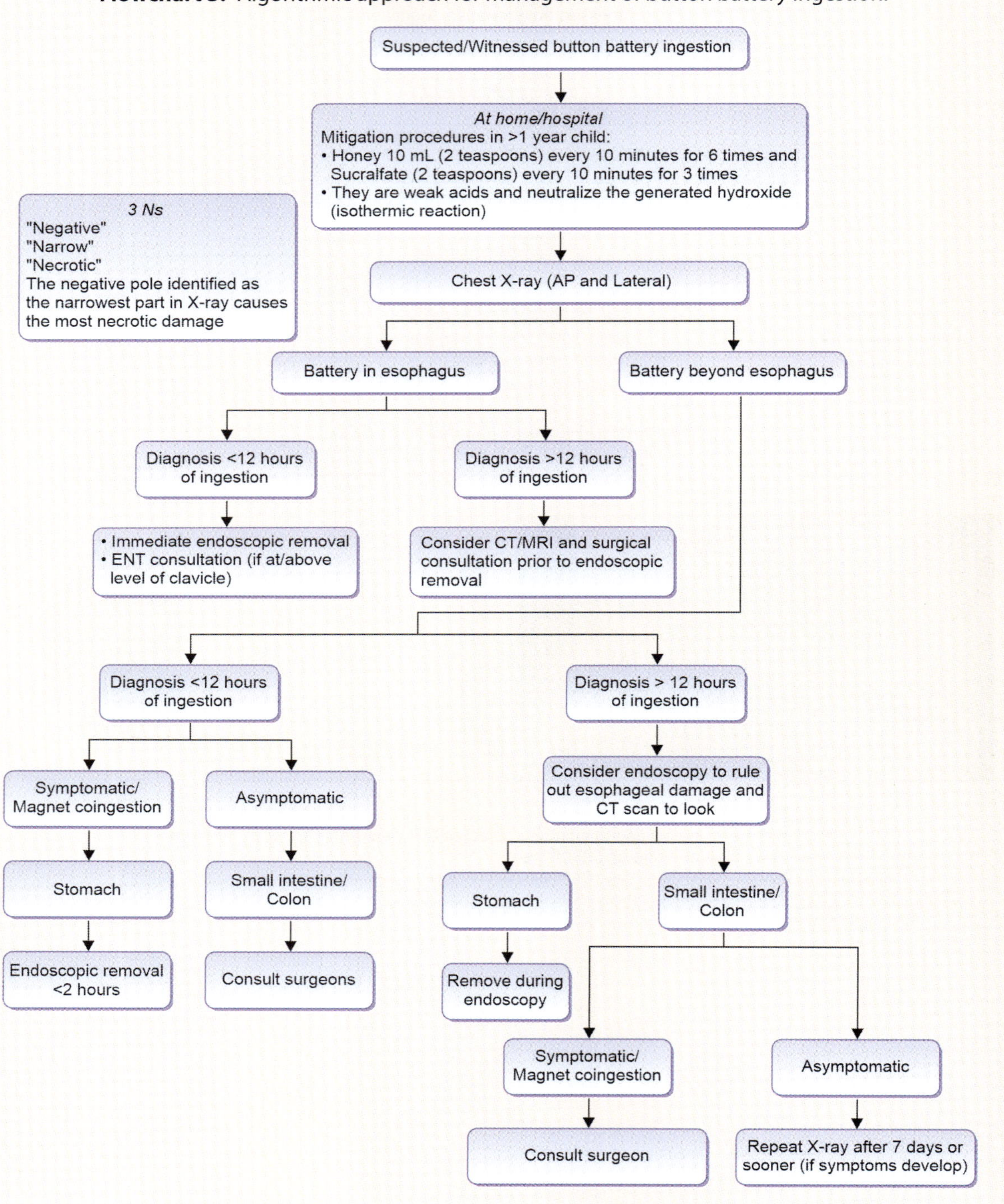

Endoscopy

Endoscopy should be the *gold standard* for BB removal as it allows direct visualization of the BB, site of impaction, and negative pole (side without the "+" sign and imprint) as this is the site of severe damage.

In case of significant mucosal damage, a nasogastric tube should be carefully placed endoscopically to maintain patency of the lumen and the patient should not receive any food by mouth until it is definite that no perforation or other complications have occurred.

If there is no evidence of perforation, irrigation of injured areas of esophagus with 50–150 mL 0.25% sterile acetic acid should be done to neutralize alkali.

- Even if the BB has passed beyond the esophagus, esophageal injury should be looked for, especially when it has magnet coingestion as it can cause entrapment of the battery to the wall of the stomach/intestine and cause necrosis/perforation.
- Concurrent direct laryngoscopy and bronchoscopy should be done to evaluate for airway injury and presence of fistula, especially when the negative pole of BB is facing anteriorly.

DIFFERENTIALS

Differential diagnoses involve:

- BB ingestion can be confused with a coin ingestion; however, the chest X-ray showing "double ring" or "halo sign" and "step off" sign **(Flowchart 2)** differentiates the two.
- Unwitnessed BB ingestion can present as vague symptoms and can mimic a viral/bacterial illness
- Posteriorly impacted negative pole of the BB can lead to aortoesophageal fistula and can present as severe acute massive upper GI hemorrhage.

POSTREMOVAL MONITORING AND FOLLOW-UP

- All patients with mucosal injury after battery removal should be admitted to the hospital and monitored closely for any associated complications.
- A clear liquid diet may be started if there are no signs of perforation on the esophagogram, which can be performed 1–2 days after removal of BB. When a clear liquid diet is tolerated, the diet can progress to soft foods.
- The plan for repeat endoscopies and imaging (CT/MRI) to look for damage to nearby structures should be individualized **(Flowchart 4)**.

Flowchart 4: Plan for repeat endoscopies and imaging.

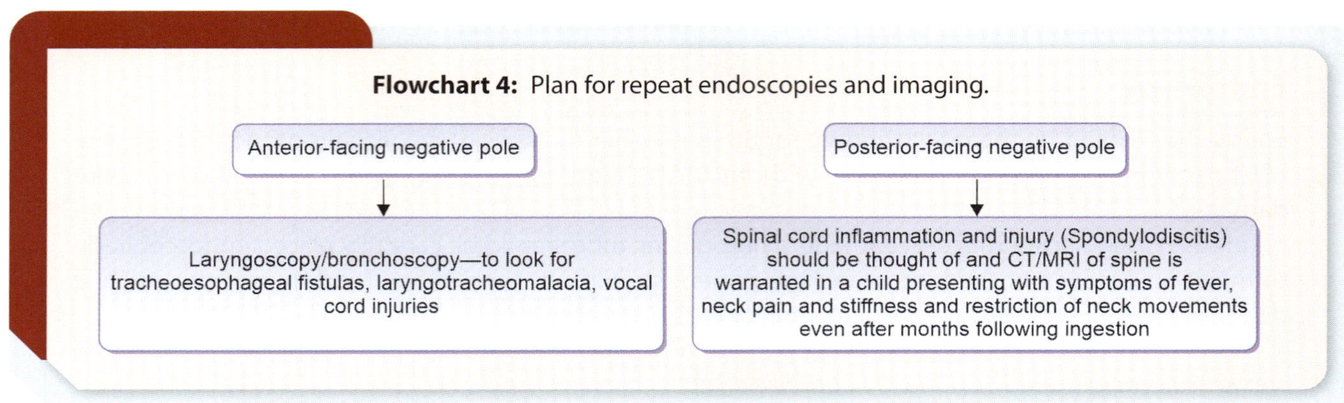

KEY LEARNING POINTS

- Prevention is always better than cure. Hence, health education of parents and caregivers regarding hazards of BBs is a must to make sure that they are inaccessible to children at home.
- BB ingestion is usually unwitnessed and may present with vague symptoms mimicking a viral/bacterial infection, hence clinical suspicion should be high.
- Parents should be educated about honey/sucralfate as mitigation procedures once they suspect BB ingestion in their child.
- The presence of BB beyond the esophagus, should not exclude esophageal injury.
- In all button battery ingestions, esophageal injury should be assumed as a rule, unless proved otherwise.

SUGGESTED READING

1. Burns H, Park SJ. Button battery injury: An update. AJGP. 2022;51(7):471-5.
2. Jatana KR, Rhoades K, Milkovich S, Jacobs IN. Basic mechanism of button battery ingestion injuries and novel mitigation strategies after diagnosis and removal. Laryngoscope. 2017;127(6):1276-82.
3. Lorenzo C, Azevedo S, Lopes JC, et al. Battery ingestion in children, an ongoing challenge: Recent experience of a tertiary centre. Front Pediatr. 2022;10.
4. Machta J, Hyer W. Diagnosis, management and prevention of button battery ingestion in childhood: A European Society for Paediatric Gastroenterology Hepatology and nutrition position paper. Arch Dis Child Educ Pract Ed. 2023;108(4):292-5.
5. Semple T, Calder A, Ramaswamy M, McHugh K. Button battery ingestion in children—a potentially catastrophic event of which all radiologists must be aware. Br J Radiol. 2018;91(1081):20160781.
6. Sethia R, Gibbs H, Jacobs IN, Reilly JS, Rhoades K, Jatana KR. Current management of button battery injuries. 2021;6(3):549-63.

Hydrocarbon Poisoning in Children

Javed Ismail, Syed Ahmed Zaki

INTRODUCTION

- Accidental poisoning remains a significant cause of morbidity and mortality among children globally. Within this spectrum of pediatric poisonings, hydrocarbon ingestion has emerged as a particularly concerning public health issue.
- Hydrocarbons were among the top 10 most frequently reported substances associated with fatalities in children younger than 6 years in the United States.[1]
- Among developing countries like India, Bangladesh, and Nepal, commonly available hydrocarbons like kerosene and paint thinners account for up to a significant proportion of all pediatric poisonings.[2-5]
- The widespread availability of hydrocarbon-containing products in domestic environments, coupled with young children's natural curiosity and exploratory behavior, contributes to the high incidence of accidental exposure.
- This chapter provides an overview of the pathophysiology, clinical presentation, assessment, and management of hydrocarbon poisoning in children.
- Hydrocarbons are a common constituent of many household chemicals, including cleaning agents, disinfectants, cooking fuels, and insect repellents.
- This widespread presence in domestic environment makes them a readily accessible potential toxic substance.
- The storage of these products in inappropriate containers, such as soft-drink bottles or water-storage cans, further increases the risk of accidental exposure, particularly for young children who are naturally curious and prone to mouthing objects.
- In a small percentage of patients, especially adolescents, intentional exposure from recreational inhalant misuse can occur.

TYPES OF HYDROCARBONS

Hydrocarbons are a heterogeneous group of organic substances that are primarily composed of carbon and hydrogen molecules. They come in four structural classes:[6]

1. *Aromatic hydrocarbons:* These contain a benzene ring and are among the most toxic hydrocarbons. They are used in solvents, glues, paints, and paint removers.
2. *Aliphatic hydrocarbons:* These are derived from petroleum distillates and are found in polishes, lamp oils, and lighter fluids.
3. *Halogenated hydrocarbons:* These contain fluorine, chlorine, or bromine, and are used in refrigeration (freon) and as insecticides and herbicides.
4. *Terpene hydrocarbons:* These are found in turpentine and pine oil.

Some hydrocarbons may be present in mixed forms like kerosene, which is a mixture of aliphatic, aromatic, and cycloparaffins in differing amounts, and some are used as aerosol spray propellants.

PATHOPHYSIOLOGY

Hydrocarbons exert their toxic effects through various mechanisms. The severity of hydrocarbon poisoning can vary depending on several factors, including:

- *Type of hydrocarbon:* Different hydrocarbons may have varying toxicities. Unlike the aromatic or aliphatic hydrocarbons, the halogenated hydrocarbons tend to cause a wider range of toxicity.
- *Viscosity:* The viscosity of a hydrocarbon can influence its aspiration risk; lower the viscosity deeper is the lung penetration.
- *Volatility:* The volatility of a hydrocarbon can affect its rate of absorption. Volatile hydrocarbons have an increased risk for pulmonary absorption.
- *Surface tension:* The surface tension of a hydrocarbon can influence its spread; lower surface tension allows for easy spread.

The most common route of exposure in children is accidental ingestion, leading to aspiration into the lungs. The aspiration of hydrocarbons can cause chemical pneumonitis, characterized by inflammation and damage to the lung tissue. This inflammatory process can result in alveolar collapse, hypoxemia, and respiratory distress. Cardiotoxicity can manifest as dysrhythmias, often secondary to catecholamine-induced myocardial sensitization. Gastrointestinal manifestations such as throat pain, abdominal pain, nausea, and vomiting are due to irritant effects. Hepatic: The chlorinated hydrocarbons, in particular carbon tetrachloride, are hepatotoxic and can cause free radical formation, lipid peroxidation, and centrilobular (zone III) necrosis. Dermal irritation may be caused after prolonged contact with the skin or mucosa, and partial- or full-thickness burns may also be caused. Hemolysis has been reported following the acute ingestion of various types of hydrocarbons. Neurological complications may include euphoria, depression, lethargy, convulsions, and coma. The volatile nature of many hydrocarbons allows for their rapid absorption through the lungs and gastrointestinal tract, leading to central nervous system (CNS) depression and other systemic effects.

CLINICAL FEATURES

The clinical presentation of hydrocarbon poisoning can vary depending on the type of hydrocarbon, type of exposure, the amount ingested, and the child's individual factors. However, common symptoms include:

- *Respiratory:* Cough, tachypnea, dyspnea, chest pain, cyanosis, and hypoxemia
- *Gastrointestinal:* Vomiting, abdominal pain, and nausea
- *Cardiovascular:* Arrhythmias
- *Neurological:* Lethargy, drowsiness, altered mental status, seizures, and coma
- *Renal:* Acute kidney injury
- *Skin:* Skin irritation or burns
- *Hematological:* Anemia and thrombocytopenia

EVALUATION

The evaluation of suspected hydrocarbon poisoning requires a thorough history and physical examination. Key elements of the history include the type of exposure, type of substance ingested, the amount consumed, the time of exposure, and the presence of any symptoms. Ingestion of even small amounts can result in aspiration pneumonitis. The physical examination should focus on assessing the child's cardiorespiratory status, neurologic function, and gastrointestinal symptoms.

EMERGENCY CARE

Initial Assessment and Management

The evaluation of suspected hydrocarbon poisoning requires a comprehensive history and physical examination, focusing on the type of substance ingested, the amount consumed, the time of exposure, and the presence of any symptoms. Cardiorespiratory status, neurologic function, and gastrointestinal symptoms should be assessed.

Decontamination

To prevent ongoing exposure, contaminated clothing should be removed expeditiously. Affected skin and hair should be thoroughly cleansed to eliminate residual hydrocarbons, as many of these substances can induce cutaneous irritation. In case of prolonged exposure to hydrocarbons like gasoline or methylene chloride, which can cause cell membrane injury and lipid dissolution, initial treatment should prioritize pain control and copious water irrigation. Importantly, external decontamination should not delay critical life-saving interventions.

Activated charcoal has limited binding capacity for hydrocarbons and increases risk of aspiration, therefore it is not recommended. Given the risk of inducing emesis and subsequent pulmonary aspiration, gastric emptying procedure, such as nasogastric lavage is *contraindicated*. Nasogastric lavage should only be considered in rare cases of ingestion of large quantities of aromatic hydrocarbons (less likely in children) where the risk of systemic toxicity from gastrointestinal absorption of the hydrocarbon exceeds the increased risk of pulmonary aspiration associated with this procedure. Furthermore, nasogastric lavage should be withheld in patients with a depressed mental status who may not be able to protect their airway, unless endotracheal intubation is performed first.

SPECIFIC MANAGEMENT

Specific management typically involves:

- *Asymptomatic patients:* Asymptomatic patients should be observed with continuous pulse oximetry for at least 6 hours. If they remain asymptomatic, a chest radiograph can be obtained after 4–6 hours of exposure to evaluate for aspiration. Radiological changes may not be apparent if the X-ray is done immediately after exposure. In patients with electrocardiography (ECG) changes, monitor electrolytes and correct if abnormal. Hypokalemia is common in hydrocarbon exposure, and can rarely present as periodic paralysis.[7] Continue to replace fluid losses with maintenance intravenous fluids; fluid resuscitation may be considered in patients with hemodynamic instability.
- *Patients with respiratory distress:* Patients with mild tachypnea can be supported with low-flow or high-flow nasal oxygen or noninvasive ventilation as appropriate. Those exhibiting signs of progressive respiratory failure or impending respiratory failure despite supplemental oxygen may require rapid sequence intubation and positive pressure ventilation. High-frequency ventilation might be helpful in patients with severe hypoxic respiratory failure. Extracorporeal membrane oxygenation may be lifesaving in selected patients who fail advanced modes of ventilation.[8]
- *Role of antibiotics:* Antibiotics are used to treat secondary infections, although there is no evidence supporting prophylactic use.[9] Antibiotic therapy may be considered in cases of recurrent fever after the initial 48 hours, increasing infiltrate on chest radiograph, leukocytosis persisting beyond 48 hours, or a positive bacterial culture of sputum or tracheal aspirate.

- *Management of arrhythmias:* If arrhythmias occur, electrolytes, including magnesium and potassium, should be checked. For patients presenting with ventricular arrhythmias with cardiac arrest (ventricular fibrillation or pulseless ventricular tachycardia), early administration of lidocaine should be considered. Avoidance of catecholamines like epinephrine infusion in cases of ventricular fibrillation is recommended.
- *Patients with seizures and altered mental status:* Blood sugar should be checked. Benzodiazepines (e.g., diazepam or lorazepam) are recommended to abort seizures. In patients presenting with status epilepticus, arrhythmogenic anticonvulsants (e.g., fosphenytoin and phenytoin) may be avoided. Other etiologies of altered mental status should be investigated as clinically appropriate.
- *Role of steroids and surfactants:* Steroids and surfactants have not been shown to be beneficial in hydrocarbon poisoning.[9]
- *Renal and hepatic effects:* Exposure to hydrocarbons like toluene can result in severe metabolic acidosis. Other renal complications, including renal tubular damage, acute kidney injury, and renal calculi can occur. Rhabdomyolysis can occur secondary to hypokalemia and hypophosphatemia. Biliary tract injury occurs out of proportion to hepatocellular damage, which is reflected as elevated alkaline phosphatase and gamma-glutamyl transpeptidase.[10]

The algorithm approach to the management of hydrocarbon poisoning is given in **Flowchart 1**.

Flowchart 1: Algorithm on management of hydrocarbon poisoning.

Hydrocarbon ingestion

→ *Asymptomatic*
- Decontamination
- Cardiorespiratory monitoring
- Chest radiograph after 4–6 hours of ingestion

→ *Continues to remain asymptomatic:* Can be discharged after 6 hours of monitoring

→ *Symptomatic*

→ *Decontamination:*
- Remove contaminated clothing, wash skin and exposed areas
- Activated charcoal and gastric lavage are contraindicated

→ *Respiratory:*
- Oxygen therpy to treat hypoxia
- Blood gas and vitals monitoring
- Respiratory support as indicated
- Steroids and antibiotics not routinely indicated

→ *Other systems:*
- Neurological monitoring and treat seizures with benzodiazepines
- ECG monitoring for arrhythmias
- Supportive care for gastrointestinal manifestations

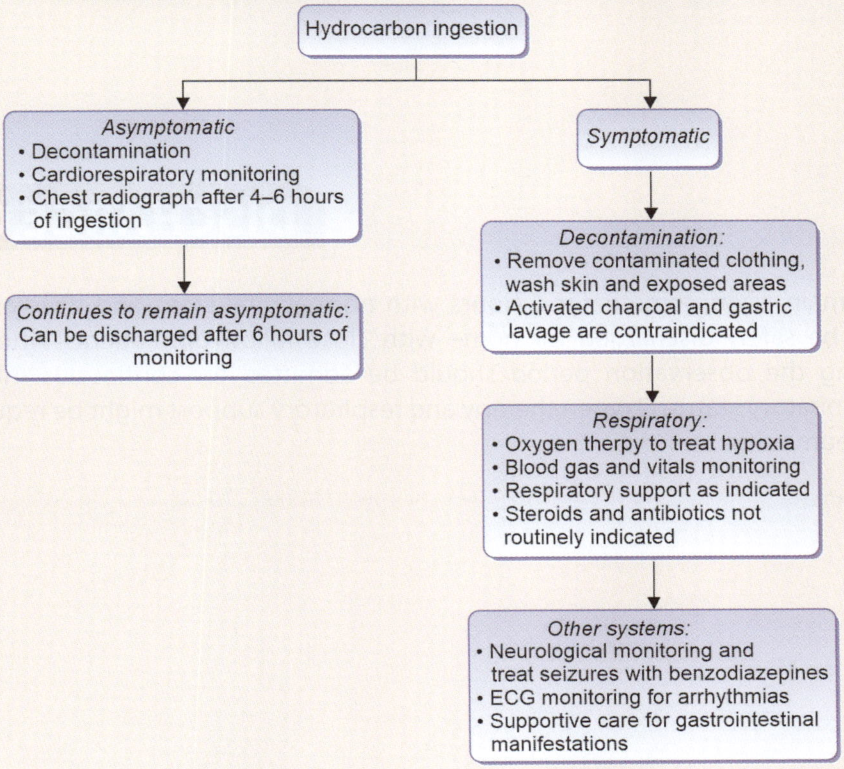

MONITORING

Continuous monitoring of vital signs, oxygen saturation, and cardiorespiratory status is essential. Serial chest X-rays may be obtained to assess for pneumonitis, if respiratory symptoms worsen.

Specific Considerations for Kerosene and Gasoline

Kerosene and gasoline, being highly volatile, low-viscosity, and low-surface tension substances, pose a greater risk of aspiration and lung injury. These characteristics contribute to their rapid absorption and potential for causing severe respiratory complications.

While the management of kerosene and gasoline poisoning is generally similar to other hydrocarbons, specific considerations may include:

- *Aspiration risk:* Due to their physical properties, kerosene and gasoline are more likely to be aspirated into the lungs, increasing the risk of pneumonitis and other respiratory complications.
- *Rapid onset of symptoms:* These hydrocarbons can often cause a more rapid onset of symptoms, requiring prompt medical attention.
- *Long-term effects:* In severe cases, aspiration of kerosene or gasoline can lead to long-term pulmonary sequelae, such as pulmonary fibrosis.

DISCHARGE CRITERIA

Patients who remain asymptomatic for 6 hours with normal vital signs and have a normal chest radiograph can be safely discharged for home with close follow-up. Patients who develop any symptoms during the observation period should be admitted for continuous monitoring and evaluation of respiratory status. Oxygen therapy and respiratory support might be required for those with signs of pneumonitis.

KEY LEARNING POINTS

- Hydrocarbon poisoning remains a significant health problem in children.
- Respiratory, neurological, and cardiac manifestations are the main adverse effects. Nasogastric lavage or activated charcoal are contraindicated.
- Respiratory symptoms can manifest up to 6 hours after exposure.
- While most cases have a favorable outcome with appropriate management, severe complications can occur.
- Early diagnosis, prompt intervention, and supportive care are crucial for optimizing patient outcomes.

REFERENCES

1. Gummin DD, Mowry JB, Beuhler MC, Spyker DA, Rivers LJ, Feldman R, et al. 2022 Annual Report of the National Poison Data System® (NPDS) from America's Poison Centers®: 40th Annual Report. Clin Toxicol (Phila). 2023;61(10):717-939.
2. Gupta P, Singh RP, Murali MV, Bhargava SK, Sharma P. Kerosene oil poisoning–a childhood menace. Indian Pediatr. 1992;29(8):979-84.
3. Vuppala AK, Nelakurthi R, Akunuri S, Arif A, NM A. Clinico-demographic profile and outcome of acute pediatric hydrocarbon poisoning in South India. Public Health Toxicol. 2024;4(2):1-6.
4. Anwar S, Rahman A, Houqe SA, Moshed AA, Yasmin L, Saleh A, et al. Clinical Profile of Kerosene Poisoning in a Tertiary Level Hospital in Bangladesh. Bangladesh J Child Health. 2014;38(1):11-4.
5. Dhakal AK, Shrestha D, Shakya A, Shah SC, Shakya H. Clinical Profile of Acute Poisoning in Children at a Teaching Hospital in Lalitpur. J Nepal Paediatr Soc. 2014;34(2):100-3.
6. Curtis J, Metheny E, Sergent SR. Hydrocarbon Toxicity. StatPearls [Internet]. Treasure Island (FL): StatPearls Publishing; 2024 Available from: http://www.ncbi.nlm.nih.gov/books/NBK499883/ [Last accessed September, 2024].
7. Anitha A, Selvaraj V, Kandasamy SK, Ismail J. Hypokalemic periodic paralysis associated with glue-sniffing. Indian J Pediatr. 2016;83(8):870.
8. Di Nardo M, Alunni Fegatelli D, Marano M, Danoff J, Kim HK. Use of Extracorporeal Membrane Oxygenation in Acutely Poisoned Pediatric Patients in United States: A Retrospective Analysis of the Extracorporeal Life Support Registry From 2003 to 2019. Crit Care Med. 2022;50(4):655-64.
9. Das S, Behera SK, Xavier AS, Selvarajan S. Prophylactic Use of steroids and antibiotics in acute hydrocarbon poisoning in children. J Pharm Pract. 2020;33(1):90-5.
10. Camara-Lemarroy CR, Rodríguez-Gutiérrez R, Monreal-Robles R, González-González JG. Acute toluene intoxication–clinical presentation, management and prognosis: A prospective observational study. BMC Emerg Med. 2015;15:19.

45 Iron Poisoning

Poovazhagi V

INTRODUCTION

Iron is widely available leading to accidental poisoning which can be fatal in children. It is the prenatal iron supplements or the supplement for school children which serve as the source of iron. Timely recognition and appropriate management are essential for survival. Iron poisoning can be accidental in young kids or suicidal in older children. The bright color, sugar coating, and the appearance of that of a candy appeal the kids for ingestion.

PATHOLOGY

The dose of ingestion is associated with severity of poisoning. Elemental iron ingested has to be calculated for the dose per kilogram. Ingestion up to 20 mg/kg is nontoxic. Moderate ingestion is 20–60 mg/kg and severe ingestion is >60 mg/kg. However, there is literature evidence for severe toxicity after 40–60 mg/kg. Ferric iron (Fe^{3+}) is toxic to tissues leading to free radical injury. Following acute iron ingestion, it causes corrosive injury or cellular injury. Corrosive injury causes gastrointestinal mucosal cell necrosis features. Free iron crosses cell membranes and concentrates in the mitochondria and acts as an electron sink leading to anaerobic metabolism and lactic acidosis by cellular injury. These excess free radicals cause peroxidation of lipids and proteins and lead to organ damage. Lung injury leads to acute respiratory distress syndrome (ARDS). Elemental iron content is more important than iron salt. The following iron salts are commonly found over the counter: Ferrous sulfate (20% elemental iron), ferrous gluconate (12% elemental iron), and ferrous fumarate (33% elemental iron).

CLINICAL FEATURES

Iron poisoning presents as five clinical stages[1,2] and are summarized in **Table 1**.

TABLE 1: Clinical features of iron poisoning.

Stage	*Time*	*Clinical features*
1	30 minutes to 6 hours	Gastrointestinal symptoms like anorexia, nausea, vomiting, pain in abdomen, and diarrhea. Hemorrhagic necrosis of the mucosa leads to hematemesis*
2	6–24 hours—latent phase	Stage of no symptoms; child looks stable and is false reassuring
3	6–72 hours	Multiorgan involvement with liver necrosis, myocardial dysfunction
4	12–96 hours	Elevated liver enzymes will be noted leading to acute liver cell failure
5	2–8 weeks	Gastrointestinal scarring causing gastric outlet obstruction

*In children with enteric-coated tablet ingestion, there may be a delay of clinical presentation up to 12 hours. Persistent vomiting for more than 4 times indicates severe poisoning.

Not all children will pass through these stages in succession. Children may present without gastrointestinal symptoms.

MANAGEMENT

History will help in identifying the ingested dose per kilogram. However, serum levels confirm ingestion, guide treatment, and give prognostic information. It is done at 4–6 hours of ingestion. Iron is rapidly cleared from the serum by 6 hours and deposited in the liver. Blood sample obtained beyond 6 hours may not give reliable information about the degree of intoxication from serum. In time-release formulations or enteric-coated preparations, the sample can be taken at 6–8 hours of ingestion due to delayed absorption. Serum iron levels below 350 μg/dL are indicative of minimal toxicity, 350–500 μg/dL of moderate toxicity, and beyond 500 μg/dL of severe systemic toxicity. Iron tablets are radio-opaque and may be seen in X-ray abdomen but not always. Blood counts may reveal leukocytosis, blood sugar may show hyperglycemia, and blood gases reveal metabolic acidosis. Monitor liver enzymes, urea and creatinine after 24 hours of ingestion. Get blood grouping typing done.

DIFFERENTIAL DIAGNOSIS

It includes poisoning with drugs which cause gastrointestinal symptoms predominantly with other system involvement. Differential diagnosis of iron poisoning is summarized in **Table 2**.

TABLE 2: Differential diagnosis of iron poisoning.

Diagnosis	*Clinical features*
Salicylates	Vomiting, tinnitus, liver cell failure, coagulopathy, neurological features, pulmonary edema, hyperglycemia/hypoglycemia, metabolic acidosis, respiratory alkalosis
Organophosphorus	Bradycardia, bradycardia, pinpoint pupils, increased sweating, lacrimation, salivation, diarrhea, pulmonary edema, fasciculations lethargy, and respiratory failure
Nicotine	Nausea and vomiting, abdominal pain, salivation, tachycardia, hypertension, bronchorrhea, bronchospasm, wheeze, agitation, fasciculation, and seizures of rapid onset
NSAIDs	Tinnitus, drowsiness, nausea, vomiting, headache, pain in abdomen, depressed sensorium
Mushroom poisoning	Pain abdomen, vomiting, feeling sick, watery diarrhea or bloody diarrhea

(NSAIDs: nonsteroidal anti-inflammatory drugs)

History and laboratory findings will help to rule out other poisoning.

SUPPORTIVE THERAPY

Decontamination with gastric lavage is indicated in the following: (1) If the child is seen in <1 hour of ingestion, (2) If the child has ingested >60 mg/kg, (3) Ingestion of sustained release tablets, (4) If X-ray abdomen reveals iron tablets in the stomach.

There is no role of activated charcoal. Whole-bowel irrigation is an alternative at 150–250 mL/hr and is indicated if X-ray abdomen shows ingestion of iron tablets of >60 mg/kg. This is given at a dose of 15 mL/kg/hr orally until the rectal effluent is clear. Whole-bowel irrigation is contraindicated if there are signs of hemorrhage.

Children with hemodynamic compromise may need fluid resuscitation including blood products. Acute liver cell failure is treated by standard protocols. Pressor therapy may be needed. Metabolic acidosis may warrant sodium bicarbonate. Acute renal failure may need renal replacement therapy.

SPECIFIC ANTIDOTE

Desferrioxamine (syn: deferoxamine) is indicated in features of clinical toxicity like lethargy, hypotonia, tachypnea, tachycardia, seizures or coma, metabolic acidosis, serum free iron >50 µg/dL or serum iron >350 µg/dL, or visualization of iron tablets in X-ray. Deferoxamine binds ferric ions in the blood leading to formation of ferrioxamine. This is excreted in urine. Desferrioxamine removes the free iron that is involved in cellular dysfunction. The iron already bound to hemoglobin or transferrin is not affected by desferrioxamine. Start intravenous infusion at a dose of 10 mg/kg/hr and gradually increase with 5-mg increments up to 35 mg/kg to avoid hypotension. Presence of vinrose color to urine, persistent or worsening metabolic acidosis, and persistent or development of organ failure should prompt increments of infusion. Desferrioxamine may lead to tachycardia, hypotension, and shock if given intravenously rapidly. Generalized flushing, erythema, and urticaria may be seen. Beyond 4 hours, reduce the dose of desferrioxamine. Total dose should not exceed 80 mg/kg/day[3] and the usual duration will be 12–16 hours. Desferrioxamine is associated with pulmonary toxicity; hence, limit the usage to <24 hours. Rare literature reports exist for infusion of desferrioxamine for >24 hours.[4] Proposed mechanisms for pulmonary injury include free radical formation and intracellular catalase depletion.[5] Urine changes to vinrose color after desferrioxamine therapy. Continue till disappearance of symptoms or resolution of metabolic acidosis and disappearance of vinrose color of urine. Urine color may be pink, reddish, or orange and it is not indicative of efficacy or lack of efficacy of the chelator. Plasmapheresis is indicated along with desferrioxamine in children with life-threatening intoxication. Continuous venovenous hemofiltration, hemodialysis, and plasmapheresis have resulted in enhanced survival in severe toxicity.[6-8] In children with acute liver failure with elevated enzymes, *N*-acetylcysteine has been tried. Liver transplant may be the option in children with liver cell failure. Management of iron poisoning is summarized in **Flowchart 1**. Watch for complications like acute renal failure, acute liver cell necrosis, ARDS, and infections with *Yersinia*. Follow-up these children with psychiatric counseling. Prevention of accidental poisoning is by storing iron tablets in areas that are not accessible to children. Child-resistant closures should be in place for storage bottles which have iron tablets.

Flowchart 1: Management of iron poisoning—admit all children with iron poisoning.

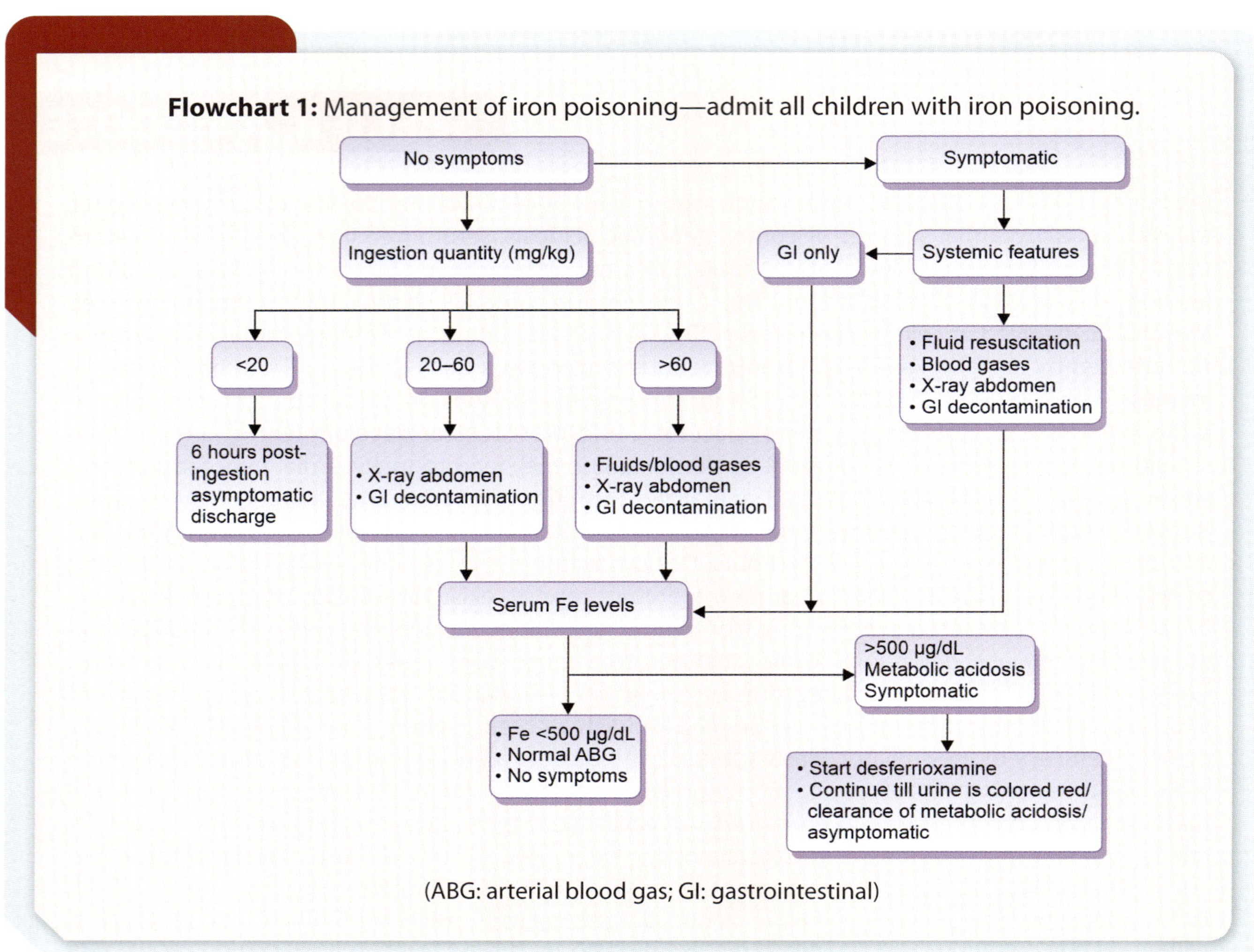

(ABG: arterial blood gas; GI: gastrointestinal)

KEY LEARNING POINTS

- Iron poisoning is dose related and can be fatal.
- Corrosive injury of the gastrointestinal system and cellular toxicity are the major pathologies.
- Gastrointestinal, cardiac, hepatic, renal involvement, and coagulopathy are the clinical features.
- History, clinical features, and serum levels of iron help in diagnosis.
- Treatment is supportive and a specific antidote is desferrioxamine.
- Prevention of iron ingestion by storing in places out of reach of children is warranted.

REFERENCES

1. Yuen HW, Becker W. Iron Toxicity. [Updated 2023 Jun 26]. In: StatPearls [Internet]. Treasure Island (FL): StatPearls Publishing; 2024 Jan-. [online] Available from https://www.ncbi.nlm.nih.gov/books/NBK459224 [Last accessed April, 2024].
2. Liebelt EL. (2024). Iron poisoning. [online] Available from https://www.uptodate.com/contents/acute-iron-poisoning [Last accessed April, 2024].
3. The Royal Children's Hospital Melbourne. Clinical practice guidelines. Iron poisoning. [online] Available from https://www.rch.org.au/clinicalguide/guideline_index/iron_poisoning/dt 10.2.2024.
4. Lança ASF, Romana ASC, Silva AC, Ferreira MG. Acute Oral Iron Poisoning in the Pediatric Emergency Department. Pediatr Oncol J. 2023;20:56-8.
5. Tenenbein M, Kowalski S, Sienko A, Bowden DH, Adamson IY. Pulmonary toxic effects of continuous administration in acute iron poisoning. Lancet. 1992;339:699-701.
6. Gumber MR, Kute VB, Shah PR, Vanikar AV, Patel HV, Balwani MR. Successful treatment of severe iron intoxication with gastrointestinal decontamination, deferoxamine, and hemodialysis, renal failure. Renal Fail. 35(5):729-31.
7. Nye R, Singh T. Use of CRRT and plasmapheresis to treat simultaneous iron and acetaminophen overdose. Blood Purif. 2022;51:292-5.
8. Chandran J, Sanketh R, Vyasam S, Chrysolyte A, Ebenezer K. Accidental iron poisoning in children—Experience from a teaching institution. J Fam Med Primary Care. 2023;12(10):2520-3.

46 Methemoglobinemia

Sibabratta Patnaik, Sumita Mishra

INTRODUCTION

- Methemoglobinemia is a life-threatening condition caused due to an abnormal hemoglobin with decreased oxygen-carrying capacity, converting the iron in hemoglobin from ferrous (Fe^{2+}) to ferric (Fe^{3+}) form.
- Thus, it can lead to histotoxic hypoxia. Medications and exposure to chemicals are the common causes of methemoglobinemia.

PATHOPHYSIOLOGY

The ferric form of iron in methemoglobinemia renders hemoglobin binding to oxygen ineffective. The allosteric bond formation shifts the oxygen-dissociation curve to the left and impairs oxygen release from hemoglobin causing tissue hypoxia.

Metabolic Processes

- *Major pathway:* This pathway primarily uses *cytochrome-b5 reductase*, an enzyme dependent on nicotinamide adenine dinucleotide (NADH) produced during glycolysis. This is the dominant system, responsible for maintaining methemoglobin levels below 1% under normal physiological conditions.
- *Minor pathway:* This pathway uses *NADPH-methemoglobin reductase*, an enzyme dependent on nicotinamide adenine dinucleotide phosphate hydrogen (NADPH), which is generated by the activity of glucose-6-phosphate dehydrogenase (G6PD) in the hexose monophosphate (HMP) shunt pathway. Although less efficient than the major pathway, it acts as a backup system to help reduce excess methemoglobin levels.

Both pathways are crucial in maintaining the balance between oxidized and reduced hemoglobin, ensuring optimal oxygen transport and delivery.

ETIOLOGY

- *Congenital:* Associated with enzyme deficiencies like cytochrome-b5 reductase, NADPH-MetHb reductase, and hemoglobin M disease (substitution of amino acid with tyrosine)
- *Acquired:* Exposure to direct oxidizing agents (e.g., benzocaine and prilocaine), indirect oxidation (e.g., nitrates), or metabolic activation (e.g., aniline and dapsone) **(Box 1)**

BOX 1: Drugs and toxins responsible for methemoglobinemia.
Drugs: • *Analgesics:* Phenazopyridine • *Antiepileptics:* Phenytoin and sodium valproate • *Anesthetics:* Benzocaine, prilocaine, and lidocaine • *Antimicrobials:* Chloroquine, dapsone, primaquine, quinine, sulfamethoxazole, rifampin, trimethoprim, and nitrofurantoin • *Antineoplastics:* Cyclophosphamide and flutamide • *Antigout:* Rasburicase • *Nitrates:* Amyl nitrate and nitroglycerine, nitroprusside, nitric oxide, and isosorbide dinitrate • *Other drugs:* Metoclopramide and methylene blue
Toxins: • Aniline dye • Naphthalene • Trinitrotoluene (TNT) • Indigo Carmine • Chlorates • Bromates • Herbicides and pesticide

CLINICAL FEATURES

Many times, the source of inciting agent may not be known, as the child may not be able to recall the sequence of events. A naphthalene ball or a common household item may be accidentally ingested by a child and can trigger symptoms, particularly in those with G6PD deficiency. The child may present with cyanosis, fatigue, depression, seizures, dysrhythmias, pallor, weakness, headache, coma, and death as part of the spectrum of methemoglobinemia. The clinical severity depends on the percentage of methemoglobin, the rate at which it was accumulated, and their capacity to naturally eliminate it, etc.

- *<13% methemoglobin (MetHb):* Asymptomatic or cyanosis; oxygen delivery intact
- *13–20% MetHb:* Light-headedness and anxiety; mild hypoxia
- *20–50% MetHb:* Headache, confusion, dyspnea; significant hypoxia
- *50–70% MetHb:* Seizures, lethargy, arrhythmias; life-threatening
- *>70% MetHb:* Fatal due to severe hypoxia and collapse

CLASSICAL CASES

- "Chocolate-brown blood" appearance is typically observed in patients with methemoglobinemia.
- The patient appears cyanotic without respiratory distress but does not improve with 100% oxygen—"refractory hypoxemia".
- Arterial oxygen tension remains normal or raised despite cyanosis. But oxygen saturation (SpO_2) will be low.
- Oxygen saturation calculated from arterial blood gas (SaO_2) is misleading. SpO_2 is usually lower than normal but does not correspond to the true degree of desaturation.
- Usually, SaO_2 and SpO_2 difference (saturation gap) is <5%. But if the saturation gap is >5%, it is suggestive of abnormal hemoglobin like MetHb.

EVALUATION

Evaluation is done by the following:

- *Blood profile:* Complete blood count (CBC), peripheral smear arterial blood gas (ABG), lactate dehydrogenase (LDH), and reticulocyte count
- *Organ function assessment:* Liver function test (LFT) and renal function test (RFT)
- Genetic testing in congenital causes
- *High-performance liquid chromatography (HPLC):* To detect abnormal hemoglobin like HbM
- G6PD activity
- *Enzyme assays:* Genetic causes

MANAGEMENT

Congenital Methemoglobinemia

- *Cyb5R deficiency:* Treatment is done with oral methylene blue (MB) after excluding G6PD deficiency. If G6PD deficiency is present, treatment can involve ascorbic acid. MB is administered intravenously at a dose of 1–2 mg/kg or orally at 100–300 mg daily. Ascorbic acid is typically given at 1,000 mg (200–500 mg/day) thrice daily. (Both are ineffective in HbM.)
- Patients at risk must avoid precipitating factors causing methemoglobinemia.

Acquired Methemoglobinemia

- *Toxins removal:* Remove the source from the patient or discontinue the offending drug.
- *Supportive therapy:* Maintenance of airway, breathing, and circulation (ABC), hydration, oxygen supply, and ventilation if required, and managing neurological complications with antiseizure drugs
- *Methylene blue:* Its chemical name is tetramethylthionine chloride.
  - *Dose:*
    - 2 mg/kg in <1 year of age
    - 1.5 mg/kg in older children
    - 1 mg/kg in adults (diluted in 1% sterile aqueous solution infused over 5 minutes). The dosage can be administered again every hour, with a maximum total of 7 mg/kg over 24 hours.
- Ascorbic acid (Vitamin C)
  - *Dose:* In cases of acute or toxic exposure resulting in symptoms or methemoglobin levels >30%, administer up to 10 grams intravenously either as a single dose or divided into multiple doses.
- *Riboflavin:* Uses the alternate pathway of MetHb reduction, effective in high doses
- *MB refractoriness and G6PD deficiency:* In cases where a patient does not respond to treatment, it is important to consider several factors such as inadequate decontamination, G6PD deficiency, unusual toxins, etc. Hyperbaric oxygen and exchange transfusion can be tried.

The algorithmic approach to the treatment of methemoglobinemia is given in **Flowchart 1**.

Flowchart 1: Treatment of methemoglobinemia.

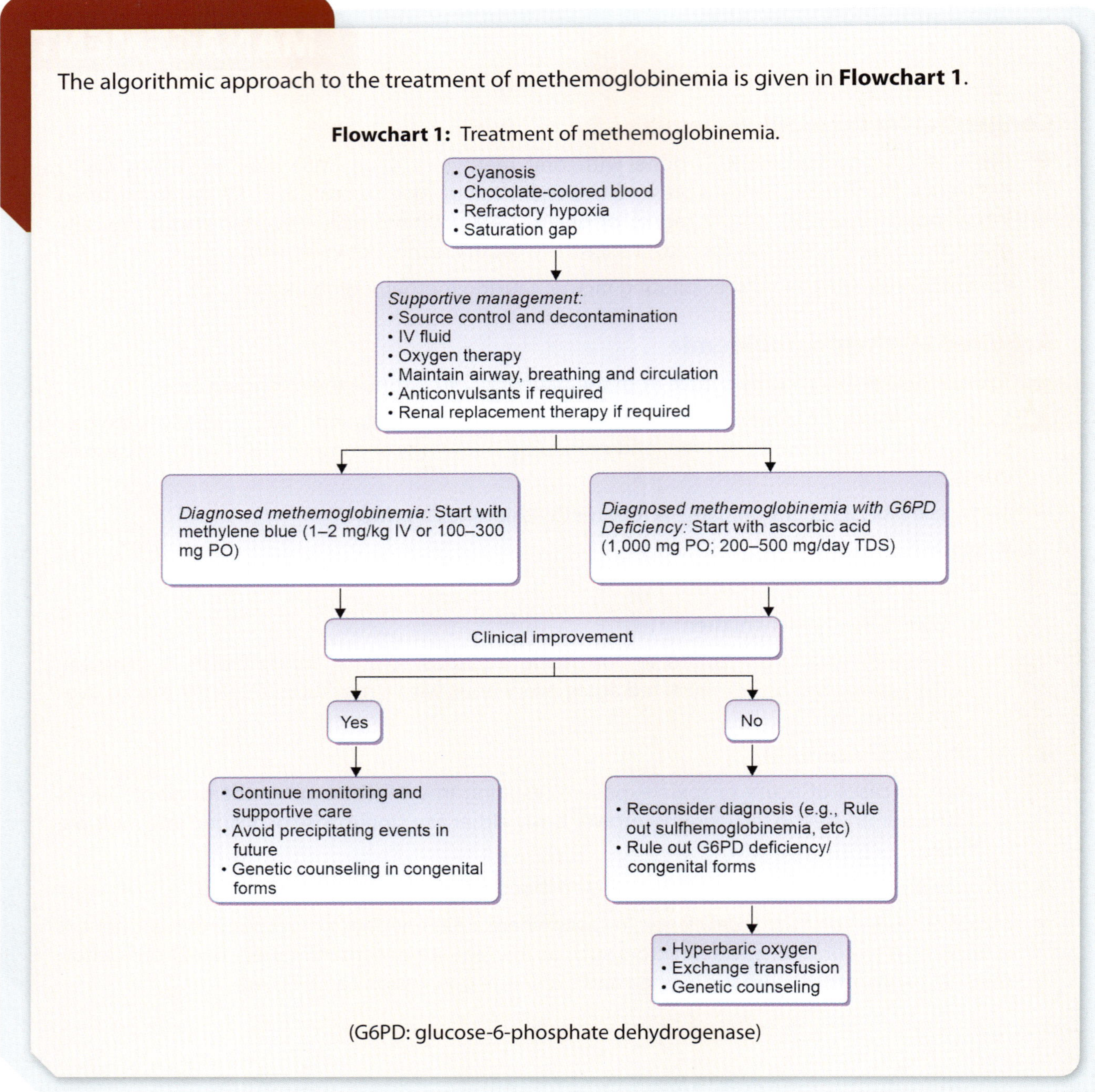

(G6PD: glucose-6-phosphate dehydrogenase)

CONCLUSION

Methemoglobinemia, though an uncommon condition, can be potentially life-threatening requiring prompt diagnosis and management. Clinical suspicion is heightened if the cyanosis does not improve even after giving oxygen, to a previously normal child. Arterial blood gas and co-oximetry are the important tests for diagnosis. MB remains the cornerstone in management of this condition, though in G6PD deficiency, it is contraindicated. Rarely exchange transfusion is an option for management.

SUGGESTED READING

1. Bradberry SM. Occupational methaemoglobinaemia. Mechanisms of production, features, diagnosis and management including the use of methylene blue. Toxicol Rev. 2003;22(1):13-27.
2. Golden PJ, Weinstein R. Treatment of high-risk, refractory acquired methemoglobinemia with automated red blood cell exchange. J Clin Apher. 1998;13(1):28-31.
3. Iolascon A, Bianchi P, Andolfo I, Russo R, Barcellini W, Fermo E, et al. Recommendations for diagnosis and treatment of methemoglobinemia. Am J Hematol. 2021;96(12):1666-78.
4. Khan Suheb M, Naaz F, Anderson TK, McClanahan A. A case of cyanosis with saturation gap: Dapsone-induced methemoglobinemia. Cureus. 2022;14(11):e31684.
5. Patnaik S, Natarajan MM, James EJ, Ebenezer K. Methylene blue unresponsive methemoglobinemia. Indian J Crit Care Med. 2014;18(4):253-5.

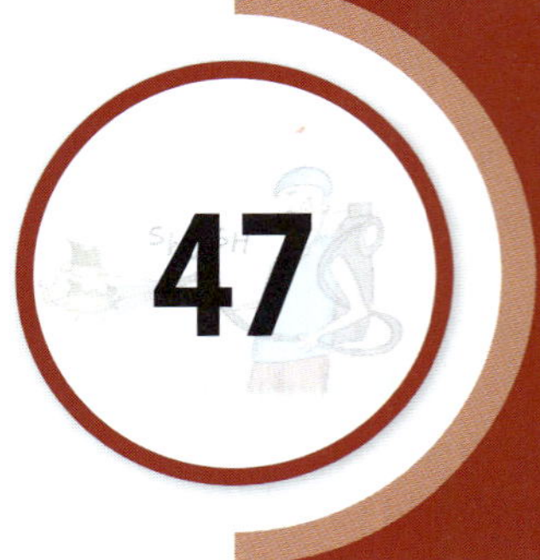

47 Organophosphate and Carbamate Poisoning

Madhu PK, Vinod H Ratageri

INTRODUCTION

Organophosphorus (OP) compounds are the most commonly used insecticides. Carbamates are similar to organophosphate pesticides structurally and both have similar mechanism of action. Both compounds are potent cholinesterase inhibitors and following overdose, they result in severe cholinergic toxicity demonstrating similar clinical manifestations, requiring similar management.[1]

Human poisoning can occur by inhalation, cutaneous exposure, or ingestion of both carbamate (aldicarb, methomyl, etc.) and organophosphate (parathion, chlorpyrifos, fenthion, diazinon, malathion, etc.) insecticides.[2] More than a hundred organophosphorus compounds are in common use. These are classified according to their toxicity and clinical use **(Table 1)**.

TABLE 1: Classification of organophosphorus (OP) compounds.

Toxicity	*Highly toxic organophosphates*	*Intermediately toxic organophosphates*	*Low toxicity organophosphates*
Clinical use	Agricultural insecticides	Animal insecticides	Household application and as field sprays
Examples	Tetraethyl pyrophosphates and parathion	Coumaphos, chlorpyrifos, and trichlorfon	Diazinon, malathion, and dichlorvos

PATHOPHYSIOLOGY

Following absorption from skin, lungs, or gastrointestinal tract, OP compounds bind to red blood cell (RBC) acetylcholinesterase (AChE). This enzyme is rendered nonfunctional resulting in excess of acetylcholine at the neuronal synapses and the neuromuscular junctions causing signs and symptoms of muscarinic and nicotinic effects. This AChE enzyme bound to OP compound undergoes a conformational change known as "aging", which renders the enzyme permanently inactivated and resistant to reactivation by oximes. This aging process might take 24–48 hours depending on whether the OP compound is diethyl or dimethyl analog.[3] Unlike OP compounds, carbamates spontaneously hydrolyze from the enzymatic site within 48 hours resulting in transient inactivation of the enzyme. Hence, toxicity due to carbamates is of shorter duration compared to equivalent doses of OP compounds, although the mortality rates are similar with both compounds.[1]

CLINICAL FEATURES

Signs and symptoms of toxicity appear within 2–3 hours of oral or respiratory exposures but are delayed by up to 12 hours from dermal absorption. Some lipophilic compounds (dichlofenthion, malathion, fenthion, etc.) result in delayed onset of toxicity, and illness may be prolonged for more than 30 days due to rapid uptake by adipose tissue and slow release from fat stores. Toxic effects can be divided into muscarinic effects, nicotinic effects, and central nervous system (CNS) effects. Acute toxicity from OP compounds presents with manifestations of cholinergic toxidrome. Nicotinic signs and symptoms include muscle fasciculations, cramping, weakness, and diaphragmatic failure **(Box 1)**.[4] Occasionally, cardiac arrhythmias, heart block, and QTc prolongation are observed.[5]

BOX 1: Clinical syndromes of organophosphorus (OP) compound poisoning.

Acute toxicity:
- Manifests in minutes to hours
- SLUDGE: Salivation, lacrimation, urination, defecation, and gastric emptying
- BBB = Bradycardia, bronchorrhea, bronchospasm (Cholinergic toxidrome)
- Muscle weakness, CNS depression, copious secretions, and bronchospasm may result in respiratory insufficiency

Intermediate (neurologic) syndrome:
- Occurs in approximately 20% of patients 1–4 days after exposure
- Bulbar, respiratory, and proximal muscle weakness are prominent features (nicotinic symptoms)
- Usually resolves in 1–3 weeks

Organophosphorus agent-induced delayed peripheral neuropathy (OPIDN):
- Occurs several weeks after exposure (usually 7–21 days)
- Primarily motor involvement but may start with paresthesia and calf pain
- Initially weakness is observed in the distal leg muscles, then small muscles of the hands, and extends proximally. May resolve spontaneously but can result in permanent neurologic dysfunction[6]

(CNS: central nervous system)

DIAGNOSIS

Diagnosis of OP compound toxicity is given in **Box 2**.

BOX 2: Diagnostic evaluation of organophosphorus (OP) compound poisoning.

Clinical findings:
- Organophosphorus compound or carbamate poisoning should be suspected if there are features of cholinergic excess
- Characteristic petroleum or garlic-like odor
- Identify the agent precisely as AChEs inhibited by diethyl analogs of OP compound reactivate and age slowly; they require prolonged oxime treatment compared to dimethyl analogs of OP compound[7]

Atropine challenge:
- If diagnosis is in doubt, 0.01–0.02 mg/kg of atropine may be administered
- Organophosphate or carbamate poisoning is suggested if there is an absence of anticholinergic signs (mydriasis, tachycardia, dry skin, etc.) after atropine challenge

Laboratory abnormalities:
- Degree of toxicity can be ascertained by measurement of RBC AChE activity
- In the acute phase of organophosphate poisoning, low plasma (or pseudo-) AChEs (>50% of minimum normal value) support the diagnosis of organophosphate poisoning but it does not show a significant relationship to the severity of poisoning, hence should not be used to guide therapy

(AChEs: acetylcholinesterase; RBC: red blood cell; OP: organophosphorus)

MANAGEMENT

Based on the severity of toxicity, patients may require treatment with oxygen, atropine, oxime, and benzodiazepine **(Flowchart 1)**.

Flowchart 1: Management of organophosphorus (OP) compound poisoning.

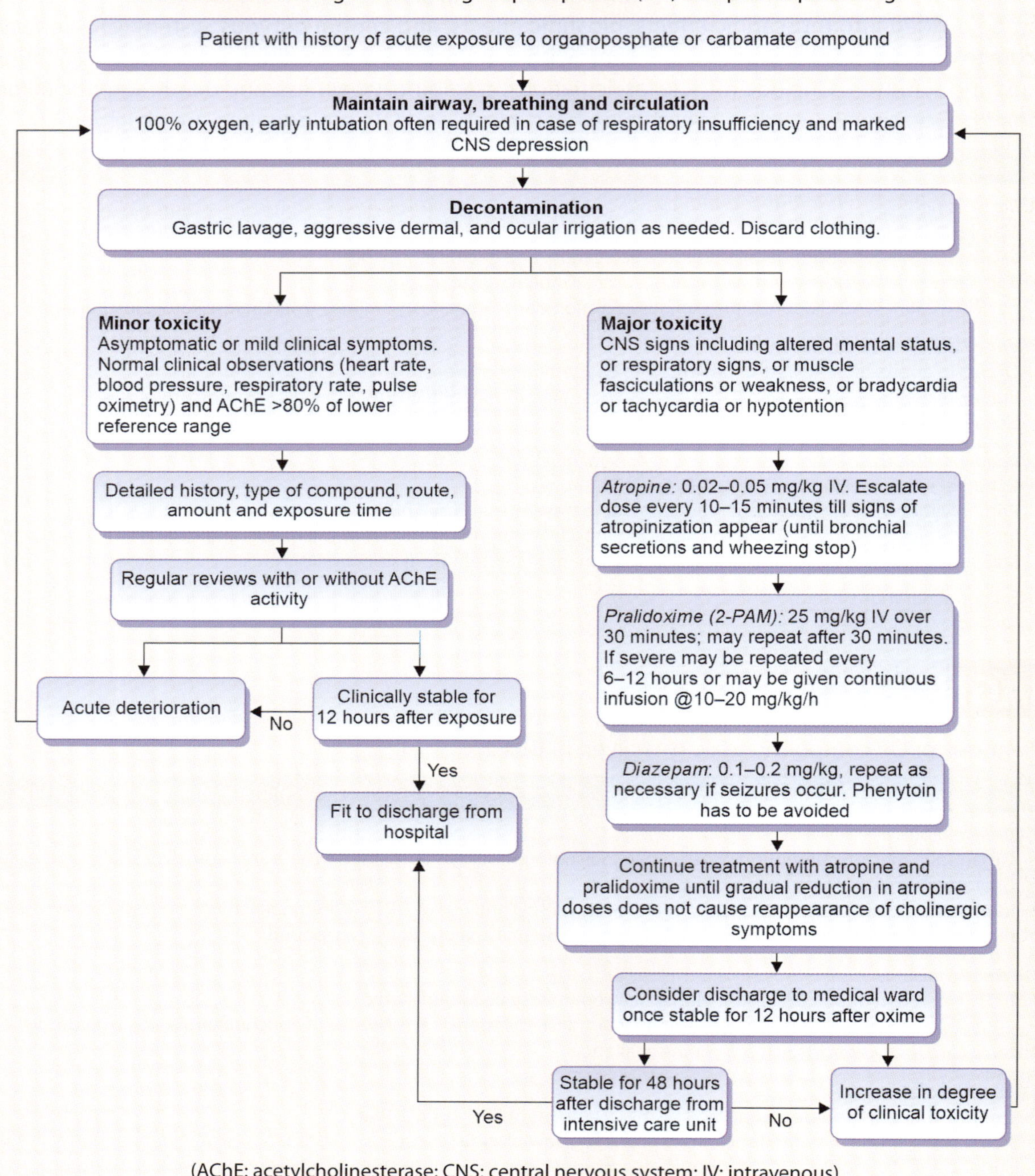

(AChE: acetylcholinesterase; CNS: central nervous system; IV: intravenous)

Initial Resuscitation

Patients, with severe muscle weakness, marked CNS depression, copious secretions, and bronchospasm, who rapidly develop respiratory insufficiency may require early endotracheal intubation. Nondepolarizing neuromuscular blocking agents (e.g., rocuronium) at higher doses must be preferred during rapid-sequence intubation. Succinylcholine may result in prolonged neuromuscular blockade; hence, it should be avoided.

Simultaneously, adequate volume resuscitation with isotonic crystalloid should be carried out. Some patients who do not respond to anticholinergic therapy might require inotropes such as epinephrine.

Decontamination

Gastric lavage performed within an hour is of maximum benefit, as these compounds get absorbed rapidly from the gastrointestinal tract. In case of exposure, eyes should be washed with clean tap water, whole body should be thoroughly washed with soap and water, and clothing should be safely discarded to prevent further absorption. Due to the risk of aspiration and seizures, forced emesis is contraindicated.

Atropine

Atropine blocks muscarinic receptors, thereby alleviating central and muscarinic cholinergic effects.

- *Children <12 years*: 0.02–0.05 mg/kg intravenous (IV) every 10–20 minutes until atropinization (decreased secretions and/or wheezing, dry flushed skin, tachycardia, mydriasis, and fever) is seen and then every 1–4 hours for at least 24 hours
    - *Maximum single dose for neonate (0–4 weeks):* 0.03 mg/kg
    - *Maximum single dose for children:* 0.5 mg
- *Children 12 years of age or older:* 1–2 mg IV initially

If no response, the dose is doubled every 5–10 minutes until tracheobronchial secretions are dry and the patient can be oxygenated.

Continue the treatment until a gradual reduction in dose does not cause the reappearance of cholinergic symptoms. In severe organophosphate poisoning, very large doses and treatment for days to weeks may be necessary. Administration by infusion in severe cases may be considered. Initial infusion rates of 0.02–0.08 mg/kg/h have been recommended. Tachycardia and mydriasis are not contraindications to atropine use.[8]

Pralidoxime

Pralidoxime neutralizes the nicotinic effects of OP or carbamate compounds. The World Health Organization (WHO) recommends 25–50 mg/kg of pralidoxime chloride in normal saline over 30 minutes, which may be repeated after 30 minutes followed by 10–20 mg/kg/h in case of severe symptoms. In situations where other salt forms, other than chloride salt, are available (e.g., iodide, mesilate and metilsulfate), doses are calculated by converting the recommended pralidoxime chloride dose into equivalent dosing units.[9] Since AChEs inhibited by diethyl analogs of OP compound reactivate and age slowly, they require prolonged oxime treatment compared to dimethyl analogs of OP compound. The effectiveness of oxime therapy can be determined by sequential measurement of RBC AChE activity. Atropine therapy to counter CNS and muscarinic effects should be continued along with pralidoxime therapy to counter nicotinic effects. Pralidoxime is generally not indicated for carbamate poisoning.[10]

Supportive Measures

Seizures should be treated with benzodiazepines. As arrhythmias may be precipitated, phenytoin has to be avoided while treating seizures.

KEY LEARNING POINTS

- Acute toxicity from OP agents presents with manifestations of cholinergic excess. The dominant clinical features of acute cholinergic toxicity include defecation, urination, miosis, bronchorrhea/bronchospasm/bradycardia, emesis, lacrimation, and salivation (DUMBELS).
- Organophosphate or carbamate poisoning is diagnosed clinically. If the diagnosis is doubtful, absence of anticholinergic signs (mydriasis, tachycardia, and dry skin) after administration of 0.01–0.02 mg/kg of atropine suggests poisoning.
- Intermediate syndrome occurs in approximately 20% of patients 1–4 days after exposure. Bulbar, respiratory, and proximal muscle weakness are prominent features (nicotinic symptoms). It usually resolves in 1–3 weeks.
- Identify the agent precisely as AChEs inhibited by diethyl analogs of OP compound reactivate and age slowly; they require prolonged oxime treatment compared to dimethyl analogs of OP compound.
- Based on the severity of toxicity, patients may require treatment with oxygen, atropine, oxime, and benzodiazepine.

REFERENCES

1. Aman S, Paul S, Chowdhury FR. Management of organophosphorus poisoning: Standard treatment and beyond. Crit Care Clin. 2021;37(3):673-86.
2. Eddleston M, Phillips MR. Self poisoning with pesticides. BMJ. 2004;328:42-4.
3. Khurana D, Prabhakar S. Organophosphorus intoxication. Arch Neurol. 2000;57(4):600-2.
4. King AM, Aaron CK. Organophosphate and carbamate poisoning. Emerg Med Clin North Am. 2015;33(1): 133-51.
5. Wang MH, Tseng CD, Bair SY. Q-T interval prolongation and pleomorphic ventricular tachyarrhythmia ('Torsade de pointes') in organophosphate poisoning: Report of a case. Hum Exp Toxicol. 1998;17(10): 587-90.
6. Sevim S, Aktekin M, Dogu O, Ozturk H, Ertas M. Late onset polyneuropathy due to organophosphate (DDVP) intoxication. Can J Neurol Sci. 2003;30(1):75-8.
7. Eyer P. The role of oximes in the management of organophosphorus pesticide poisoning. Toxicol Rev. 2003;22(3):165-90.
8. Atlantic Canada Poison Centre. (2015). Atropine–Pediatric. [online] Available from https://atlanticcanadapoisoncentre.ca/atropine-pediatric.html [Last accessed on January, 2024].
9. World Health Organization. (2008). Pralidoxime. [online] Available from https://list.essentialmeds.org/recommendations/939 [Last accessed January, 2024].
10. Rajendiran C, Ravi G, Thirumalaikolundu Subramanian P. Organophosphate, carbamate and rodenticide poisoning in children. IJPP. 2009;11(1):6-14.

48

Opioid Poisoning in Children

Daisy Khera, Lokesh Kumar

INTRODUCTION

- Opioids are used in the treatment of pain but are often sold illicitly and misused for their euphoric effects. Opioid poisoning remains a significant public health concern globally, particularly in the pediatric population due to accidental ingestion, with young children more vulnerable due to their curiosity and lack of understanding about the dangers of medication.
- Opioid overdose is a preventable and potentially lethal condition. Opioids, while effective in managing pain, can cause life-threatening respiratory depression and altered consciousness when ingested in excessive amounts.

TERMINOLOGIES AND DEFINITIONS

Some terminologies and definitions are as follows:

- *Opioids:* An opioid is any synthetic or natural agent that stimulates opioid receptors and produces opium-like effects (pain relief, euphoria, and sedation).[1] It includes morphine, codeine, semi-synthetic drugs like oxycodone and hydrocodone, and synthetic opioids like fentanyl and methadone.
- *Opioid dependence:* Opioid dependence is a clinical syndrome characterized by physical and psychosocial dependence, resulting in tolerance, withdrawal symptoms, and addiction.
- *Opioid intoxication:* It is defined as a condition of transient and clinically significant disturbances in consciousness, perception, behavior, cognition, affect, or coordination that develop during or shortly after the consumption or administration of opioids.[2]
- *Opioid overdose/ poisoning:* It is a life-threatening condition induced by consumption (ingestion, inhalation, or injection) of excess amounts of opioids, which is characterized by pinpoint pupils, unconsciousness, and respiratory depression.[2]
- *Naloxone:* It is a competitive opioid receptor antagonist used as an antidote to reverse the effects of opioid toxicity.

ETIOPATHOLOGY

The pharmacokinetics of particular opioid analgesic agents (absorption, onset of action, clearance, and biologic half-life) are often irrelevant in overdose. Children who ingest opioid formulations usually ingest a higher dose than adults per kilogram of body weight, and therefore develop more severe symptoms and require larger doses of naloxone to reverse the effects of overdose.[3]

Opioids bind to specific receptors in the central nervous system (CNS), particularly the mu, kappa, and delta receptors, which mediate their analgesic, euphoric, and sedative effects. The binding of opioids to mu receptors leads to the inhibition of pain transmission and the slowing of respiratory drive, which can be fatal in overdose. **Table 1** lists various forms of opioids, their onset of action, duration of action, and dosage in children.

TABLE 1: Various forms of opioids, their onset of action, duration of action, and dosage in children.

Opioid	*Onset of action*	*Duration of action*	*Intermittent dosage*	*IV infusion dosage*
Morphine	5–10 mins (IV) 30–60 minutes (oral)	3–4 hours (IV) 4–5 hours (oral)	0.05–0.2 mg/kg/dose (IV) 0.01–0.3 mg/kg/dose (oral) (max. 10 mg)	0.01–0.04 mg/kg/h
Fentanyl	1–2 minutes (IV)	30–60 minutes	1–4 µg/kg dose IV (max. 100 µg/dose)	1–4 µg/kg/h
Hydromorphone	5–10 minutes (IV) 30–60 mins (oral)	3–4 hours	0.01–0.015 mg/kg/dose (IV) (max 2 mg) 0.03–0.08 mg/kg/dose (oral) (Max. 5 mg)	0.003–0.005 mg/kg/h
Methadone	30–60 minutes (oral)	4–12 hours	0.1– 0.2 mg/kg/dose (IV/PO) (max 10 mg)	NA
Remifentanil	1–3 minutes (IV)	3–10 minutes	N/A	0.1 µg/kg/min
Oxycodone	30–60 minutes (Oral)	3–6 hours	0.1–0.2 mg/kg/dose (Oral) (max: 5–10 mg/dose)	
Tramadol	30–60 minutes (oral)	6–8 hours	*>12 years:* 1–2 mg/kg/dose (oral) (max: 100 mg/dose)	
Codeine	30–60 minutes (oral)	4–6 hours	*>12 years:* 0.5–1 mg/kg/dose (oral) (max 60 mg/dose)	

Source: Anderson CC, Kapoor S, Mark TE (Eds.) The Johns Hopkins University, American Academy of Pediatrics. The Harriet Lane Handbook, 23rd edition. Philadelphia, PA: Elsevier; 2023)

CLINICAL FEATURES

Although the classic toxidrome of apnea, stupor, and pinpoint pupil suggests the diagnosis of opioid toxicity, all of these findings are not consistently present.[4]

At the bedside, however, the most easily recognized abnormality in cases of opioid overdose is a decline in respiratory rate culminating in apnea. Bradypnea in a child who is not in physiologic sleep strongly suggests acute opioid intoxication, particularly when accompanied by miosis or stupor.[5]

Miosis alone is insufficient to infer the diagnosis of opioid intoxication because overdose from antipsychotic drugs, anticonvulsant agents, ethanol, and other sedative–hypnotic agents can cause miosis and coma.[6,7] **Table 2** enlists the systems affected and their clinical features.

TABLE 2: The classic signs and symptoms of opioid poisoning.

System affected	*Clinical features*
Central nervous system (CNS) depression	Pinpoint pupil, seizures, drowsiness, stupor, and coma
Respiratory depression	Chest rigidity, bradypnea, apnea, hypoxia, respiratory failure
Cardiovascular effects	Bradycardia and hypotension
Gastrointestinal effects	Nausea, vomiting, and constipation

Physical Examination

The physical examination should assess the level of consciousness, pupillary reaction, respiratory status (rate, depth, and pattern), and cardiovascular function (pulse rate, rhythm, and blood pressure).

DIAGNOSIS

In most situations, a child with poisoning will present like an unknown emergency.

When to suspect poisoning?

- Sudden onset of altered consciousness or coma or breathing difficulty or apnea
- There is a vacuum in history, for example, apparently well child playing in the room unsupervised, is found drowsy or comatose after few hours.

The presence of hypopnea or apnea, miosis, and stupor should lead the clinician to consider the diagnosis of opioid poisoning. Dramatic clinical response to naloxone in a patient who also fits the clinical picture is diagnostic.

DIFFERENTIAL DIAGNOSIS

While opioid poisoning presents with characteristic symptoms, several conditions may mimic the clinical picture. Clinical assessment and laboratory investigations, as necessary, should be used to include or rule out other conditions. **Table 3** enlists various differential diagnoses and their clinical features.

TABLE 3: Differential diagnosis for opioid poisoning.

Diagnosis	*Clinical features*
Meningitis/encephalitis	Altered sensorium and respiratory signs and symptoms but miosis is not seen usually
Head injury	Altered sensorium, abnormal breathing, and pupillary abnormality; pontine hemorrhage can present with pinpoint pupils
Metabolic etiologies	Altered mental status, seizures but miosis is not seen. For example, hypoglycemia, metabolic encephalopathies, diabetic ketoacidosis, or electrolyte disturbances
Benzodiazepine /barbiturate poisonings	Cause central nervous system (CNS) depression and respiratory symptoms, but miosis is usually not seen
Organophosphate (OP) poisoning	Presents with coma and pinpoint pupils but is associated with tachypnea and other systemic symptoms of OP poisoning

INVESTIGATIONS

Investigations include the following:

- *Toxicology screen:* Blood or urine toxicology tests are done to detect the presence of opioids. However, routine screens may not identify all opioids, especially synthetic or novel compounds.
- Qualitative analyses of urine for drugs of abuse (toxicology screens) rarely affect decisions about patient care and have little role in the immediate evaluation and management of opioid intoxication.[8]
- *Other tests like* arterial blood gas, chest X-ray, ECG, serum glucose, electrolytes, and liver and kidney function tests.

MANAGEMENT

Emergency Care

ABCDE of emergency care

Airway, if not clear: Suction, position, and intubate

Breathing, if not appropriate: Oxygenate and intubate

Circulation, if signs of poor perfusion: Give bolus and assess for inotropes

Disability: Assess GCS, pupil size, and reaction

Exposure: Look for injection sites, other clues to the poisoning, and RBS

Fig. 1: Approach to management in emergency care. (GCS: Glasgow Coma Scale; RBS: random blood sugar)

Specific Management

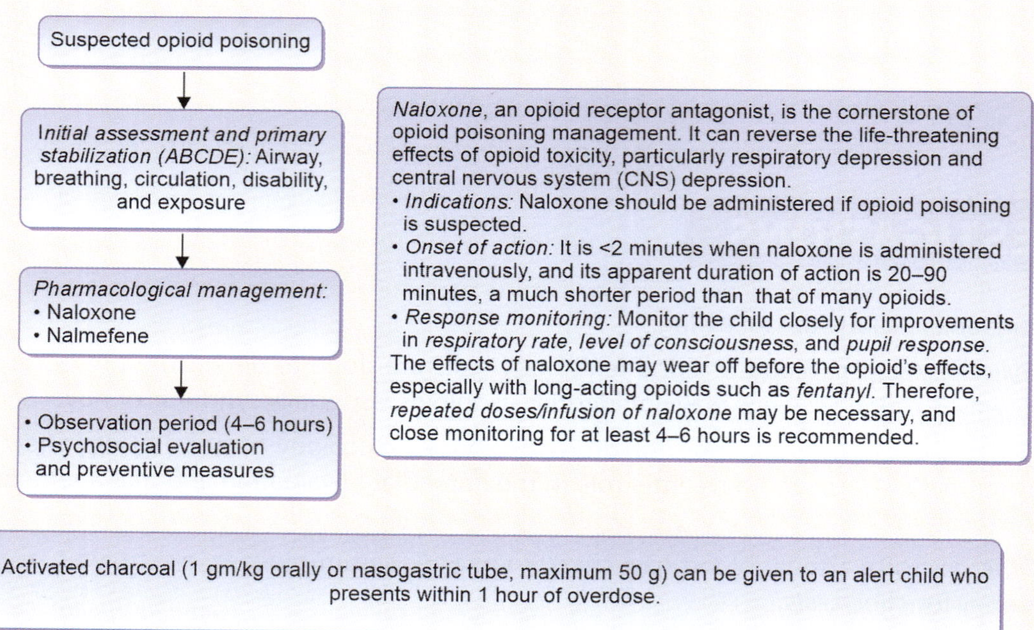

Naloxone Dosage[2]

- *Initial dose:* For children, the recommended starting dose of naloxone is *0.1–0.2 mg/kg* IV, with a maximum initial dose of *2 mg*. When patients show improvement with naloxone, the improvement occurs within 2–3 minutes in the form of pupillary dilatation and increase in the respiratory rate.
- If no response is observed within 2–3 minutes, repeat the dose every 2–3 minutes as needed until the child responds or the total dose reaches 10 mg.
- If no IV access is available, naloxone can be administered *intramuscularly (IM)* or *intranasally* (IN), using similar dosages.
- In case of response to naloxone, IV infusion should be considered in patients with overdose from longer acting opioids (e.g., buprenorphine) because the patient can fall back into coma as the effect of naloxone decreases. For naloxone infusion, two-thirds of the reversal dose should be given hourly (2/3 × total reversing effective dose in mg × weight in kg). Half of this dose should be administered over the first 15 minutes and the remaining over the next 45 minutes.

Nalmefene

Nalmefene, an emerging drug, 6-methylene analog of naltrexone, is an opioid antagonist that prevents or reverses the effects of opioids (including respiratory depression, sedation, and hypotension). Nalmefene has a longer duration of action than naloxone at fully reversing doses and has no opioid agonist activity.[9]

DISPOSITION AND FOLLOW-UP

- *Observation period:* Once the respiratory rate improves after the administration of naloxone, the patient should be observed for 4–6 hours before discharge is considered.
- Psychosocial and preventive measures:
  - If opioid poisoning is suspected to result from intentional exposure or parental misuse, it is important to consider *psychosocial evaluation* and *safeguarding measures.*
  - Families should receive education about *opioid safety* and the *proper storage* of medications to prevent future incidents and counsel patients and families on the signs of opioid overdose and how to respond to an overdose.

KEY LEARNING POINTS

- *Opioid poisoning in children* requires rapid recognition and intervention, particularly focusing on securing the airway and supporting ventilation along with trial of naloxone.
- *Naloxone* is the first-line treatment, and its effects should be closely monitored as the duration of action may be shorter than some opioids.
- *Synthetic opioids like fentanyl* pose significant challenges due to their potency and long half-life, necessitating higher doses of naloxone and prolonged monitoring.
- *Airway management* and *respiratory support* are the cornerstones of initial management.
- *Toxicology screens* are helpful but may not detect all opioids, especially synthetic ones.
- *Prevention is key:* Educating families on safe medication practices and ensuring proper storage of opioids can help prevent accidental poisoning.

REFERENCES

1. BMJ Best Practice. (2024). Opioid overdose. [online] Available from https://bestpractice.bmj.com/topics/en-gb/339 [Last accessed December, 2024].
2. Sarkar S, Bhatia G, Dhawan A. Clinical practice guidelines for assessment and management of patients with substance intoxication presenting to the emergency department. Indian J Psychiatry. 2023;65(2):196-211.
3. Boyer EW. Management of opioid analgesic overdose. N Engl J Med. 2012;367(2):146-55.
4. Hoffmann RS, Goldfrank LR. The poisoned patient with altered consciousness: Controversies in the use of a "coma cocktail". JAMA. 1995;274(7):562-9.
5. Hoffmann JR, Schriger DL, Luo JS. The empiric use of naloxone in patients with altered mental status: A reappraisal. Ann Emerg Med. 1991;20(3):246-52.
6. Alberto G, Erickson T, Popiel R, Narayanan M, Hryhorczuk D. Central nervous system manifestations of a valproic acid overdose responsive to naloxone. Ann Emerg Med. 1989;18(8):889-91.
7. O'Malley GF, Seifert S, Heard K, Daly F, Dart RC. Olanzepine overdose mimicking opioid intoxication. Ann Emerg Med. 1999;34:279-81.
8. Boyer EW, Shannon MW. Which drug tests in medical emergencies? Clin Chem. 2003;49(3):353-4.
9. Edinoff AN, Nix CA, Reed TD, Bozner EM, Alvarez MR, Fuller MC, et al. Pharmacologic and clinical considerations of nalmefene, a long duration opioid antagonist, in opioid overdose. Psychiatry Int. 2021;2(4):365-78.

49

Paraquat Poisoning

Namrata Das, GV Basavaraja

INTRODUCTION

- Paraquat (1,1-dimethyl-4,4-bipiridylium chloride) is a toxic herbicide belonging to the chemical family of Bipyridilium quaternary ammonium herbicides.
- This liquid herbicide was primarily used for weed and grass control, and because of its low cost and easy availability, it is being widely used in India.
- It is very lethal to human beings and even a minor amount (10–20 mL) of 20% paraquat can be life-threatening.

TERMINOLOGIES AND DEFINITION

- *PQ:* Paraquat compound.
- *Redox reaction:* A chemical reaction that involves the transfer of electrons between two species—oxidation and reduction.
- *Hemoperfusion:* It is an extracorporeal technique that removes toxins by a process called adsorption, using activated charcoal or resin.
- *Paraquat tongue:* Extensive ulceration of the tongue occurs on paraquat ingestion due to the highly corrosive nature of the substance. It is one of the first signs of paraquat poisoning and may be predictive of more threatening mucosal erosions in the gastrointestinal tract.

ETIOPATHOLOGY

The herbicidal activity of paraquat as well as its toxicity to humans has been found to be linked to its redox potential.

The mechanism of toxicity of paraquat can be well explained by:

- Generation of free radicals and oxidative stress
- Secondary effects of oxidative stress

The mechanism of toxicity of the PQ compound involves cyclical reduction–oxidation reactions, which produce reactive oxygen species (ROS) and depletion of nicotinamide adenine dinucleotide phosphate (NADPH), which in turn, is a source of ATP and an essential electron donor for several cellular reactions.

- **Flowchart 1** shows the redox cycling reaction of Paraquat ion and pathophysiology of organ injury in paraquat poisoning.

Flowchart 1: Redox cycling reaction of paraquat ion and pathophysiology of organ injury in paraquat poisoning.

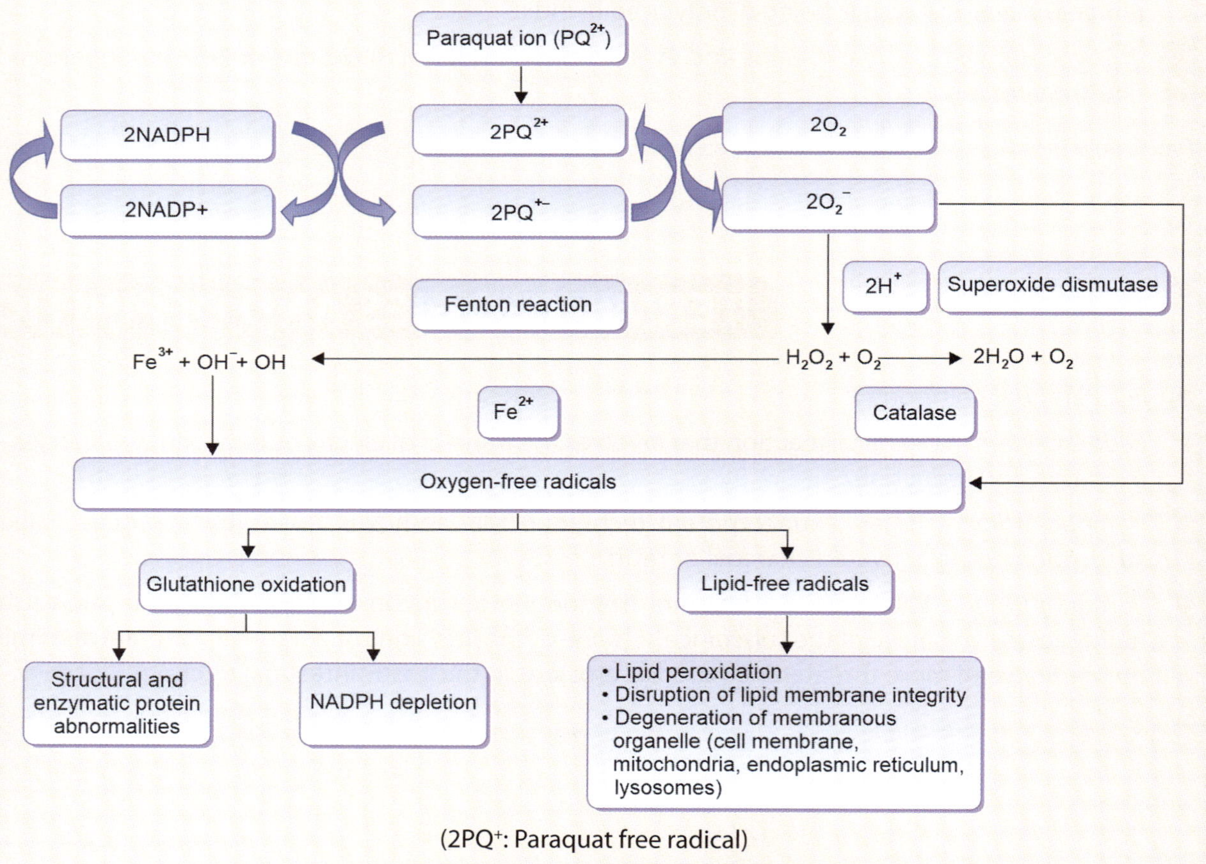

($2PQ^+$: Paraquat free radical)

- PQ is reduced enzymatically to PQ^+ mainly by NaDPH cytochrome 450 reductase.
- The PQ^+ is then oxidized to its original form in the presence of oxygen with subsequent generation of O^{2-}.
- This sets up a cascade generating free radicals that cause peroxidation of lipid and protein, causing mitochondrial damage and also activating nuclear factor-kappa B (NF–kB) **(Flowchart 1)**.
- Once activated, it induces inflammatory genes, causing translation of inflammatory enzymes, cytokines, and chemokines.

The elimination of PQ is mostly renal—glomerular filtration and tubular secretion with very minimal reabsorption. However, when high doses of paraquat are ingested, it causes vacuolation in the cells of the proximal convoluted tubules, causing renal tubular necrosis, a rapid decline in GFR, and further accumulation of the substance.

TOXICOKINETICS OF PARAQUAT

Paraquat has a large volume of distribution on ingestion. Paraquat is rapidly absorbed from the gut after ingestion, which then gets rapidly distributed to other tissues, with maximum tissue levels reached after about 6 hours of ingestion.

Within 12–24 hours of ingestion, 90% of the paraquat is excreted unchanged in urine, as it undergoes no or minimal metabolism in the body.

There is time-dependent elimination from the central compartment (blood) by the kidneys. Lungs behave as a third "toxic" compartment that can actively take up paraquat, by an energy-dependent polyamine uptake system, even against a concentration gradient **(Flowchart 2)**.

Flowchart 2: Distribution of Paraquat after ingestion.

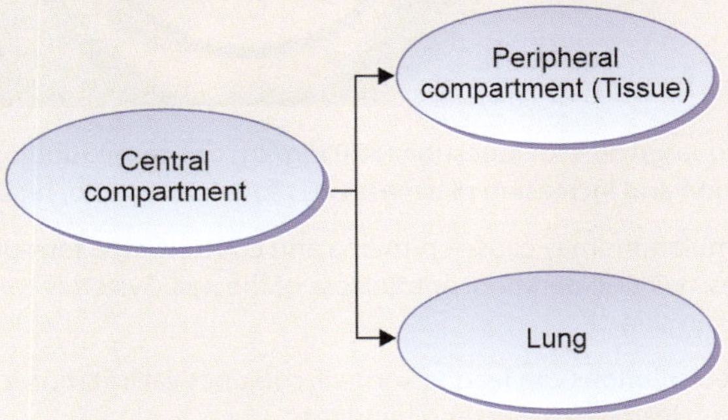

Central compartment → Peripheral compartment (Tissue)

Central compartment → Lung

CLINICAL FEATURES

The clinical features of paraquat poisoning are dose-dependent and can be classified into mild, moderate, and severe.

Principal target organs are lungs, gastrointestinal system, and kidney **(Table 1)**.

TABLE 1: Organs involved and clinical features.

Organ	*Clinical features*
Lung	The paraquat concentration in lung is 10–20 times more than in plasma. The symptoms of lower respiratory tract involvement sets in within 24–48 hours after exposure. On being taken up by the alveolar cells, it leads to redox cycling and leads to production of reactive oxygen species. This oxidative stress leads to pulmonary damage in 3 phases: 1. *Acute destructive phase (acute pulmonary alveolitis):* 1–3 days 2. *Proliferative phase:* Vascular proliferation, attachment of platelets and PML to endothelium, fibroproliferation 3. *Pulmonary fibrosis:* Ground glass appearance, collagen and ECM deposition, and type II respiratory' failure
Gastrointestinal	• Paraquat is a caustic herbicide and can cause corrosion of the oral, esophageal, and gastrointestinal mucosa within hours of ingestion even at small doses of ingestion (<20 mg/kg) • Mucosal lesions can occur in oral cavity and tongue can become red and swollen, which is classically called as the "*Paraquat tongue*" It can also cause esophageal ulceration, perforation, mediastinitis, and pneumomediastinum 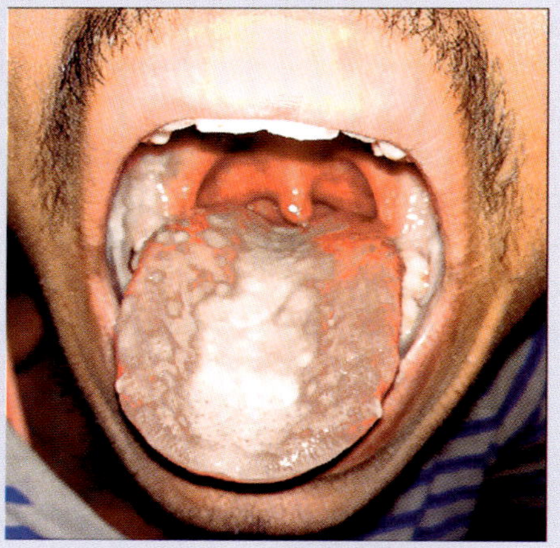
Renal	Moderate-to-large dose of ingestion (>20 mg/kg) can cause tubulopathy and necrosis, preventing renal excretion and increasing plasma levels of the compound, requiring dialysis
Skin	Diluted formulations may cause erythema and concentrated formulations may cause blistering, burn injuries, nail discoloration, or total loss of the nail. Systemic toxicity is rare, but can occur when there is broken skin
Eye	Concentrated solutions can lead to corneal, conjunctival irritation, uveal inflammation and eventually can lead to scarring and blindness
Other organ systems	Very large doses (>40 mg/kg) can cause liver failure by hepatic necrosis, myocardial necrosis, cerebral edema, adrenal insufficiency, pancreatitis with pancreatic dysfunction, and severe metabolic acidosis

EVALUATION

The main key to diagnosis is a circumstantial history and a good examination. Careful history should be taken about the mode of poisoning (ingestion, inhalation, and contact) and the amount of substance ingested. In toddlers or unwitnessed consumption, eliciting the above might still be challenging. The steps for evaluation of any child with suspected paraquat poisoning are cited in **Flowchart 3**.

Flowchart 3: Approach to suspected Paraquat poisoning.

Suspected paraquat consumption

↓

Amount consumed?
Hours since consumption?

↓

- Mild (<20 mg/kg)
- Moderate (20–40 mg/kg)
- Severe (>40 mg/kg) >30 mL (20%)

↓

Qualitative testing:

Beside urine sodium dithionate test: To 10 mL of urine in a test tube, add 0.1 g NaOH/1g $NaHCO_3$. Then add 1 g of sodium dithionate and mix gently. A color change to blue indicates presence of paraquat and the degree of color change give a semiquantitative assessment

0 | 3 | 10 | 30 | 100 µg//mL

↓

- No change in urine color → Unlikely systemic toxicity. If doubt persists, can repeat after 6 hours
- Plasma levels (If available) → SIPP score (time from ingestion in hours × serum levels in mg/dL) → <10—good predictive score
  - → ***Blood investigations:*** CBC, electrolytes, RFT, LFT, pancreatic enzymes, lactate, blood gas. Chest X-ray, CT chest

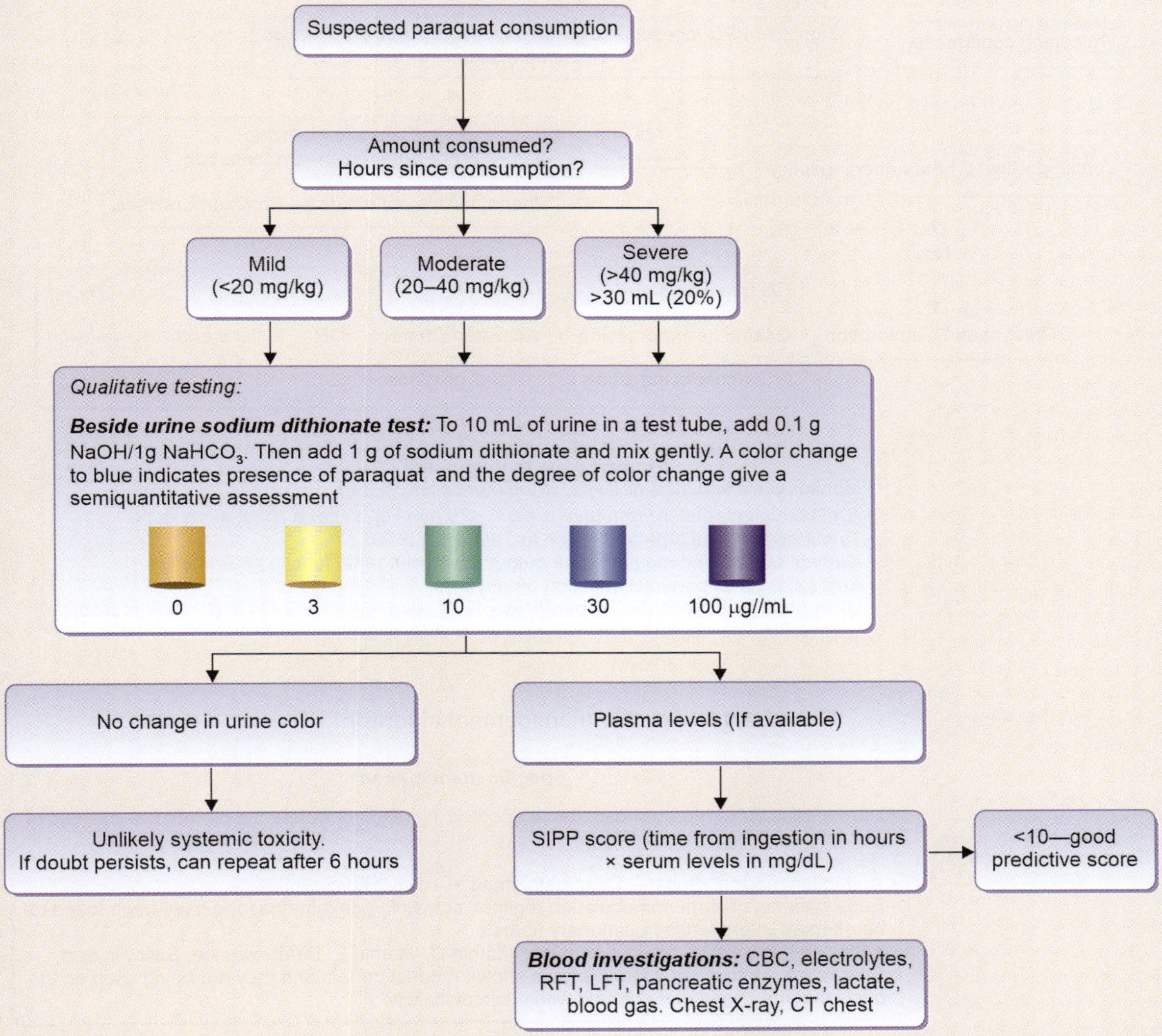

(CT: computed tomography; CBC: complete blood count; LFT: liver function test; RFT: renal function test)

The emergency management is well-illustrated in **Flowcharts 4 and 5**.

Flowchart 4: Emergency management algorithm.

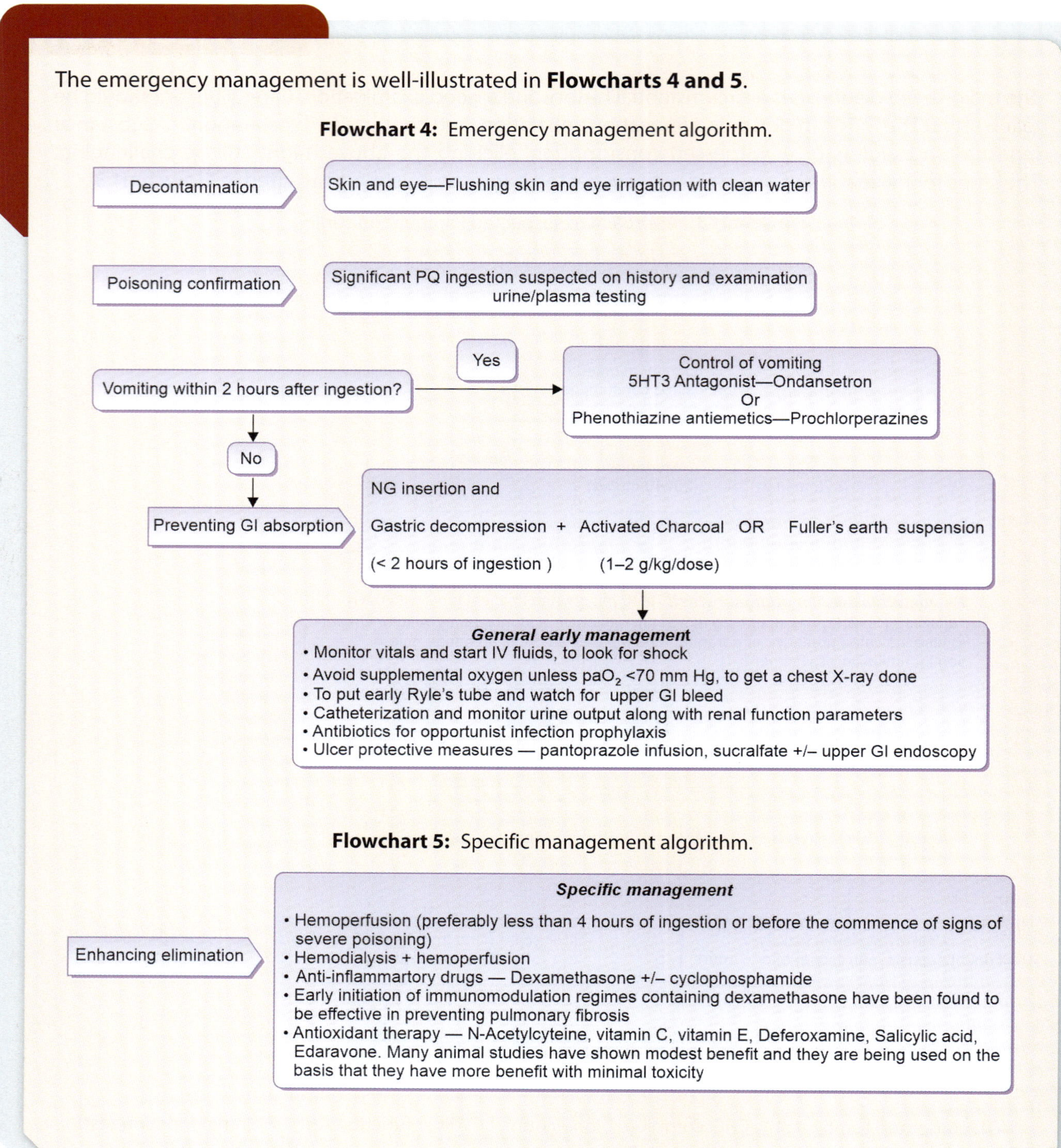

Flowchart 5: Specific management algorithm.

WHAT TO MONITOR?

Symptoms and signs of paraquat poisoning usually manifest within first 12 hours of ingestion, so patient should be monitored accurately during this period.

At admission:

- *Respiratory:*
  - To look for tachypnea, saturation, crepitations, or bronchial breathing on auscultation
  - Arterial blood gas (ABG) analysis to look for hypoxia (to be careful to not start oxygen unless PaO_2 <70 mm Hg)
  - *Imaging:* Baseline chest X-ray to look for infiltrates (direct pneumonitis or aspiration or pneumomediastinum).
    - To repeat chest X-ray or CT chest, if there is clinical suspicion of progressive lung involvement—reticulonodular opacities or ground glass appearance
- *Hemodynamic:* Look for tachycardia and hypotension. Shock can be multifactorial—hypovolemic, hypoxic, or hemorrhagic. Adequate fluid resuscitation and monitoring of end-organ perfusion should be done—lactate, urine output, sensorium.
- *Renal function:* To anticipate acute kidney injury and monitor urine output, electrolytes, and renal function parameters and to assess the need for hemodialysis.
- *Other organ systems:*
  - *Gastrointestinal:* To examine for oral mucosal ulcerations, to anticipate upper GI bleeds, and to assess the need for upper GI endoscopy
  - *Hepatic:* To monitor for right hypochondriac pain, jaundice, deranged liver enzymes, and coagulopathy
  - *Pancreatic:* To monitor pancreatic enzymes and watch for pancreatitis.
  - *Severe poisoning:* Severe metabolic acidosis with severe myocardial dysfunction and consumptive coagulopathy can occur with severe poisoning which has a very poor prognosis.

Signs of severe poisoning include tachypnea and hypoxia on room air, refractory hypotension despite fluid resuscitation, clinical and X-ray features of mediastinitis or pneumomediastinum, severe metabolic acidosis, and rapid decline in GFR.

KEY LEARNING POINTS

- Paraquat is a very lethal compound and ingestion of a small amount can lead to severe systemic toxicity.
- Early hemoperfusion (<4 hours) and early initiation of immunomodulation may help in drug elimination and preventing pulmonary fibrosis, respectively.
- The likely outcome of paraquat poisoning becomes evident in a day or two of ingestion and once manifestations of systemic toxicity set in, palliative care is a better option due to its irreversible damage to organs.
- There is no antidote for paraquat, hence, prevention is always better than cure.

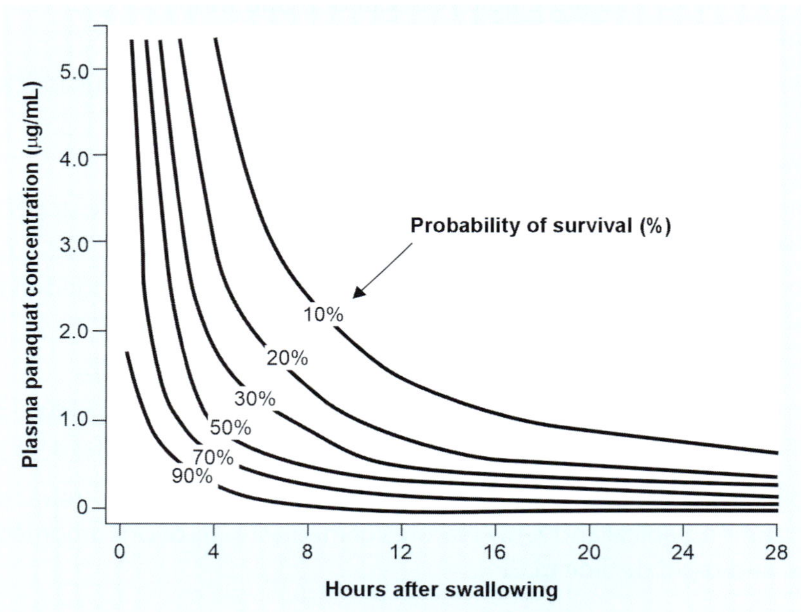

Fig. 1: Relation between plasma paraquat concentrations (µg/mL), time after ingestion, and probability of survival. *Source:* Hart TB, Nevitt A, Whitehead A. A new statistical approach to the prognostic significance of plasma paraquat concentrations. Lancet. 1984;2(8413):1222-3.

SUGGESTED READING

1. Dinis-Oliveira RJ, Duarte JA, Sánchez-Navarro A, Remião F, Bastos ML, Carvalho F. Paraquat poisonings: Mechanisms of lung toxicity, clinical features, and treatment. Crit Rev Toxicol. 2008;38(1):13-71.
2. Roberts DM, Buckley N. (2023). Paraquat poisoning. In: Burns MM, Ruha M (Eds). UptoDate [online] Available from https://www.uptodate.com/contents/paraquat-poisoning [Last accessed January 2025].
3. Rupesh KA, Ghosh V. Paraquat poisoning: A growing homicidal threat: Insights and strategies. JME. 2024; 5(3): 232-7.
4. Sukumar CA, Shanbhag V, Shastry AB. Paraquat: The poison potion. Indian J Crit Care Med. 2019;23(4):S263-6.

Management of Acetaminophen Poisoning

Reshmi Mishra, Sibabratta Patnaik

INTRODUCTION

- The easy accessibility of paracetamol (acetaminophen) over the counter and the perception of its safety has led to unintentional overdoses and toxicity.
- Its potential for harm has been underestimated, especially when taken in higher doses or combined with other medications that contain paracetamol.[1]
- Paracetamol is widely used for its analgesic and antipyretic properties, yet its exact mechanism of action remains somewhat unclear.

MECHANISM OF ACTION OF PARACETAMOL

Paracetamol primarily works in the central nervous system, where it inhibits cyclo-oxygenase (COX) enzymes, which synthesize prostaglandins—compounds that promote inflammation, pain, and fever. Paracetamol can effectively lower fever and alleviate pain by reducing prostaglandin production in the brain.

Additionally, paracetamol may influence the hypothalamus directly, which plays a crucial role in regulating body temperature. This direct action contributes to its antipyretic effects.[2]

PHARMACOKINETICS AND PHARMACODYNAMICS

Paracetamol has high bioavailability and is well absorbed, reaching peak blood concentration within about 90 minutes. Food in the stomach may delay the peak absorption time but does not affect the overall extent of absorption. It is not highly bound to plasma proteins, therefore, it exerts its effects quickly. Under normal dosing, its plasma half-life ranges from 1.5 to 2.5 hours. However, in cases of overdose, metabolic pathways become impaired, prolonging the half-life to approximately 4.5 hours, finally leading to significant hepatic impairment.[3]

Acetaminophen is primarily metabolized in the liver through multipathways, which makes it generally safe at therapeutic doses but can be dangerous when taken in excess:[4]

- *Conjugation:* Approximately 85% of a therapeutic dose undergoes conjugation to sulfated and glucuronidated metabolites. The conjugated metabolites (glucuronides and sulfates), which are metabolically inert, get excreted in the urine.
    - *Glucuronidation (40–65%):* Acetaminophen is conjugated with glucuronic acid to form acetaminophen glucuronides.
    - *Sulfation (20–40%):* Sulfate conjugation occurs, mainly as acetaminophen sulfate.
- *Oxidation:* Up to 10% of acetaminophen undergoes oxidation via the cytochrome P450 enzyme and N-acetyl-p-benzoquinone imine (NAPQI) reactive metabolite is formed. Under normal conditions, NAPQI is rapidly detoxified by conjugation with glutathione to produce mercapturic acid, a nontoxic product, and is eliminated in the urine.

Toxicity: In cases of overdose, the liver's store of glutathione is depleted. This depletion results in an accumulation of NAPQI, which binds to hepatocytes and causes liver injury. Once glutathione stores are depleted by approximately 70%, NAPQI attaches to cellular proteins, leading to significant cellular damage **(Flowchart 1)**.

Flowchart 1: Summary of the key steps in acetaminophen metabolism.

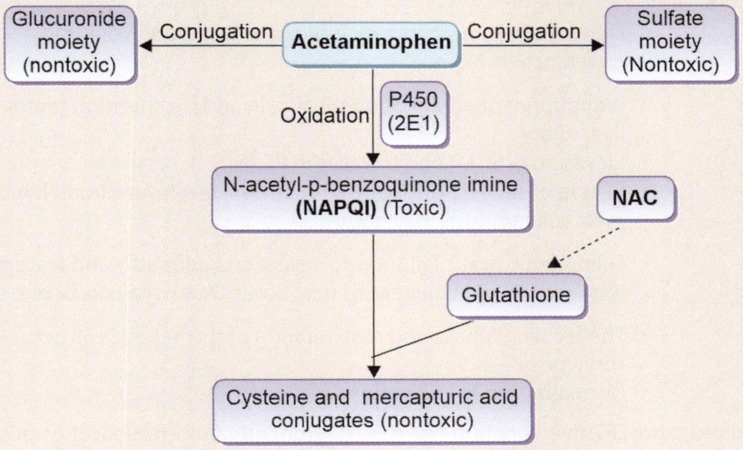

(NAC: N-Acetylcysteine)

DOSAGE OF PARACETAMOL

Dosage of paracetamol in different age groups is given in **Table 1**.

TABLE 1: Dosage of paracetamol in different age groups.

Age group	*Dose*	*Dosing interval*	*Maximum dose per 24 hours*	*Maximum daily dose (mg)*	*Normal serum concentration (mcg/mL)*
Children <12 years	10–15 mg/kg/dose	Every 4–6 hours	5 doses	75 mg/kg	10–20 µg/mL
Children >12 years and adult	325–1,000 mg per dose	Every 4–6 hours	5 doses	4,000 mg	10–20 µg/mL

Toxic Doses

Toxicity occurs when a single dose exceeds 150 mg/kg in children and when daily intake surpasses 7.5–10 grams in adults. In case of acute overdose, the majority of the acetaminophen is absorbed within 2 hours of ingestion and the peak plasma concentration occurs within 4 hours. The risk of hepatic toxicity increases in case of acute febrile illnesses, poor nutritional status, and with the use of enzyme inducers like rifampicin or phenobarbitone.

CLINICAL FEATURES

According to the clinical signs and symptoms, paracetamol toxicity is generally divided into four phases **(Table 2)**.[5]

TABLE 2: Stages of acute paracetamol poisoning.

Stage	*Postingestion time*	*Clinical features*
Stage 1	0–24 hours	• Nonspecific symptoms like anorexia, nausea, and vomiting • *Liver function:* Normal
Stage II	24–36 hours	• Right upper quadrant abdominal pain and hypotension represent the onset of liver injury • Elevation of SGOT and increase in PT/INR • In case of severe poisoning, bilirubin will be elevated, and hypoglycemia and metabolic acidosis may occur
Stage III	72–96 hours	• Fulminant hepatic failure with severe coagulopathy and features of encephalopathy; renal failure and pancreatitis may occur. Death may occur due to multiorgan failure
Stage IV	>5 days	• The recovery phase and regeneration of the hepatic cell occur in this stage in the survivors • Normalization of LFT occurs

(INR: international normalized ratio; LFT: liver function test; SGOT: serum glutamic–oxaloacetic transaminase; PT: prothrombin time)

INVESTIGATIONS

The diagnosis of paracetamol toxicity relies on measuring serum levels of the drug, even in the absence of symptoms. As coingestions are very common, a urine drug screen, electrocardiogram (ECG), and metabolic panel, along with an arterial blood gas analysis, may be beneficial. Additional laboratory tests include serum amylase and lipase, kidney function test (KFT) with electrolytes, liver function tests (LFTs), and a coagulation profile [prothrombin time (PT)/ international normalized ratio (INR)]. In cases of severe ingestion, LFTs may begin to rise within 8–12 hours and persistently remain high in the second and third stages.[6]

TREATMENT

Assessment of the patient's general condition along with airway, breathing, and hemodynamic status is crucial while initiating treatment for suspected paracetamol overdose. It is important to evaluate for other potentially life-threatening coingestants.[7] Supportive care with oxygen therapy and intravenous fluid and correction of hypoglycemia, if present, is highly required.

Activated charcoal administration should be done for the patients who present within 1 hour of acetaminophen ingestion. The dose is 1 gm/kg body weight orally. It should be avoided in mentally compromised patients or those who do not have an intact or protected airway.[8]

A serum paracetamol concentration should be measured after 4 hours of ingestion to evaluate the risk of hepatotoxicity. In patients who have ingested extended-release preparations, a repeat sample should be sent to see the additional increase in serum drug concentration. Rumack–Matthew nomogram should be utilized for assessment and to start treatment with N-acetylcysteine (NAC).[9] NAC restores glutathione levels by replenishing its stores, enabling the detoxification of NAPQI, and helps in preventing hepatotoxicity and requirement of liver transplantation.

Early administration of NAC after a suspected acetaminophen overdose is nearly 100% effective in protecting the liver and should be administered within 8 hours.[10] **(Flowchart 2)**.

N-acetylcysteine can be given orally or by intravenous (IV) infusion and both routes are effective. IV administration is favored if the patient is having any of the following:

- Intractable vomiting
- Contraindications to oral administration (e.g., aspiration risk due to altered mental status, pancreatitis, bowel ileus or obstruction, and bowel injury)
- Hepatic failure
- Refusing oral administration

Flowchart 2: Management algorithm of paracetamol poisoning.

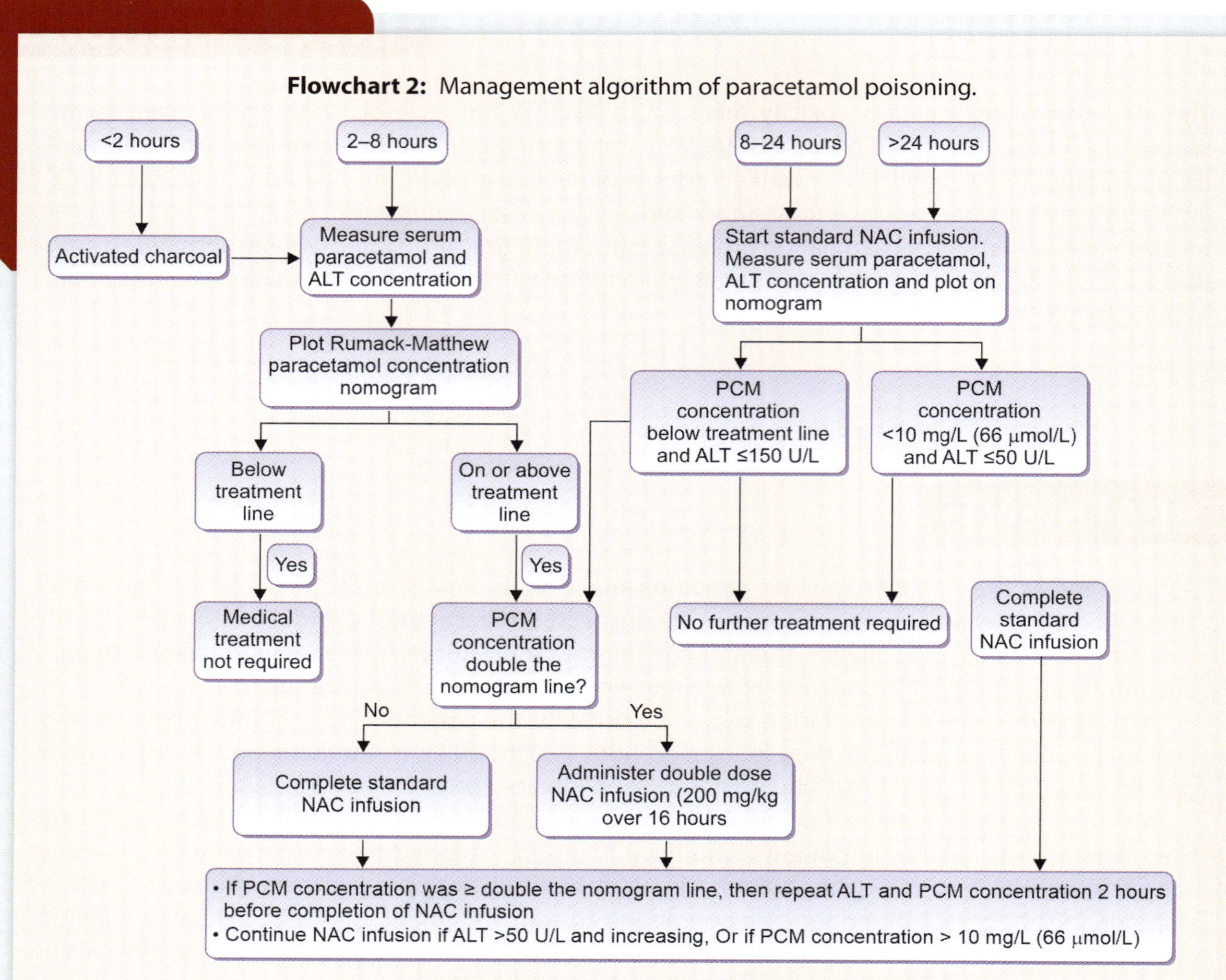

Nomogram for acute single-dose immediate-release paracetamol poisoning is given in **Figure 1**.

A two-stage infusion of NAC, total 300 mg/kg over 20 hours is recommended (recently changed from three-stage infusion).[11]

- *Stage 1:* 200 mg/kg over 4 hours (maximum 22 g) followed by
- *Stage 2:* 100 mg/kg over 16 hours (maximum 11 g)

Do not exceed the maximum recommended doses (22 g for stage 1, 11 g for stage 2).

The calculated dose should be diluted with normal saline or half normal saline or 5% dextrose solution, but we have to be careful about the sodium level.

If the treatment endpoint is not achieved, NAC should be continued in the stage 2 with the infusion rate of 100 mg/kg over an additional 16 hours.

Massive acetaminophen ingestion (more than double the height of the treatment nomogram line), requires higher stage-2 infusion rates, i.e., 200 mg/kg over 16 hours.[12]

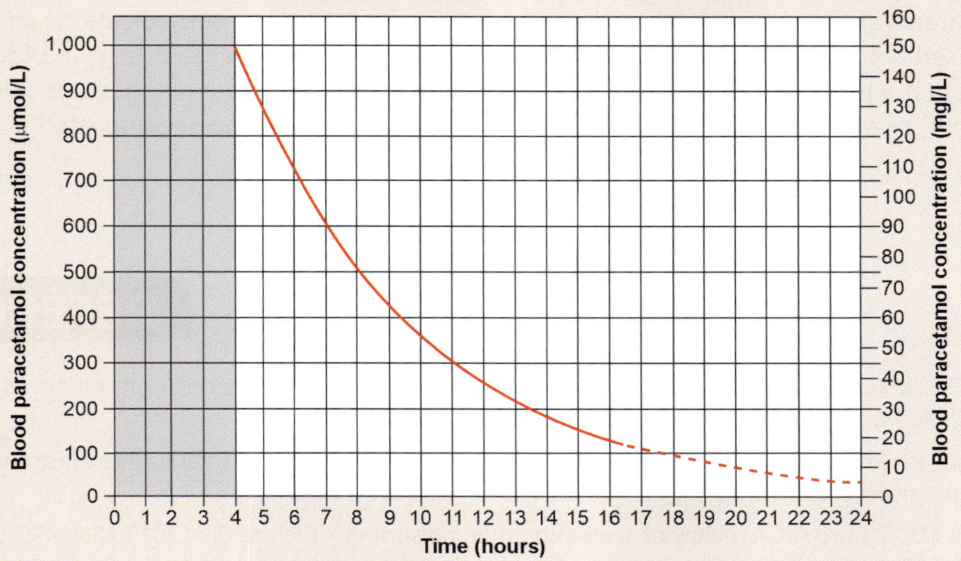

Fig. 1: Nomogram for acute single-dose immediate-release paracetamol poisoning.

All the investigations should be repeated after 18 hours of starting NAC infusion and it can be stopped once the patient is clinically well with:

- Acetaminophen concentration <10 μg/mL
- INR <2.0
- Alanine aminotransferase (ALT) and aspartate aminotransferase (AST) levels are normal or decreased 25–50% from peak

Injectable NAC infusion may cause non-IgE-mediated anaphylactoid reactions, which can be severe and require management similar to anaphylaxis. In such cases, the infusion should be immediately discontinued, and after stabilizing the patient, it can be restarted at a slower rate after a few hours.

Criteria for liver transplantation include the following:

- Metabolic acidosis unresponsive to resuscitation (pH <7.3 and arterial lactate >3 mmol/L)
- *Kidney failure:* Oliguria and/or creatinine >2.25 mg/dL
- Coagulopathy (INR >3.0 at 48 hours OR >4.5 at any time)
- Encephalopathy [Glasgow Coma Scale (GCS) <15]

CONCLUSION

Most single, accidental ingestions in children do *not require treatment* unless the ingested dose exceeds toxic thresholds. Early administration of NAC is nearly 100% effective in preventing liver damage. Parents should be advised on the importance of safe storage of medications and the need for supervised access to prevent accidental. In cases of intentional overdose (e.g., in older children or adolescents), a psychiatric evaluation is recommended to address underlying issues. It is crucial to assess for other potentially life-threatening substances that may have been coingested.

REFERENCES

1. Rajaram P, Subramanian R. Management of acute liver failure in the intensive care unit setting. Clin Liver Dis. 2018;22(2):403-8.
2. Ghanem CI, Pérez MJ, Manautou JE, Mottino AD. Acetaminophen from liver to brain: New insights into drug pharmacological action and toxicity. Pharmacol Res. 2016;109:119-31.
3. Hodgman MJ, Garrard AR. A review of acetaminophen poisoning. Crit Care Clin. 2012;28(4):499-516.
4. Wang YX, Du Y, Liu XF, Yang FX, Wu X, Tan L, et al. A hepatoprotection study of Radix Bupleuri on acetaminophen-induced liver injury based on CYP450 inhibition. Chin J Nat Med. 2019;17(7):517-24.
5. Farrell SE, Defendi GL. (2024). Acetaminophen toxicity clinical presentation. [online] Available from https://emedicine.medscape.com/article/820200-clinical?form=fpf [Last accessed January 2025].
6. McGill MR, Jaeschke H. Biomarkers of drug-induced liver injury: progress and utility in research, medicine, and regulation. Expert Rev Mol Diagn. 2018;18(9):797-807.
7. Alempijevic T, Zec S, Milosavljevic T. Drug-induced liver injury: do we know everything? World J Hepatol. 2017;9(10):491-502.
8. Chyka PA, Seger D, Krenzelok EP, Vale JA. Position paper: Single-dose activated charcoal. Clin Toxicol (Phila). 2005;43(2):61-87.
9. Fontana RJ, Liou I, Reuben A, Suzuki A, Fiel MI, Lee W, et al. AASLD practice guidance on drug, herbal, and dietary supplement-induced liver injury. Hepatology. 2023;77(3):1036-65.
10. Whyte IM, Francis B, Dawson AH. Safety and efficacy of intravenous N-acetylcysteine for acetaminophen overdose: Analysis of the Hunter Area Toxicology Service (HATS) database. Curr Med Res Opin. 2007;23(10):2359-68.
11. Chiew AL, Reith D, Pomerleau A, Wong A, Isoardi KZ, Soderstrom J, et al. Updated guidelines for the management of paracetamol poisoning in Australia and New Zealand. Med J Aust. 2020;212(4):175-83.
12. Royal Children's Hospital Melbourne. (2021). Clinical practice guideline: Paracetamol poisoning. [online]. Available from https://www.rch.org.au/clinicalguide/guidelineindex/Paracetamol_poisoning/ [Last accessed January 2025].

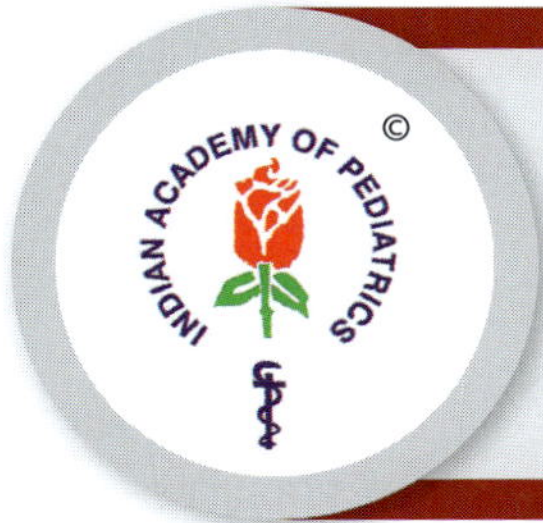

Index

Page numbers followed by *b* refer to box, *f* refer to figure, *fc* refer to flowchart, and *t* refer to table.

A

B

C

D

E

F

I

J

K

L

O

P

Q

R

W

X

Y

Z